T0280382

# The Essence of Nursing Practice

**Hesook Suzie Kim, PhD, RN**, is a professor emerita of nursing at the University of Rhode Island, from which she retired after a tenure of 31 years where she held academic positions, including the deanship of the College of Nursing from 1983 to 1988. She has held the position of professor II at the Institute of Nursing Science, University of Oslo from 1992 to 2003 and a professor at Buskerud University College in Norway from 2004 to 2008, where she currently holds the position of professor II. She has published extensively in the areas of nursing epistemology, theory development in nursing, the nature of nursing practice, and collaborative decision making in practice, as well as in various areas of clinical nursing research. She is the author of *The Nature of Theoretical Thinking in Nursing* (in its third edition), and the coeditor with Dr. Ingrid Kollak of Berlin, Germany, of the book, *Nursing Theories: Conceptual and Philosophical Foundations* (in its first and second editions). She has been the project director of two research projects funded by the Norwegian Research Council to Buskerud University College from 2007 to 2011; one on post-stroke fatigue and the other on crisis resolution and home treatment in community mental health care.

# The Essence of Nursing Practice

## *Philosophy and Perspective*

Hesook Suzie Kim, PhD, RN

SPRINGER PUBLISHING COMPANY
NEW YORK

Springer Publishing Company, LLC
11 West 42nd Street
New York, NY 10036
www.springerpub.com

*Acquisitions Editor*: Joseph Morita
*Composition*: MPS Ltd, India

*ISBN*: 978-0-8261-9428-2
*e-book ISBN*: 978-0-8261-9429-9

15 16 17 18 / 5 4 3 2 1

The author and the publisher of this Work have made every effort to use sources believed to be reliable to provide information that is accurate and compatible with the standards generally accepted at the time of publication. Because medical science is continually advancing, our knowledge base continues to expand. Therefore, as new information becomes available, changes in procedures become necessary. We recommend that the reader always consult current research and specific institutional policies before performing any clinical procedure. The author and publisher shall not be liable for any special, consequential, or exemplary damages resulting, in whole or in part, from the readers' use of, or reliance on, the information contained in this book. The publisher has no responsibility for the persistence or accuracy of URLs for external or third-party Internet websites referred to in this publication and does not guarantee that any content on such websites is, or will remain, accurate or appropriate.

**Library of Congress Cataloging-in-Publication Data**

Kim, Hesook Suzie, author.
The essence of nursing practice : philosophy and perspective / Hesook Suzie Kim.
p. ; cm.
Includes bibliographical references and index.
ISBN 978-0-8261-9428-2—ISBN 978-0-8261-9429-9 (e-book)
I. Title.
[DNLM: 1. Nursing Care—methods. 2. Nursing Process. 3. Philosophy, Nursing. WY 100.1]
RT84.5
610.7301—dc23

2014049278



Printed in the United States of America by McNaughton & Gunn.

# Contents

# Preface

This book has been in the making for the past 30 years or so. It has brewed from the countless hours spent with students and colleagues regarding "nursing practice" as a concept and an area of study. I designed and taught courses on theories of nursing practice in the master's and PhD programs in nursing at the University of Rhode Island, College of Nursing from the beginning of the 1980s. During my years teaching these courses on theories of nursing practice and delineation of concepts in the nursing practice domain, I have struggled with my students and colleagues regarding how best we could characterize the essential features of nursing practice in a normative stance. I believed then and continue to believe that the construct of nursing practice has to be specified by extracting elements encompassed within it, which are necessary for the practice of nursing to be of the highest quality. This means it is imperative to describe nursing practice in terms of how it *should* be practiced. Developing nursing practice either for beginning practitioners or advanced clinicians requires a guidepost toward which nurses' practice has to move to achieve the highest quality possible.

An analytical model of nursing practice is presented in this book as this guidepost and as a framework to delineate critical and essential elements of nursing practice. The literature is lacking in these sorts of comprehensive and analytic models to illustrate and examine features of nursing practice, and this has perhaps led education of nurses for nursing practice to be generally compartmentalized in relation to clinical problems. The model of nursing practice advanced in this book includes five structural levels—*perspective, knowledge, philosophy of practice, dimension,* and *process*—as the interconnected analytical structures that provide guidelines for how nursing practice needs to be configured and what elements are to be integrated to formulate nursing practice. Reed states that "the practice of nursing is an art of combining the contingencies of the moment, including diverse patterns of knowing, with systematic and scientific knowledge to create a caregiving situation" (2011, p. 20). In order for nurses to practice nursing in this sense, they have to rely not only on the knowledge, patterns of knowing, and the situational contingencies but more critically have to know the way to integrate these aspects to make their practice to be *nursing*. This integration does not occur naturally, but through an "intentional" application of various processes involved in human practice to make it nursing. The model is applied to delineate and examine factors that go into this integration for nursing practice. The major aim for the book is to sensitize nurses, both at the beginning and advanced levels, to the complexities involved in the practice of nursing, and to provide material necessary for an in-depth understanding and analysis of nursing practice in order to advance their practice.

The book is designed primarily for graduate students in nursing, especially those in advanced practice nursing programs at the master's and doctoral (DNP) programs who are engaged in clarifying the process of advanced nursing practice, and those in PhD programs who are interested in addressing epistemic questions related to nursing practice as generic subject matter. Senior-level undergraduate nursing students can benefit from this book if it is incorporated into their senior-level courses dealing with professional nursing, as it will provide a base with which they can begin to examine clinical practice in beginning practitioner roles. It will also be useful to nurses in practice in reflecting upon their own practice to develop their practice further. The book will be a resource to nursing educators in course designs and teaching of nursing practice regardless of clinical specialization.

I have been fortunate to be associated with many colleagues and graduate students who have stimulated and contributed to my thinking contained in this book. Among them, I must acknowledge three individuals specifically. Dr. Donna Schwartz-Barcott who, as a colleague at the University of Rhode Island, College of Nursing for nearly 30 years, has been a tireless sounding board and support for me. Dr. Inger Margrethe Holter of Norway has encouraged me over the years to continue with the line of thinking I hold about nursing practice, and has asked me to write an abridged version of my model for publication in a Norwegian nursing textbook. Also, Dr. Björn Sjöström of Sweden is acknowledged and fondly remembered. He was a wonderful colleague who had challenged me to work through various philosophical underpinnings of nursing practice in many hours of discussions at our meetings in all parts of the world, including one on a cold winter evening at a railway station in a small village in Sweden on our way to a conference. He helped greatly in crystalizing my thinking, especially in relation to pragmatism for the study of nursing practice. In addition, many of the ideas contained in this book have been expressed at various presentations made at annual meetings of the Eastern Nursing Research Society, at the New England Knowledge Conferences for Nursing Knowledge Development held at the University of Rhode Island from 1990 to 1994 and at Boston College from 1996 to 2001, and at other seminars for graduate students and faculty in Norway and Korea. The audiences at these presentations have been of great help through voicing their ideas and debates in clarifying my thinking.

Finally, I acknowledge the constant support provided by my husband, Hyung G. Park, who has encouraged me relentlessly to continue with this project even in our "retirement." It is to him that I dedicate this book.

My hope is that the book can serve as a springboard for lively discussions and debates regarding the nature and essence of nursing practice in our pursuit to advance nursing practice.

—Hesook Suzie Kim

CHAPTER 1

# Introduction

NURSING AS A FORM OF SERVICE has a long history, dating back to informal caregiving in ancient times to the current, highly organized, and disciplined professional practice. Although nurses hold various positions and roles within the health care system being engaged in direct patient care, administration, quality assurance, education, and research, it is what nurses do in direct patient care that constitutes the core of nursing as a practice discipline. Nurses in direct patient care are engaged in their practice as staff nurses, clinical specialists, master clinicians, advanced practitioners, or clinical supervisors in acute-care hospitals; long-term care institutions such as, nursing homes, chronic-care hospitals, or rehabilitation centers; home-care situations; community health care settings such as, group homes, schools, and health centers; clinics/ambulatory settings; and private offices. Although how nurses practice varies greatly across these settings depending on what patients generally require, which other professionals and nonprofessionals are there together with the nurses, and what the purposes of the settings are in relation to patient services, nurses are invariably the major players responsible for ensuring patients receive the care and treatments necessary to manage their health.

As occurs in many different fields and settings within the health care system, nursing practice encompasses many different sorts of actions and relationships. These range, for example, from deciding upon the best way to help a patient become competent doing his own colostomy care, to arranging for a patient's discharge to a nursing home after a stroke. However, it is not such actions or relationships per se as discrete entities that make nursing practice what it is, but it is in how they are put together by a nurse in the context of the patient as a person in need of assistance and service. Claire Fagin, in her introduction to Suzanne Gordon's book *Life Support,* articulates this by stating that even "emptying a bedpan" by a nurse, just as any other aspect of nursing practice, must be considered in "the context of a larger focus on the total patient" (Gordon, 1997, p. xviii). Nursing practice should not be equated with discrete actions such as assessing patients, giving medications, teaching patients, comforting, and discharge planning, however valuable and essential these are as segments of nursing practice. Such discrete actions are "techniques" unto themselves, which can be performed skillfully by anyone who is given training or has experience. And because techniques are only tools and methods applicable in the context of a goal, design, or production, it is the context of application that is of utmost importance. In nursing practice, various "techniques" are brought forward and applied in the context of patient care with the goal of enhancing healthful living or peaceful dying for patients. A nurse-midwife sits with a woman in labor, "doing nothing" as Kennedy (1999) puts it, but this "sitting" as a technique is a part of carefully constructed nursing practice for patients in labor, which involves noticing the progress, constant vigilance and surveillance of abnormal presentations, and bringing supportive presence. Sitting as a technique certainly is simple enough for anyone to perform; however, it becomes an essential aspect of nursing practice in this context not for its technical complexity but in its meaning and goals.

Often when teaching beginning nursing students nursing faculty may emphasize skill development in nursing "techniques" in isolation from the context of total nursing practice, which may be a necessary approach in teaching. However, it is not until such skills are put into a total package of nursing care that they come to have "nursing" meanings. Moreover, in the pressure-driven, time-constraining situations of the current health care arena, nurses sometimes are technique-oriented, often working with a list of activities to be carried out within a given span of time, with the completion of tasks as their primary focus. Tasks and techniques that are carried out by nurses with no relation to the meaning structure of nursing practice stand as separate strands dangling without being woven into what Baer and Gordon (1994) called "the tapestry of nursing." Gordon describes nursing "as a tapestry of care woven from countless threads into an intricate whole" (1997, p. 20). The nature and essence of nursing practice described and specified in this book is based on the notion of this tapestry not in the conventional, one-dimensional form, but in a complex, multidimensional work of integration and coordination. To begin with, nursing is a socially mandated form of human service, of which the nature and the demands change along with the changes that occur at larger social institutions and culture. Hence, the practice of nursing cannot be presumed to remain static in its character, but should be considered to evolve and change.

## THE DEFINITION OF NURSING PRACTICE

Writing in the cultural, scientific/technological, and societal backdrop of Europe and England in the 19th century, Florence Nightingale in her *Notes on Nursing* (1859/1946) considered human suffering, not of diseases themselves but suffering in diseases, the primary focus of nursing attention and suggested nursing to be critical in assisting the reparative process of nature. She wrote, "It [nursing] ought to signify the proper use of fresh air, light, warmth, cleanliness, quiet, and the proper selection and administration of diet—all at the least expense of vital power to the patient" (1859/1946, p. 6), and referred to it as *sanitary nursing*, differentiating this aspect of nursing from what she called *the handicraft of nursing* practiced in "surgical nursing" (1859/1946, p. 71). However, her notion of nursing expressed in these *Notes* addressed nursing in the context of "personal charge of health in others" in a generic sense rather than as a professionalized notion. Although Nightingale's ideas and her work have revolutionized the societal approaches to nursing and nursing education, the current ideas regarding the meaning of nursing reflect a great deal of change from this notion of *sanitary nursing*.

Henderson defined nursing more than four decades ago by stating that "the unique function of the nurse is to assist the individual, sick or well, in the performance of those activities contributing to health or its recovery (or to peaceful death) that he would perform unaided if he had the necessary strength, will or knowledge, and to do this in such a way as to help him gain independence as rapidly as possible" (1961, p. 42). This became the cornerstone for nursing practice in the second half of the 20th century, especially in the United States. Henderson, reflecting on her earlier writing in 1991, expanded this notion by putting more emphasis on primary health care as an expanding nursing responsibility, and nurses' role in helping patients with "a good death" (1991, p. 33).

In the background of Henderson's definition, and in reflection of the current situation of health care and nursing, the World Health Organization (WHO) Expert Committee on Nursing Practice, which convened in Geneva in 1995, proposed a functional definition of nursing. This definition emphasizes nursing's role in helping individuals, families, and groups in addressing and achieving their physical, mental, and social potential in the context of their everyday lives. Nursing functions encompass promotion and maintenance of health; prevention of ill health; and care during illness, rehabilitation, disability, and dying. It furthermore specifies that nursing has to uphold the values of self-determination and people's involvement in all aspects of health care. Nursing as an art and a science requires both specialized knowledge and knowledge from related fields applied to carry out its functions (WHO Expert Committee on Nursing Practice, 1996).

These statements in the definition reflect the current ideas of professional nursing practice and circumscribe the general characteristics of nursing. The definitions of nursing from that of Florence Nightingale to the most recent one by the WHO panel suggest the evolving nature of nursing practice in the context of both the internal and external forces that shape the nature of nursing practice in societies. However, there are major threads that remain constant regardless of the time and place. These are nursing's focus on people's health and illness, not on diseases, and its service orientation and person orientation.

Nursing practice is a form of human service, which is specifically anchored on the benefit of others (i.e., clients, patients, or service users), requiring the practice to be intentional, thought-out, and goal-directed. Nursing practice is a complex of online engagement in human actions, oriented to helping patients live their lives as well as possible in the context of health, illness, and dying. It is totally person-specific and established activities of nurses as agents of specific responsibilities. This means that each nursing situation involving a patient is unique in its demand for nursing actions. A patient in a specific time and context requires of the nurse in practice to respond to the patient- and situation-specific demands, needs, and considerations. Nursing situations vary within a broad spectrum of acuteness, complexity, seriousness, and meaning, ranging, for example, from a patient at a clinic who is newly diagnosed with diabetes having only a few problems of living to a patient in an intensive care unit who has gone through an extensive bypass surgery to deal with a coronary arterial obstruction, and to an elderly patient in a nursing home who is frail, confused, and dependent. Nursing practice occurs with patients who are located in various situations of living, including short-term or long-term institutions within the health care system, as well as in their homes. Nursing practice involves human beings both as recipients of nursing care (the patient) and as agents of nursing acts (the nurse). Because nursing practice is a special class of human actions, having a normative goal orientation as its starting point, our consideration of nursing practice must be framed within a normative model. That is, when we talk about nursing practice, we must deal with what it *ought to be*, which then can be used as the basis for examining what it is (i.e., how it is actually practiced). Nursing practice is defined as the following, encompassing several key ideas to identify nursing as a specific form of human service:

> *Nursing practice is a goal directed, deliberative, action oriented, and coordinated work for and with patients for enhancing healthful living or peaceful dying, in which patients and nurses share the ontological realities of human*

*features and life, and of human agency. Nursing practice is an intentionally coordinated process consisting of scientific, technological problem solving, human-to-human engagement, and services to patients with specific needs. It occurs in social situations of health care in which nurses assume particular sorts of responsibilities. (Kim, 2010, pp. 48–49; see Figure 1.1)*

*Nursing practice is goal directed*, meaning it is oriented to helping patients to deal with problems and issues pertaining to their health, both in times of health and illness. This goal is socially and legally mandated, as nurses are licensed to practice in accordance with the law that specifies what the practice must entail. The goal orientation of nursing practice is also articulated in the mandates advanced by professional nursing organizations such as the American Nurses Association (ANA). The ANA in its Social Policy Statements specified that nursing "is the protection, promotion, and optimization of health and abilities, prevention of illness and injury, alleviation of suffering through the diagnosis and treatment of human responses, and advocacy in the care of individuals, families, communities, and populations" (ANA, 2003, as quoted

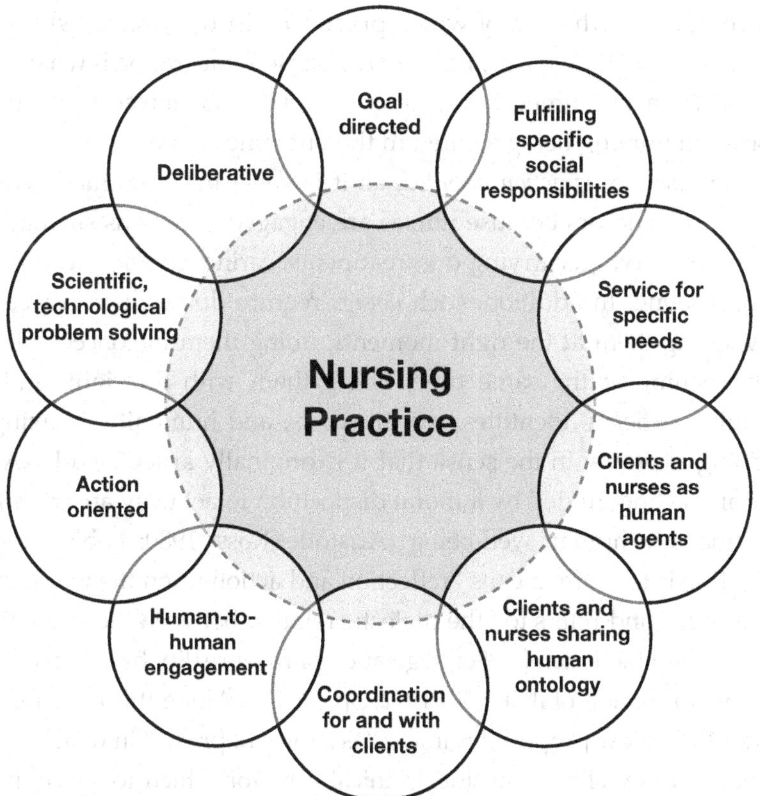


**FIGURE 1.1** Components of nursing practice embedded in the definition of nursing practice.

in ANA, 2010c, p. 10). Nurses themselves, patients and their families, professionals such as physicians, nonprofessionals, as well as laypersons expect nursing practice to be oriented to goals related to patients' health. The goal is related to enhancing patients to gain or sustain healthful living or peaceful dying.

*Nursing practice is deliberative*, in that it is designed and intentional to address the goals for patients. It requires nurses to know how to mobilize their own resources, both instrumental and cultural (such as knowledge, skills, techniques, attitudes, and values), and resources in patients and the environment deliberatively and intentionally. In practice, nurses need to be aware of and take into consideration the consequences of their actions in patients through their deliberations. Deliberation is making choices; Aristotle says that we deliberate about things that are in our power and that could be done in one way or another in order to achieve a given end. Aristotle, in his *Nicomachean Ethics*, articulates the characteristics of excellence in deliberation as that is aimed at an end, involving an inquiry into "a particular kind of thing," as "a kind of correctness," and involving reasoning, thus summarizing this by stating that "excellence in deliberation in a particular sense is that which succeeds relatively to a particular end ... [*and*] will be correctness with regard to what conduces to the end of which practical wisdom [*phronesis*] is the true apprehension" (Aristotle /Ross, 1980). In this sense, deliberation is what occurs in a situation of practice aimed at a goal or an end that is viewed to be "good"—"goodness" in nursing being located in the outcomes of patients.

*Nursing practice is action oriented*, as it is *doing* that eventually counts in practice. Practice occurs because nurses are engaged in actions such as assessing patients, observing, carrying out treatments, caring, communicating, teaching, or counseling. In addition, such *doings* require doing them correctly and skillfully, doing them at the right moments, doing them in concert with other things happening at the same time, doing them with foresight, and doing them valuing patients' identities, worth, wants, and humanity. Nursing practice as doing is praxis, in the sense that it is originally articulated by Aristotle as doing and acting guided by a moral disposition to act truly and rightly with a commitment to human well-being (Aristotle/Ross, 1980; Lobkowicz, 1967, pp. 9–15). Praxis to Freire means "reflection and action upon the world in order to transform it," and refers to "the dialectic relation between the subjective and the objective in which men [sic] engage and confront reality by critical intervention for transformation of it" (1970/1992, pp. 36–37). Along this line of thinking, Holmes and Warelow proposed nursing "as a form of praxis" in which it is "seen as a standard of excellence, an ideal ethical goal for which to strive; it is also what Marxists would describe as an attempt to make an irrational world more rational, or a way of making useable sense of one's practice world" (2000, p. 175).

Nursing practice as doing in this sense transcends the mere acting or performing and elevates it to the realm of morally committed human actions of nurses.

*Nursing practice is a coordinated work for and with patients.* Nurses are responsible for coordinating various sectors and players in the health care system to bring about the goals for patients. Nursing, in general, is not practiced in an isolated, separated, solo format, but is practiced in concert with others engaged together within a same time period or connected in a network of relationships. Nurses in hospitals, even under the primary nursing format of organized nursing service, work with other nurses on a same unit during a given shift, nurses from other shifts assigned to same patients, and nurses on other units who may have cared for the same patients or who will be caring for them later. Nurses not only coordinate the work of each other, as many nurses are involved in providing care to patients at different times and are responsible for different things, but also coordinate the work of physicians, various therapists, para-professionals, and other assistive workers so that patients receive appropriate care, therapy, and attention from these people. More importantly, nurses coordinate with patients and their families so that patients' needs, wants, and resources are brought into patient care. Nursing practice is primarily "working with" patients not upon patients, as patients are not receptacles of care provided by nurses but are coparticipants in the process of care. As coparticipants in the process of care, patients are involved in transforming their lives and actualizing their potentials for healthful living in concert with nurses. Therefore, the coordination required in nursing practice is encompassed within the notion of collaborative practice.

*Nursing practice involves patients and nurses sharing the ontological realities of human features and life.* This means that nursing practice as a form of life needs to be understood to involve patients and nurses, involving both as humans embodying strengths and weaknesses of humanness, such as (a) bounded physicality and consciousness, (b) unbounded imagination and creativity, (c) discursiveness, (d) social, cultural, and historical situatedness, (e) interpersonal dependence, and (f) solitary, independent existence. Humans are complex beings ontologically, encompassing various forms of paradoxes. On one hand, humans cannot deny their bodies as providing the concrete basis of existence, but, on the other hand, humans transcend their bodies in their existence as it has meanings stretching beyond the matters of body, as selfhood is an essential aspect of humans determining what it means to be individual human beings. Humans use language and other symbols to communicate with each other, and engage in thoughts and activities that are based on imagination and creativity.

Humans are also social, historical entities, each with a unique biography and at the same time also sharing social and historical backgrounds with many others. Nurses encounter each patient as a human being, who presents a human body and selfhood all at once that are framed by one's unique biography, social, cultural, and historical situatedness, and possibilities for consciousness, transformation, and relationships. Likewise, nurses are in practice as human beings with the same qualities. This means that as patients rejoice birth, recovery, and physical and emotional triumphs, nurses exult in success, competence, and collaboration; at the same time, as patients suffer and endure pain, are in a state of disability or dependence, or face impending death, nurses in practice also suffer and endure fatigue, irritation, disappointments, or helplessness. Individual human beings are unique in their makeup, existence, and experiences, although there are some aspects of individuals that express the shared qualities of humanness. Each nursing practice occasion is a meeting of at least two human beings with their complexities, similarities and differences, and commonness and uniqueness. In this sense, nursing practice is a part of life, that of both the patient and the nurse.

Ontological realities of humanness in patients within the perspective of nursing practice must encompass the idea of the human body as the seedbed of health, disease, and illness—not as a separate entity but one that is encased with other nonbodily aspects such as selfhood, history, sociality, and culture. The locus of nursing practice begins in patients with such realities, which are connected in a complex web of sensations, meanings, and expressions, and which nurses must respond to and address in their practice.

*Nursing practice involves patients and nurses as human agents.* "Human agency" is a term that refers to a human's autonomy, freedom, and responsibility in relation to one's own actions. Humans as agents are viewed to be entrusted with choice and deliberation (Dewey, 1922/1957), having the power and right to make decisions regarding one's actions and being responsible for one's conduct and participation in social life. Human agency refers to having the power to act, that is, "to intervene in the world, or to refrain from such intervention, with the effect of influencing a specific process or state of affairs," and having the "transformative capacity" for human action (Giddens, 1984, pp. 14–15). Human agency requires making choices and acting based on moral and ethical responsibility, and making a fine balance between self-interest and communal interests in social life. Nursing practice viewed in terms of human agency refers to the participation of nurses and patients in care as agents of autonomy, freedom, and responsibility. This means that both nurses and patients are to be held accountable for their choices and actions, but, at the same time, such accountability must emerge from a careful coordination of interests and choices. Imperative in this notion is the moral grounding with which human agency plays out in practice to produce a coordinated and effective social life.

The concepts of human agency differ among many philosophers and social scientists, ranging from a view that human agency is strictly contained within the self as an independent, autonomous being open to freedom to a postmodern view of human agency embedded through and through in culture, power, language, and history. For our purpose, human agency is conceived to be both free and constrained in dialectic relations to each other for the control of human actions and in the pursuit of a coordinated life. Hence, in nursing practice from the human agency perspective, it is neither the nurse nor the patient who wields final choices, but both as engaged agents. Because of this feature, nurses are called upon to act as moral agents in upholding the human agency of patients (Liaschenko, 1994), at the same time being responsible moral agents themselves.

*Nursing practice encompasses an aspect of scientific/technological problem solving*. Nursing within the current scientific/technological culture and the culture of economic efficacy and accountability has been entrusted with the responsibility of providing solutions for a set of human problems of health and illness. This has occurred both within nursing, as the nursing profession has sought to identify its social and instrumental identity as a worthwhile and necessary health care profession, and from external pressures to account mostly for the costs of its services within the health care system. Hence, nursing is responsible for providing solutions to problems presented by patients from the nursing perspective, utilizing scientific knowledge and technological instrumentation. Outcomes of nursing practice are measured in the context of expected results of nursing treatments, strategies, and interventions applied to solving patients' problems.

Thus, nurses are engaged in identifying problems, thinking through possible solutions based on available knowledge and techniques, and applying such solutions in order to achieve the most possible effectiveness and efficacy in situations. Problems that nurses are responsible to address include situational problems experienced by patients such as discomfort associated with prolonged bed rest to problems of living associated with illness such as dealing with dietary and activity requirements from being a diabetic or managing chronic fatigue and weakness in a cancer patient on long-term chemotherapy.

In addition, nurses often practice within the context of medical problem solving that focuses on diagnosing and treating diseases, participating as supporters and partners in the application of medical technologies and therapeutics. Nursing practice involves, for example, giving medications and monitoring the effects of drugs on patients, adjusting oxygen flow rates depending on patients' oxygen-saturation levels, instituting medical therapeutic regimes, or helping patients get x-rays. Liaschenko considers "monitoring patient responses to medical treatment the most visible, well-defined and, perhaps, common understanding of nursing practice" (1998, p. 13). Although nurses exercise a great deal of freedom in solving problems such as adjusting medication dosage or changing the timing of therapy, their work is circumscribed within the perspective of medical therapeutic effectiveness in this respect. However, this aspect of nursing practice is ancillary to the problem solving regarding patients' nursing problems.

In both of these sorts of involvement in problem solving, nursing practice relies on scientific knowledge and technology to attend to problems in rational, instrumentally oriented processes of decision making, critical thinking, and project design. This aspect of nursing practice is prescriptive and involves strategic actions. However, solving patients' problems in practice situations is a complex process in which presenting problems need to be contextualized and interpreted, and often "managed" or "attended to" rather than "solved" or "removed." The notion of scientific problem solving in nursing does not necessarily mean applying standardized solutions, but approaching a patient's problem as an individual, unique problem requiring an application of general theories and techniques fashioned for such uniqueness and individuality.

*Nursing practice involves human-to-human engagement.* Nursing practice occurs among people, with nurses and patients being the major players. It is a relational practice as Gadow (1995) and Bishop and Scudder (1999) suggest, in which nurses and patients are engaged with each other as humans, interacting and sharing. In human engagements, people present their selves and reveal their individualities through bodily and discursive acts. Through these acts, people arrive at constructions regarding others' and their own wants, needs, desires, and meanings, and formulate interpersonally valid and appropriate approaches to each other regarding such constructions. Human engagements are means through which humans gain access to each other's resources. However, patient-to-nurse engagements as relationships and interactions have a different character from that of the usual, personal engagements people establish in ordinary lives, as the patient-to-nurse engagement is framed within the respective roles of patients and nurses in the context of health care. Nortvedt (2001b) suggests that patient–nurse engagements as relationships are guided by moral responsibilities on the part of the nurse for attending to the needs and suffering of patients. Furthermore, patient–nurse engagements are akin to Freire's view of dialogical engagements of teacher–student in learning (Freire, 1970/1992), in which the climate of mutual trust is created for growth and transformation based on humility, love of life, the world, and other humans, and faith in human power. This relational character and mutuality in nursing practice can be threatened by power domination that is possible in all human relationships. Therefore, nursing practice as a form of human-to-human engagement needs to be founded upon mutual understanding attained through emancipatory insights and actions as suggested by Habermas (1983/1990).

*Nursing practice is a service to patients with specific needs.* Nursing practice is a form of human service aimed at helping patients with specific needs related to their health and illness. As a form of human service, it is guided by a set of ethical and moral principles and standards that shape the normative basis for the practice. Nursing's professional organizations such as the ANA or the International Council of Nurses (ICN) set the standards of ethical conduct in nursing practice, and formulate guidelines for moral sensibility desired in practice. Hence, besides nursing practice being guided by legal mandates, it is also guided by such ethical and moral standards and guidelines to be service-oriented and patient-oriented.

*Nursing practice occurs in social situations of health care in which nurses assume particular sorts of responsibilities.* Nursing practice is assumed by nurses who are social actors with the knowledge of their specific role obligations and expectations. This means that although each instance of nursing practice is unique and individualistic because of the singularity and uniqueness of the patient, the nurse, and the situation present in that instance, nursing practice constituting human activities has the character of continuity, routineness, and reproducibility. This makes nursing practice to be social practice contextualized both within each individual social situation and within the continuing structure of practice situations. Giddens (1984) suggests that social practice is founded upon "knowledgeability" as practical consciousness of social actors regarding the conditions and consequences of their conduct, and that such knowledge "provides for the generalized capacity to respond to and influence an indeterminate range of social circumstances" (p. 22). The key characteristic of social practice in this sense is the reproducibility of institutionalized practices in social situations. This is put somewhat differently by Bourdieu (1990) who suggested that an individual's practice is an on-the-spot coordination of situational knowledge and the habitus, through which there is a continuous shaping and reshaping of the habitus of the individual and of the social institution. An individual nurse's practice occurs in an environment of a health care situation in which her or his practice must be coordinated within the history and structure of the setting, and both influences and is influenced by other nurses' practice. This makes nursing practice a form of social practice that is bound both to specific time-space and to contiguous time-space contexts.

These key characteristics and elements together illustrate nursing practice in the contemporary world. Each characteristic by itself does not depict nursing practice, but all of these as a complex set of characteristics are present in nursing practice. Nursing, whether practiced in a neighborhood health clinic or in a highly critical tertiary care unit, involves an intricate weaving and putting together of these elements for each occasion of practice and for each patient so that the goal of improving patients' living in the context of health and illness is attained. For such weaving to occur successfully, efficiently, and finely (or beautifully), it is necessary that such weavings be guided by a normative model, a stencil, or signposts. The following chapters provide a detailed description of a model for nursing practice.

## NURSING PRACTICE IN THE CONTEXT OF THE HEALTH CARE SYSTEM, SOCIETY, AND CULTURE

Nursing in modernity has developed as a profession having its place of service within organized health care systems, especially hospitals as the main location. While the increasing complexity of current health care systems requires nursing to be practiced in various settings, nursing continues to be practiced as a part of an organized service delivery system. The ANA estimates that more than 90% of nurses in practice in the United States work at hospitals, long-term care institutions, and home-care agencies. Only a small fraction of nurses works independently in private practice. This means that nurses in practice are members of organized nursing care delivery systems, which are components of health care institutions. Within such systems, nurses assume specific organizational positions as "staff nurses," "clinical managers," and so forth. Each position is identified with its role obligations and job description. As members of health care organizations, nurses are obligated to adhere to various forms of institutional mandates, policies, and processes. For example, in a hospital where each nursing role is composed of responsibilities in direct patient care, education, and leadership, nurses must be able to identify their practice in these three areas of service. On the other hand, if a hospital has an established formula for a clinical ladder for advancement in clinical positions, nurses in such a hospital would be required to assess their practice and experience with respect to such formula in considering advancement. Nurses in institutions work within the institutions' nursing service departments that are organized to have specific structures, control processes, and personnel.

In addition, because hospitals and other health care institutions are organized in different matrices for patient care mostly influenced by "medical" schemes for classifying patients, they have units or wards identified for specialized medical services as medical (or more specialized as cardiovascular, neurological, respiratory, etc.), surgical (or more specialized as general, orthopedic, neurosurgical, cardiac, etc.), critical (or more specialized as medical intensive care, surgical intensive care, newborn and infant intensive care), pediatric, maternity, or psychiatric. This means that nursing practice comes to have a specific clinical character as nurses on different units or wards are exposed to clinical problems and patients typical of the units' specific service orientations. This has partly influenced the emergence of nursing specialties during the past several decades, such as cardiovascular nursing, oncology nursing, critical care nursing, or family nursing.

Because nursing practice mostly occurs in complex organizations, such as hospitals and long-term care institutions, the impact of the organizational characteristics on nurses' experiences within health care systems and in their practice is an important issue in relation to quality of practice and patient outcomes. The report by the American Academy of Nursing (McClure, Poulin, Sovie, & Wandelt, 1983) that identified key characteristics of the so-called "Magnet hospitals" that were successful in recruiting and retaining professional nurses provided the base for serious attention to the effects of practice environment on nurses and their practice. The study identified 14 "forces of Magnetism" in terms of (a) organizational features including the quality of leadership, management style, and organizational structure; (b) organizational practices related to staffing, orientation, education, personnel policies/programs, and career development; and (c) organizational culture in relation to professional practice models, quality of care, autonomy, and the image of nursing as factors that together influence the attraction and retention of nurses in hospitals. These became the base for the development of the ANA's Magnet Recognition Program offered by the American Nurses Credentialing Center (ANCC) that was established in 1990. Currently, ANCC offers the Magnet Recognition Program to hospitals and long-term care facilities in the United States and internationally. ANCC functions within a conceptual framework of the Magnet Model that include five components for assessing organizational quality: (a) a transformational leadership component that encompasses quality of nursing leadership and management style; (b) a structural empowerment component that is represented by organizational structure, personnel policies and programs, community and the health care organization, image of nursing, and professional development; (c) an exemplary professional practice component that represents professional models of care, consultation and resources, autonomy, nurses as teachers, and interdisciplinary relationships; (d) a new knowledge, innovation, and improvement component encompassed by the aspect of quality improvement; and (e) an empirical quality outcomes component referring to quality of care (ANCC, 2014). The assumption is that these forces of Magnetism are the elements that shape organizations of practice not only to attract and retain professional nurses within its organizations, but also to foster higher quality of nursing practice eventually affecting patient outcomes. Such a model was developed by Stone, Hughes, and Dailey (2008) extending the work of Stone et al. (2005) in which the linkages among the facets of the health care environment to the quality of professional practice and patient outcomes are suggested. In the model, outcomes in the staff, patients, and organization are viewed to be influenced by two forces: (a) the health care organization's structural characteristics and (b) the microclimate embedded within staff, patients, and the organization. Structural characteristics of the organization enable such factors as leadership, technologies, communication, and financial resources, while the microclimate influences actions of staff and patients. Stone et al. (2008), in their review of the research literature, suggest that there is a consistently positive relationship between organizational climate and outcomes in patients and workers, especially in relation to patient safety outcomes and staff job satisfaction. Lundmark's review of the literature (2008) on the Magnet quality for nursing in hospitals shows a positive relationships between Magnet qualities and nurse outcomes, such as job satisfaction, burnout, turnover, and perceived quality of care, and Magnet characteristics and patient outcomes in aggregate, such as mortality rates and patient safety, as well as in individuals, such as patient satisfaction. Although the research evidence up to date is only tentative, the evidences from organizational sciences and sociology on the impact of social environment on people's actions suggest the importance of organizational qualities in affecting nursing practice, which, in turn, will affect patient outcomes.

Nursing practice is furthermore influenced by the economic forces and health care financing that shape the dynamics of the health care system. The introduction of diagnosis-related groups (DRGs) in the United States in the 1980s as the basis for reimbursing the costs of hospital care and prospective financing has changed the structure and management of hospital care fundamentally, causing the shortening in the average lengths of hospitalization and introducing the concept of managed care and other forms of financial control in institutional management of health care. There continues to be a controversy regarding the impacts of health care financing on nursing staff shortages, work overload, and high turnover rates. This health care financing structure also has been attributed to an increase in the acuity and intensity levels of patient care not only in hospitals but also in nursing homes and home-care institutions. As the clinical characteristics of the patient population change in this context, the demands for the types of nursing services change. This has been especially evident in the changes in home-care or community-care nursing practice, as many patients who would have stayed at hospitals were being discharged to homes for complex nursing care. Such shifts have influenced nursing practice to become more complex.

The environment of nursing practice is also a social milieu within which social patterning in practice behaviors gets established. For example, nurses' practice behaviors, such as pain assessment, have been shown to be patterned differently according to the culture of specific nursing units (Lauzon Clabo, 2008). The influence of the nursing practice environment on the shaping and patterning of the modes with which nurses on specific units practice has been examined by social science frameworks such as the work of Blau on structural effects (1964), Bourdieu's theory of practice (1977, 1990), Gidden's structuration theory (1984), and Atkinson's culturation of medical discourse (1995). Although the orientations of these theorists are quite different, their theoretical works suggest the influence of a social unit by having established somewhat stable sets of structures, patterns, norms, and values on the actions of its members. This does not mean that individual practitioners do not have unique, individualistic ways of practice, but means that individuals contribute to the patterning within social fields as well as adopt the general patterns that are established within the fields. There would tend to be more similarities than differences in the ways nurses practice within one unit compared with nurses across different units. As long as nursing is practiced in organizational settings such as hospitals, nursing homes, and clinics, it is critical to view the effects of organization of practice on individual nurses' practice.

At the societal level, nursing practice is influenced by developments and changes in societal demands for health care, scientific and technological advancements, forms of division of labor for health care, and overall economic level. There are different types of nursing services required for special populations or special clinical emphases that arise in societies at any given time, for example, in an epidemic, or in responding to a shift in the societal focus on different sorts of health care. Nursing throughout the modern period has been influenced greatly by the scientific and technological advancements in general and particularly in the medical sector. Nursing practice continues to assimilate such advances in its practice protocols, to develop specific nursing techniques utilizing scientific and technological knowledge, and to accommodate changes in medical technology in general. An increase in nursing research and knowledge development at the national and international levels as a societal development in recent decades also has had a critical impact on knowledge use in nursing practice.

On the other hand, the scope of nursing practice expands or constricts as the dynamics in the distribution of health care personnel resources change in societies. For example, the demand for primary health care services that were not met by physicians adequately was the impetus for the development of the role of nurse practitioners in the United States beginning in the late 1970s, while an increase in the use of certified nursing assistants in health care institutions during the 1990s was a response to the nursing shortage and financial constraints within the health care system.

Culture as a sustaining and continuing but at the same time evolving symbolic force on social life is the seedbed of customs, rules and norms, prevailing ideologies, and beliefs. Nursing practice, similar to any other social practice, develops within a cultural environment that provides general directions and choices in social life. Dominant cultural themes of a general nature such as utilitarianism, self-determination, gender differentiation, ageism, and various forms of discrimination have influenced people's conduct and production in general as well as the form and content of nursing practice as a social practice. For example, the change to casual, free-form attires of nurses in practice today from the starched, regulation white uniform of earlier days is a reflection of a more fundamental cultural change regarding rules, individual choices, and self-expression. A leaning toward the acceptance of nursing as a gender-neutral profession in many societies is also a reflection of cultural belief systems regarding gender and work.

From a contextual perspective, the WHO Expert Committee on Nursing Practice (1996) identified four sectors within the force field for nursing practice: (a) economic resources; (b) political, social, and cultural factors; (c) demography and epidemiology within societies; and (d) environment of practice. These sectors shape and influence nursing practice and nursing, in turn, influences them. In addition, social processes that exist in the context of nursing practice as leadership and management, working conditions, legislation and regulation, education, and research are viewed also as forces that affect how nursing is practiced in different situations. Therefore, the nature of nursing practice has to be examined and understood from the perspective of not only human action but also social and cultural contexts.

## A MODEL FOR NURSING PRACTICE

A model for nursing practice is necessary to examine the nature and essence of nursing practice comprehensively and to establish the concept of nursing practice as a professional, human-service practice. For this purpose, a model that incorporates five structural components (perspective, knowledge, philosophy, dimension, and process) has been developed and is presented here as the organizing framework for the following chapters in this book regarding the essences of nursing practice. The model of nursing practice presented in this book is a normative model rather than a descriptive model, specifying how and what nursing practice *ought to be,* rather than what it is.

The development of models of nursing practice has its beginning with the ideas of Nightingale. Nightingale (1859/1946) specified nursing in terms of what nurses must do in order to enhance health, prevent disease, and care for the sick. She classified these into four distinctive actions: (a) management of the environment and provision of food and feeding, (b) management of self and others for coordinated activities for the sick, (c) communication with the sick, and (d) observation. Her pioneering ideas set into motion the development of modern nursing practice in the following decades, and the concept of the nursing process became the epitomized model for nursing practice since the 1960s beginning in the United States. Nursing process as the model for nursing practice was developed within the culture of rationalistic problem solving as the basis for professional work, and had its beginning in Orlando's work (1961) on disciplined professional practice. The model of nursing process formally elucidated by Yura and Walsh (1978) is based on a rational, deliberate process involving assessment, planning, intervention, and evaluation, and was endorsed by the ANA (1980) as the model for nursing practice. Following this development in the United States, the nursing process has become the major organizing model for nursing practice globally with the endorsements by the ICN and the WHO. As the institutionalized method for nursing practice, many nursing theorists including Henderson, Roy, Orem, and Neuman, as well as their followers, have illustrated how their nursing theories can be specified within this model, especially in terms of providing frameworks for patient assessment. The key aspect of the nursing process is a formulation of the nursing care plan based on systematic assessment and deliberation, which is then used as the guide for nursing care. The model of the nursing process is seen to have gone through various transformations from its beginning to the present, with the most recent transformation of the model being the incorporation of nursing diagnoses (North American Nursing Diagnosis Association [NANDA]), nursing interventions (Nursing Interventions Classification [NIC]), and nursing outcomes (Nursing Outcomes Classification [NOC]) as a way to systematize nursing practice and nursing documentation (Lunney, 2009).

Departing from the nursing process model are the proposals from the phenomenological perspective for nursing practice such as those by Parse (1997, 1998) and Newman (1994) for whom nursing practice is a mutually evolving process of human-to-human engagement in the context of nursing. In addition, many expositions on description or specification of nursing practice that deviate from the concept of nursing process focus mostly on the meanings and types of nursing actions in practice such as clinical reasoning (Benner, 2009), interaction (Peplau, 1952; Travelbee, 1964), and caring (Watson, 2012) rather than providing a comprehensive model for describing nursing practice as a set of organized, goal-directed activities. Such expositions and the nursing process model do not provide us with a comprehensive view of nursing practice specifically for the extraction of essential characteristics of nursing practice. The model presented in this chapter and used as the framework for this book has been developed to remedy this shortcoming by incorporating five critical components that are viewed to make up the total nature of nursing practice.

The model is an extension and elaboration of a model presented in an earlier work (Kim, 2010). It is configured by five sets of structures: (a) the perspective, (b) the knowledge, (c) the philosophy, (d) the dimension, and (e) the process, as shown in Figure 1.2. The model is the framework by which the essence of nursing practice can be extracted and the essential characteristics of nursing practice can be fully illustrated. It is different from the model of nursing process that focuses on the process of carrying out patient care, as the model extracts the structural elements that shape nursing practice as it *ought to be practiced.*

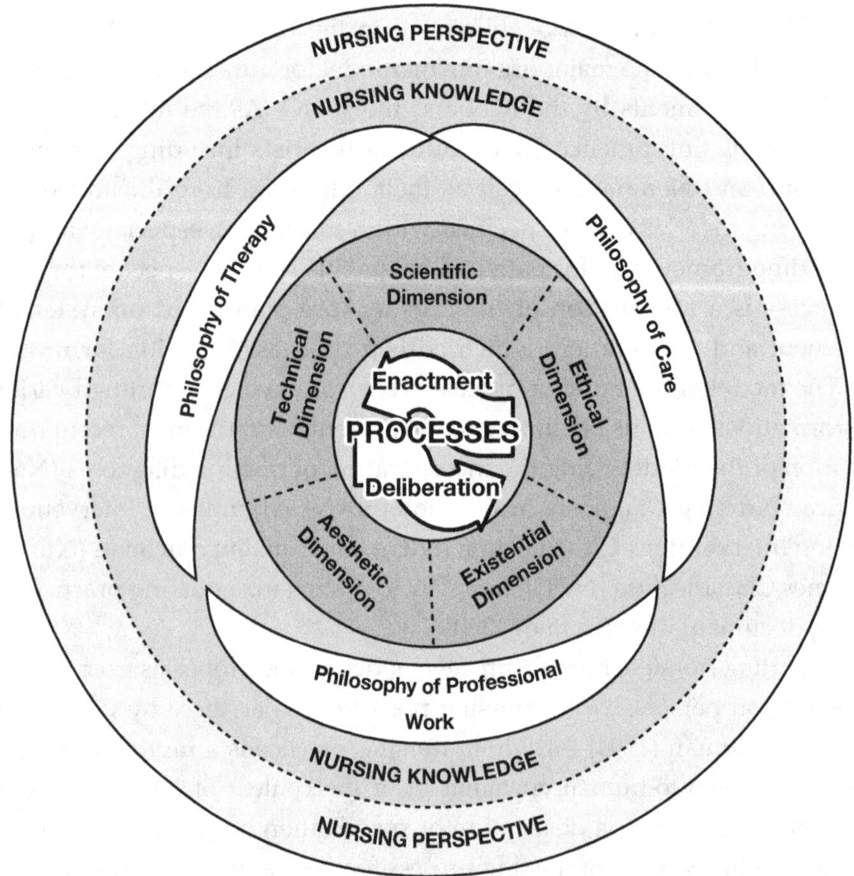


**FIGURE 1.2** An analytic model of nursing practice.

The *structure of perspective* is the base upon which all aspects of nursing practice are determined, as it identifies the guiding value systems for nursing practice. This structure of perspective consists of four value systems: (a) holism, (b) health orientation, (c) caring, and (d) person-centered practice. The guiding value systems, although evolving, provide the base for all other structures that determine the nature of nursing practice. The perspectives point to the nursing-specific ways of seeing the world, and establish the nursing frames of reference for practice. The *structure of knowledge* determines the nature of knowledge necessary for nursing practice. This structure is preconfigured by the structure of perspective but at the same time is the foundation upon which the structure of perspective can develop. The *structure of philosophy* provides the philosophical underpinnings for how nursing practice is to be carried out, and consists of three philosophical orientations: (a) the philosophy of care, (b) the philosophy of therapy, and (c) the philosophy of professional work. The *structure of dimension* refers to the characteristics that make up the nature of nursing practice and is based on five organizing rationalities to characterize nursing practice. It is constituted by the scientific, technical, ethical, aesthetic, and existential dimensions guided by five organizing rationalities, which specify five different forms of modus operandi in nursing practice. The *structure of process* encompasses how nursing practice is actualized, specifying human processes that produce actual contents and modes of nursing practice. It is composed of two processes: deliberation and enactment. The actual content of nursing practice is therefore guided by how the two processes of nursing practice are integrated into the five modus operandi of nursing practice. This means that while the structures of perspective, knowledge, and philosophy are the foundations undergirding the practice, the structures of dimension and process determine actual contents and characteristics of nursing practice. Nursing practice is thus organized about and constructed by integrating the essential elements in these five structures (as layers) to result in what nurses do for their clients.

In Chapter 2, the conceptualization of client from the nursing perspective is discussed, as the client is the central figure in nursing practice. Detailed descriptions and comprehensive expositions regarding the structures of perspective, knowledge, philosophy, dimension, and process of the model of nursing practice are presented in Chapters 3 through 7.

Chapter 8 identifies, describes, and examines the essential general tools of practice specific to nursing, which are required for and applied in nursing practice. These are behavioral and cognitive repertoires that are applicable to various sorts of nursing practice situations, and that have nursing-specific utility, meaning, and application. Chapter 9 addresses the concept of collaborative practice in terms of intra-, inter-, and cross-agency collaboration in the context of person-centered practice.

In Chapter 10, knowledge application in practice is examined applying a model of knowledge application in nursing practice. The concept of knowledge-based practice is discussed vis-à-vis evidence-based practice, and critical reflective inquiry as a generative mode of development in practice is presented. Chapter 11 deals with excellence in practice and the meaning of good practice in relation to the concept of quality of practice. In Chapter 12, the future directions for ways of advancing and developing nursing practice to meet the demands of advancing technology, of differentiated client needs, and of institutional, societal, and cultural changes are discussed.

## SUMMARY AND QUESTIONS FOR REFLECTION AND FURTHER DELIBERATION

Nursing practice as human service practice involves actions that are (a) goal directed toward and deliberative for clients' healthful well-being; (b) based on specialized knowledge, skills, attitudes, and ethics; and (c) guided by professional standards and social mandates. Nursing practice involves many different actions carried out in nursing care situations, and such diverse actions come to have the significance of nursing only when they are woven and integrated together with the *nursing* orientation. A model of nursing practice with five components is presented as the framework to design and evaluate nursing practice, and also as the organizing structure for the book in discussing what it would entail to produce best practice. The model, as a normative one, is composed of five integrative structures: (a) the perspective, (b) the knowledge, (c) the philosophy of nursing practice, (d) the dimension, and (e) the process. The model is applied to extract the essence of nursing practice and to illustrate the weaving of the best nursing practice.

- What are your worldviews relevant to your practice of nursing?
- What is your definition of nursing practice and in what ways is it different from the generic definitions given by the ANA, the ICN, and the author? What are the key concepts embedded within your definition? How is your definition of nursing practice reflected in your practice?
- A model of nursing practice as an analytical tool is presented in this chapter to be used as a framework to examine the essential features of nursing practice. What is your reaction to this model? Can you think of another approach to examine nursing practice analytically?
- The model is structured by five components: perspective, nursing knowledge, philosophy of practice, dimension, and process. Can you describe your own practice in terms of these five components?

# CHAPTER 2

# The Client of Nursing

Because nursing is a human service profession, the centerpiece of nursing practice is the client. In the tradition of nursing developed within the context of "sick care," the term "patient" has been used to identify the nursing client in general. However, because this term has often come to connote sickness, dependency, and vulnerability, there has been a shift to use "client" as a term replacing "patient" during the past three decades. Another term to replace "patient" is "service user," which has become a neutral term most often used in mental health care in a similar way as the term "client" has been used in nursing. This development aligns with the idea that nursing and health care, in general, are practiced not only with sick people but also with healthy persons, and also with the belief that people in health care should be endowed with self-determination and independency as much as possible. In this book, the terms "client" and "patient" are used interchangeably while referring to people who receive nursing care, because although I believe the generic term of client to be more neutral in general, the term patient is more natural and fitting in some contexts.

"Nursing client" refers to an individual (or an aggregate of individuals such as family or population) designated to be a recipient of nursing service in a health care situation. A person in a health care situation may be the client of nursing, medicine, physiotherapy, social work, and so forth, indicating that he or she receives care and services from several health care providers for different needs and purposes, but all having significance in the context of health. Nursing client may refer to groups of people such as families who receive nursing care as groups, or as aggregates such as a community or population especially in the context of public health and community health nursing.

Nursing is principally concerned with helping people in their experiences in the context of health and illness in various health care situations. When we talk about health regardless of how it is conceptualized, we cannot deny its relation to the human body because a bodily injury, disease, or malfunction brings about the most obvious threat to health. However, health is not simply a matter of the human body, as it refers to a fundamental state of being "good," "happy," "intact," "functioning," which goes beyond the conditions of human body, and "experiencing" as human persons. Humans conceptualized as nursing clients, therefore, are persons who experience and live with physical bodies and selfhoods in specific but contiguous situations. In nursing, the emphasis is not on any specific aspect of a person, such as bodily, psychic, or spiritual, but on the total being as an experiencing and living human person.

There have been many ways of viewing humans as composites of various compartments, parts, or aspects throughout history. Human beings are thought to be composed of body and mind in the Cartesian dualist's tradition (Wozniak, 1995), or have physiological, psychological, social, and spiritual aspects in what Parse (1987) called a totality paradigm, or are considered by many holists to be indivisible wholes. I have taken the position that humans are living entities of body and selfhood that are intricately interconnected and integrated to become constituted into humans' living (Kim, 2010).

The human body is concrete in its appearance, shape, and makeup, is experienced in time and space as an existential being, and is embodied symbolically to have specific meanings not necessarily tied to its materialistic, concrete nature. The human body is characterized by its materialistic and biologic features such as those that emerge from its genetic origins or from the processes and mechanisms for maintenance, generation, growth, regeneration, degeneration, and decay as a biologic entity. However, it is not a simple configuration of physical, materialistic, or biologic elements, but also constitutes the physical/material, the psychic/spiritual, and the symbolic/cultural elements. The human body is a vehicle through which humans are social beings, capable of symbolizing and interacting as well as being controlled and controlling. The human body exists and has meaning for its capacity to have relations with space and time, and to perform both mechanistic and expressive activities, and also for its ability to project messages and identity in a cultural context (Benoist & Cathebras, 1993). Human existence and living are concretized through the body, and the body mediates living in its many particular forms such as eating, sleeping, talking with friends, working, or loving, and in its entirety in a holistic sense such as being a specific person, an employee, a woman, or elderly.

On the other hand, selfhood is identified with its unique biography and history, and is acknowledged for its existential reality inwardly within the person as well as through external validation. Selfhood is signified by an identity that is associated with being a John Smith that is different from all other John Smiths and from all other persons. Selfhood is an essential aspect of a human person that is experienced through human subjectivity that encompasses reflexivity, consciousness, and meaning making. Selfhood exists immaterially as an idea, but it is experienced concretely in human behaviors, thoughts, attitudes, and feelings interpenetrating into all aspects of living. Often the idea of "soul," "spirit," or "mind" is attached to the notion of selfhood. However, the mind as constituted in selfhood transcends the conceptualization of it in the psychological or neuropsychological sense, and refers to the ability to construct one's own being as an existential idea. As Gadow (1980) suggests, human existence may entail phenomenological relations between the body and selfhood, and humanness is revealed in an intricate interweaving of these two aspects. Thus, clients as human beings are entities established by the body, selfhood, and sociality.

## NURSING PERSPECTIVE OF CLIENTS—HUMAN LIVING

As modern nursing became shaped and progressed during the past five decades, various nursing perspectives of viewing clients have been developed and used in practice. Henderson (1961, 1966) was a pioneer who articulated a nursing perspective of primarily helping people in the performance of activities pertaining to daily patterns of living especially in relation to 14 basic human needs. She reiterated this idea later by stating that "the primary responsibility of the nurse is that of helping people with their daily patterns of living, or with the following activities that they ordinarily perform without assistance" (1991, p. 36). Following this pioneering work in the 1960s, nursing scholars began developing various conceptual and theoretical frameworks to be used as guidelines for nursing practice as well as for knowledge development. The first in this development was to identify the nature and aspects of basic human needs (Abdellah, Beland, Martin, & Matheney, 1960). This was followed by the seminal work by Rogers who developed a unique holistic nursing perspective as the science of unitary, irreducible, human beings (Rogers, 1970, 1989, 1990, 1992, 1994). Parse (1997, 1998) and Newman (1994, 2002) proposed theories of nursing oriented to human experiencing from the phenomenological and hermeneutic perspectives, claiming their orientations to be holistic. Several different versions of holism as the perspectives for viewing clients exist that range from the unitary holism of Rogers to systems orientations. In addition, the holistic view of humans has become a slogan in nursing for the past several decades without a clear conceptualization of what holism stands for in nursing (Kim, 2006). Hence, although the nursing frameworks that were developed during the 1980s mostly maintained their orientations to holistic philosophy, they shifted their foci to causality, processes, and status (conditions) such as adaptation (Roy & Andrews, 1991), system stability and integrity (Neuman, 1998), and self-care deficit (Orem, 1995). While such nursing frameworks have been instrumental in articulating nursing's unique conceptualizations of clients departing from the medical and reductionistic orientations, they were focused either on causality/processes or on experiencing as dichotomous and separate conditions of life in viewing nursing clients.

These developments, I believe, have resulted in limited views of clients, and there is a need to refocus the nature of the nursing client as *human living* that Henderson emphasized. Shifting nursing's framework to human living (Kim, 2000, 2010) allows nursing to focus on helping people to *live* as healthful a life as possible in various health care contexts. This is more critical in this new century, because the amount of time people stay in acute-care hospitals is shortening to merely a few days. What this means is that health care settings in which we will find nursing clients are mostly going to be the settings where they carry on their daily living. Therefore, we should establish human living as our foci rather than illness or responses to disease as our primary focus of attention. This directs us to the idea that nursing is responsible for helping people to carry on with their living as independently and as fulfilled as possible.

The focus of nursing attention to the client in practice, therefore, is not just the body or the selfhood, but human living as played out through the mediation between these two aspects. Nursing practice is oriented to helping clients in their living with respect to health and illness. Human living involves being of oneself linking body and selfhood in terms of (a) acting and responding to experience; (b) sustaining, growing with, and transforming one's existence; and (c) managing in situations and with others. Human living in the health context thus means to experience oneself as a person who is known and knowable as a unique composite of the body and selfhood, characterized by its condition in relation to health and illness. It also means to engage in caring for oneself for health, such as eating the right food, exercising, getting inoculations, or managing stress. Human living as it involves managing in situations means to respond to situational demands, to control environmental constraints, to maintain the integrity of oneself, and to be adaptive and integrating with changes that occur in life situations. Therefore, in practice, nurses are concerned with clients' confrontations with trauma, acute diseases, chronic illness, disability, or dying with respect to how such confrontations affect their bodily functions, selfhood, and human relationships, and what disruptions, disarrays, and disturbances in their living are brought about by them. Nurses furthermore focus on clients' living in relation to changing life situations. For example, a nurse is required to care for a patient in a hospital with a hip replacement, attending to the problems presented in that situation, such as pain, immobility, or anxiety, and at the same time to foresee that patient being at home to continue with his or her living. Hence, the nurse is concerned with both the patient's living as it occurs at the hospital and with his or her living expected after discharge from the hospital.

Human living in this sense constitutes four integrative dimensions: living with one's body, living of oneself, living with others, and living in situations (Figure 2.1). Living in these four dimensions is oriented to continuity, fulfillment, independence, cohabitation, interdependence, and feeling good. Living with one's body, in both physical and embodied senses, refers to such aspects as rhythms, intactness and appearance, capacities and limitations, bodily feelings, and sensations. Living of oneself, on the other hand, encompasses history, genealogy, desires and wants, dreams and hopes, ideas and opinions, choices, habits, and knowing. Living with others refers to connecting, interacting, relating, and communicating with instrumental, symbolic, or affective orientations, while living in situations includes responding to, accommodating to, adapting in, managing, engaging in, choosing in, and creating within many contexts of one's existence.

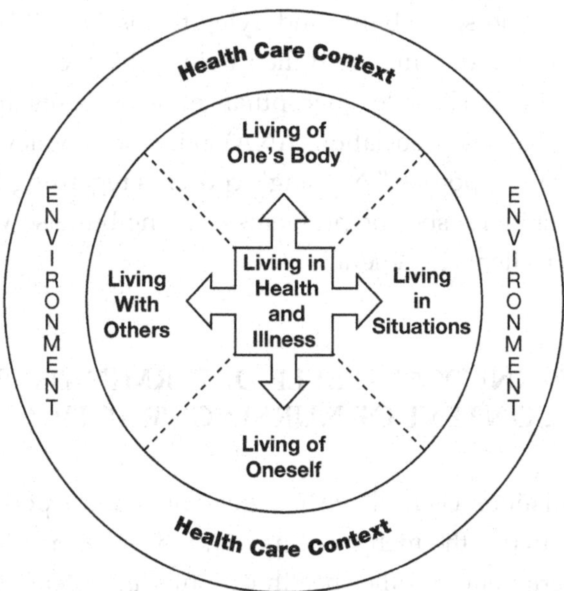


**FIGURE 2.1** A model of human living in health and illness. Adapted from Kim (2010, p. 111).

Patients' living, conceptualized in this way in this century, will be influenced greatly by limitations due to chronic disability, confinement, decreases in resources both personal and external, as well as by possibilities made available through new technologies, different settings or placements for recovery, or accessibility to information. We in nursing must begin to view patients' living and independence in it with new insights. Ryan (1997) suggests that we must shift our thinking from focusing on episodic illness and deficit thinking to health perspectives that require nursing to engage in attributional assessment, restoration, and supporting self-care.

Nursing's concern with clients is in the perspective of trajectory, and focuses on how well the patient is "living" in *this* situation of health care and how the patient is and will be progressing with his or her living throughout *this* episode of care and beyond. Nurses, as the major care providers, affect patients' living in health care situations significantly and much more than any other health care providers. Nursing affects clients' living not only at the time of care but also in relation to how ready the patient is to live the life that is open to him or her.

This is a broad conceptualization of client applicable in the nursing perspective, and is not tied to any specific philosophical or theoretical notions regarding human nature. The notions outlined earlier provide a set of generic ideas regarding how nursing must view clients and their needs for nursing care, moving away from the medical as well as a strictly psychological or social focus. Nursing's concern is health of people; it is not on the processes of trauma, diseases, illness, disability, and dying themselves. It is on the impact of such processes on individuals and their living. This focus by nursing practice on human living is a broader conceptualization of clients than that offered by the American Nurses Association (ANA) in its social policy statement that focuses on "human responses." Nursing's concerns regarding clients are thus not only associated with specific problems of living but also with enhancing healthful living in clients in general.

## HUMAN DIGNITY AND SELF-DETERMINATION IN THE CONTEXT OF NURSING PRACTICE

In health care situations, clients have to depend upon the expert powers of professionals; come under the mercy of financial powers exercised by insurance companies, government, or other health care funding agencies; become subjected to institutional regulations and mandates such as hospital rules and policies; and get confined and constrained by health care technology. Health care situations often put clients in vulnerable positions in their relations with health care professionals, institutions, and technology, leading them to be powerless. In this context, the idea of patient rights has become an important development in the present era. Patient rights in health care are, in general, related to being treated with human dignity, and with an assurance for self-determination and autonomy. During the last two decades, many countries have adopted legal mandates or principles for patient rights in health care in these regards, some as general guidelines while others focusing on specific aspects such as informed consent, or advance directives, such as the Patient Self-Determination Act for advance directives in the United States.

Human dignity is a concept that applies to an individual's worth as a human person, worthy of respect, integrity, privacy, identity, and autonomy. Clients are to be approached for their individual worth in health care. Fagermoen (1997) found human dignity as the core value in the professional practice of nurses, and suggests that human dignity as the core value in nursing practice orients nurses morally to value other related values such as security, integrity, personhood, being a fellow human, autonomy, privacy, reciprocal trust, hope, and general humanity. Upholding human dignity in nursing practice means the necessity for nurses not only to act toward clients to ensure human dignity in them, but also be aware of and astute to situations in which clients' dignity may be jeopardized and be proactive for and protective of clients' dignity as humans. Maintaining one's human dignity even in vulnerable conditions of living, as in many situations of health care (e.g., when persons have to expose their private body parts to others; are stigmatized as being abnormal, undesirable, or irresponsible; are stripped of personal identity as in being institutionalized; or lose their private space), requires support from nurses and other health care professionals.

Another prevailing value and moral guideline applicable in the conceptualization of client is the idea of self-determination. The concept of self-determination and a related concept of individual autonomy have been hailed as the major values in health care in our contemporary society. The concept, having been discussed greatly within political contexts especially in the modern era of democracy and decolonization, has been applied to individuals within the context of health care during the past several decades. The major principle of self-determination espouses the right for an individual's determination regarding choices in treatment, institutionalization, and incapacities. Although there is a commitment to the philosophy of self-determination in health care and professional caregivers uphold the philosophy in general, there are various forms and processes that seem to hinder the exercise of self-determination by clients. One major reason for this is the vulnerability of clients in health care situations. Clients of health care are often dependent on others' (i.e., professionals') knowledge, authority, and care to get better; are not always aware of choices available to them; may be incapable of decision making; or may be considered incapable of decision making. There could be various forms of aggression and impingements on freedom, either subtle or manifest, especially in the philosophy of professional dominance and social control, for example, for patients with mental illness, chronic disability, or in sudden vulnerability.

The concept of patient-centered/person-centered care has been developed in nursing as well as in medicine as an approach to uphold clients' autonomy and self-determination. The concept has been evolving within health care, especially in the United Kingdom with the term "person-centered" care to mean health and nursing care to uphold a person's individuality, the right for self-determination, and personal respect. In medicine, the concept has been developed in both the United Kingdom and the United States specifically in terms of the patient–physician relationship. Kitwood (1997) defines person-centeredness as "... standing or status that is bestowed upon one human being, by others, in the context of relationship and social being. It implies recognition, respect, and trust" (p. 7). In their review of instruments used to measure patient-centered care in medicine, Mead and Bower (2000) identified five dimensions of the concept: (a) biopsychosocial perspective for a person that expands the concept of person beyond the traditional medical model; (b) "patient-as-person" that posits the focus of attention not simply on diseases but on the person; (c) sharing power and responsibility in decision making; (d) therapeutic alliance; and (e) "doctor-as-person" that positions the doctor on an equal footing with the patient. Similarly Leplege et al. (2007) specified four dimensions of the concept of person-centeredness in the context of rehabilitation: (a) addressing the person's specific and holistic properties in terms of individual uniqueness and holistic connectedness of people's lives and identities; (b) understanding the person, especially his or her difficulties in everyday life, in the context of his or her life situation; (c) considering the person as an expert allowing for participation and empowerment; and (d) upholding respect for the person "behind" the impairment or the disease. The concept of person-centered nursing has been articulated by McCormack (2004), deriving from the concept of reflective person, which considers humans capable of seeing life as a whole and make choices that are their own, in relation to four dimensions: (a) persons existing in relationships with others; (b) persons as social beings in a social world; (c) persons living in a context through which their personhood is articulated; and (d) persons having a sense of self-actualized by recognition, respect, and trust by others. The Royal College of Nursing in the United Kingdom makes "person-centered care" as the fourth principle of nursing practice, and specifies it as "putting people at the center, involving patients, service users, their families and their carers in decisions and helping them to make informed choices about their treatment and care" (Manley, Hills, & Marriot, 2011, p. 35). The concept of person-centered practice is being incorporated into nursing practice within the collaborative practice framework.

Person-centered care (patient-centered care) is an approach for nurses and health care professionals to establish and maintain relationships with clients, which foster patients' self-determination and individual tailoring of care by equalizing personal power and professional power and by promoting partnerships (McCance, McCormack, & Dewing, 2011). Nurses as the first-line caregivers for clients have been viewed by many as patient advocates. Patient advocacy in nursing must be guided by the philosophy of human dignity and self-determination as clients need to be empowered in vulnerable situations to exercise self-determination and retain human dignity.

## CLIENT AND ENVIRONMENT

Environment as one of the four domains of interest for nursing is defined as "the entity that exists external to a person or to humanity, conceived either as a whole or as that which contains many distinct elements" (Kim, 2010, p. 220). Environment is viewed to encompass physical, social, and symbolic qualities and is organized about the temporal and spatial axes. It exists for an individual in terms of health and illness as an external reality that is both an integral part of the individual's existence and living, and the stage upon which an individual's living in health and illness occurs. Traditionally, the environment is viewed to be the source of forces that exert influences on a person's health states and the experiences of health and illness. It is the conglomeration of entities and forces that interact constantly with persons for dynamic processing, especially in human life processes that are intrinsically tied to human health states and experiences. In recent decades, the environment has been viewed as the context that shapes human life in systematic ways or that constrains human experiences via language and power.

Four distinct ways of viewing the relationship between humans and environment can be delineated to understand client states and experiences from the environmental perspective as discussed by Kim (2010). The effects approaches view environment as a whole or as specific environmental factors having effects on human beings producing specific state changes, behaviors, or experiences. From this view, the environment through its contacts (proximal or distal) with humans causes or contributes to certain responses in humans that can be temporal, long term, or permanent. From the nursing perspective, the search for causal or contributing factors in the environment that affects a client's health states, behaviors, or experiences has been one aspect of client assessment. Physical elements, such as air pollution and noise level, as well as social elements, such as social support, and symbolic elements, such as cultural belief systems, have been found to exert influences on human's health states, behaviors, and experiences. The interdependence approaches view the environment as an entity that is interdependent with humans in its existence and functioning. The unitary and systems models in nursing view human health experiences resulting from interpenetrating or interdependent processes that connect or comingle humans with environment, with changes occurring continuously in both humans and the environment. Both understanding clients and explaining client phenomena for nursing practice involve not only an understanding of the environment itself but also the interdependent processes for change in both sectors.

The environment-as-context approaches view environment as the context of human living within which the embedded conceptual/linguistic, ideational, cultural, and historical frames of reference are the orientational forces for how humans experience in life. Environment as context is contiguous and somewhat enduring rather than segmented or temporary. In nursing, this approach has encouraged the view of clients and their experiences in the contexts of enduring environments such as home, family, institutions, society, and culture. Bourdieu's work (1990) in which human practice is viewed as a function of habitus and fields of practice with a specific distributionary matrix of cultural capital is one way to understand how clients' practices of health eventuate within the maze of social relations. On the other hand, the postmodern approaches consider social environment as the site entrenched with constraining and controlling patterning and practices through language, power, and history. Humans both as collectivities and as individuals do not escape from such constraints in their social lives. Clients in this view experience health, illness, and health care reflecting the social consciousness that is thoroughly and enduringly tainted by the discursive and power practices (Foucault, 1973a, 1973b). For nursing, this view points to the possibility of false consciousness in human health experiences.

These four approaches of considering environment in relation to humans point to the complexity associated with understanding clients in relation to environment. Understanding clients means understanding clients' relationship with the environment. A model of the client for nursing practice must then include the environment as one of its constructs.

## CLIENT IN THE CONTEXT OF FAMILY

Family is the primary social environment of individuals as they go about their lives. Although the concept of family has changed over the past several decades, family remains the first-line social network through which not only the primary socialization of children occurs but also in which most intimate social interactions take place on a continuing basis. Family as a social structure and a concrete social network is the environment in which and through which individuals exchange affective, instrumental, and evaluative supports with each other as well as develop and integrate values, attitudes, and habits that form the basis for everyday experiences and activities.

The traditional Western concept of family, which is tied closely to the definition of marriage or conjugal relationships, refers to a unit constituted by a father, a mother, and a set of children, the so-called "nuclear family." In many non-Western societies, this traditional concept is broadened to include more than two generations, often referred to as "extended families." However, the diversity with which people form primary social groups and identify them as families has resulted in heated debates about, challenges with, and reformulations of the legal definitions of families in many countries in recent decades (see, e.g., Bala & Bromwich, 2002). While the recent legal debates about the constitution of family have created a great deal of confusion regarding how family should be defined from a legal perspective, the constitutions of family are quite diverse in modern societies whether they are recognized legally or not. For example, in addition to traditional families, there are childless families, single-parent families, generation-skipping families (a couple or single person with grandchildren, which emerged as one of the most common form of families in certain areas of Africa where AIDS often wiped out young adults), and families in nonmarital cohabitations including same-sex partners regardless of whether such cohabitations are legally accepted or not. There is no unified concept of family in the literature, and invariably the public and researchers define it from their own perspectives to specify the form, membership, and functioning (Trost, 1990).

Regardless of how family is formally defined from the demographic, genealogical, socio-psychological, and legal perspectives, both the common-sense and social definitions of family are closely tied to the idea of intimacy, commitment, interdependence, and continuity in relationships among family members. Family members, whether they live in a same residence or not, maintain intimate relationships, committed to each other for the members' welfare, being interdependent emotionally, physically, and economically, and are unconditionally continuous in the relationships. Family therefore is the enduring, continuous social institution for individuals to anchor their everyday lives. The breakdown or dissolution of a family often leaves an individual alienated and solitary.

Family for clients then has three specific implications: (a) family as the most immediate arena in which everyday living takes place—family is tied to "home" where clients carry on various activities of daily living in relation with members of the family, that is, family as the locus of home is the primary environmental context within which many intimate and personal activities occur and various personal habits of daily life are established; (b) family as the primary social setting within which clients develop and integrate values, attitudes, and habits regarding health, healthful living, illness, disability, health care, and so on, in that it is the primary stage where sharing of emotions, ideas, and attitudes occurs through interactions and contacts; and (c) family as the source for emotional, instrumental, economic, and evaluative support, by which its members share and are supported for their emotional, instrumental, economic, and evaluative needs.

The concepts of family functioning (Olson & Gorall, 2003), family quality of life (Summers et al., 2005), and family resilience (Lee et al., 2004) are all oriented to viewing families as social units both affecting and being influenced by individual members of the family. Thus, family as the context is central for both understanding clients and examining clients' lives. It is critical for nurses to know what daily living is like for a client in the context of his or her family; what sorts of values, attitudes, and habits are shared with his or her family members; what sorts and characteristics of support a client receives from his or her family; and how the client's health and health care affect the family.

Nursing in the context of family involves not only understanding clients and clients' problems in relation to their families in terms of structures, characteristics, and quality, but also mobilizing such understanding in the care of clients. Nurses have to gain knowledge of what influences (and what aspects of) the family has had and will have on a client's health and illness experiences as well as on health care processes in order to facilitate health maintenance and recovery or sometimes support during the process of dying. It is often possible during a course of caring for a client, that the focus of attention and care could shift between the client and family either as a unit or its members.

## CLIENT IN THE CONTEXT OF SOCIETY AND CULTURE

Society and culture from sociological and anthropological traditions have received a great deal of attention as frameworks for understanding people's illness, health-related behaviors, and health care experiences. Society and culture are viewed as the general contexts through which persons establish ideational liaisons and identities, and internalize various forms of "understandings" about the nature of human experiences including health and illness. On one hand, society and culture are viewed to be the sources of influencing forces on individuals' ways of thinking, behaving, and experiencing. The reports by the Robert Wood Johnson Foundation Commission to Build a Healthier America (2008, 2009) specifically address social disparities in health in the United States by pointing out health differences by socioeconomic status in a range of health issues birth to old age, such as infant mortality and chronic diseases. The reports specifically highlight the impact of living conditions and work environment on health disparities within the society, pointing out the impact of the environment of everyday life on health. Miller, Pollack, and Williams (2011) further point out the effects of the physical, social, and economic environments of local communities on people's health; these environments exist in differential qualities in relation to (a) economic and social opportunities and resources, and (b) living and working conditions in homes and communities. From a social–ecological perspective, immediate social environments of communities are the sites where differential exposures to harmful entities to health and varying degrees of availability in conditions supportive of healthful practices exist. Additionally, discriminatory practices present in societies are found to influence the quality of health care received by different sectors of people in societies, and specific belief systems present in a culture are found to determine labeling of diseases. On the other hand, society and culture are the "living" contexts in which humans carry on with living, including the experiencing of health and illness. It is the site of dynamic interchange of individual peculiarities with the institutionalized patterns that exist in society and culture.

From the nursing perspective, the significance of society and culture for the client may be specified in the following two areas: (a) experiences of health, illness, and suffering; and (b) experiences of health care. From the sociological and anthropological perspectives, clients' experiences of health, illness, and suffering have to be understood as social, cultural experiences reflecting the structures and patterns of values and beliefs, linguistic representations and meanings, and resources distribution. Illness representations from various perspectives offer different ways of understanding how language as the prevailing instrument of collective meanings is used to depict human experience of illness (Good, 1994). Good (1994) notes that the empirical, rationalistic tradition depicts illness experiences in the context of culture as representing belief systems, while the ethnoscientific approaches of cultural cognitivism posit illness representation basically on cultural knowledge. He adds two more explanatory frameworks as the "meaning-centered" tradition in medical anthropology, which focuses on illness experiences to be based in cultural meanings and interpretive practices, and the "critical" tradition that considers illness experiences as mystifications resulting from the relations of power (Good, 1994, pp. 37–61). Although these depict different ways in which society and culture frame and intersect with experiences of health, illness, and suffering, these views are common in their assumptions that it is not possible to understand or explain people's experiences of health, illness, and suffering separate from individuals' social and cultural contexts.

In addition, the experiences of health care are entrenched with the patterns in the distribution of power and resources, role structuring in society and culture, and the patterned meanings attached to healing, recovery, suffering, dying, and failure. The representations of health care need to be understood in terms of how power as an instrument of control is integrated into the meaning structures governing health care practices and what cultural patterns figure in the ways people act and interact in health care. The central concept within such representations is patienthood that refers to a social role related to health care seeking/receiving within a cultural context. Conceptualizations of client from the sociological and anthropological perspectives offer various ways in which patienthood is depicted in society and culture, raising issues regarding how people play out their roles in health and illness in social interactions, especially within health care. Patienthood is the label attributed within societies and cultures to have specific symbolic meanings, and is represented by different meanings evolved in cultures in relation to the social and cultural meanings of health, illness, and health care seeking; the ethos of biopower, collective survival, and control patterns for health in societies; and cultural values associated with interaction, rituals, collectivism, and individualism. Western culture has two dominant concepts of patienthood: (a) the biomedical patienthood emerging from the Western practices of health care, more specifically medical care, which is represented by specific expectations regarding people's communicative and comportment practices in medical encounters determined by sets of sociolinguistic frames such as those involved in physical examination and diagnostic authority (Harvey, 2008); and (b) the sociological patienthood integrating the notion of the sick role initially advanced by Parsons (1951) that makes individuals' health care seeking a social obligation. These two pre-/postmodernistic ideas have been challenged in the recent decades in relation to the emergent value shifts to self-determination and individualism and also to cultural relativism that emphasizes cultural variations in representing the practices of health care. The term "patient" that inherently belongs in the biomedical model has been challenged. There has been a movement to call the recipients of health care "clients" or "service users" rather than patients especially in community health, mental health care, and nursing. This shift is not a simple linguistic development, but is a reaction to the general cultural shift to delimit the characteristics of dependency in the role of "patient." Furthermore, the possession of specialized, professional medical and health care knowledge is no longer in the sole grasp of the health care professionals, becoming available widely to the public through the Internet. Thus, the notion of patienthood seems to be changing from these two prevailing notions to a cultural relativistic idea that believes it to represent cultural and linguistic variations stemming from local beliefs, meanings, and practices related to the definition of health, illness, and health care seeking. Harvey (2008) illustrates "wellness-seeking roles" instead of patient roles in different cultures that are played out with communicative practices within health care different from those depicted within the biomedical or sociological models. People participate in health care as social activities by reflecting their internalization of patienthood. From another angle, Landzelius (2006) raises an issue with the dynamic changes in the configuration of patienthood that have been resulting from what the author calls "the politics of vitality." In this view, various forms of social activism for specific diseases and health issues such as AIDS, mental illness, muscular dystrophy, chronic fatigue syndrome, multiple chemical sensitivity, breast cancer, contraceptive technologies, miscarriage and stillbirth, anti-immunization sentiments, anti-aging advocacy, the question of voluntary euthanasia, and techno-scientific invention in the care of preterm babies are bringing about changing dynamics of authorizing patienthood, mutating from patienthood and in the category of the patient. From this movement, an assignment of patienthood as a corollary of identity within a heterogeneous citizen/patient/consumer individual occurs. The consequences of a changing configuration of patienthood may be both positive and negative for individuals as their participation in health care has to be reconfigured as well. Different configurations of patienthood, which are tied to cultural practices in general and those related to health care seeking in particular, become integrated into individual experiences and practices within health care.

## SUMMARY AND QUESTIONS FOR REFLECTION AND FURTHER DELIBERATION

The client as the central focus for nursing practice has to be viewed, considered, interacted, and cared for from a multifaceted frame of reference as depicted in Figure 2.2.

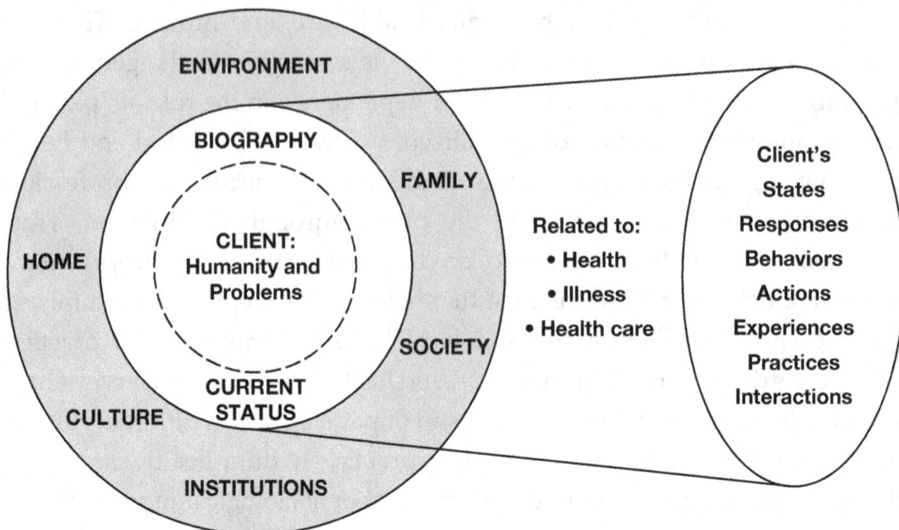


**FIGURE 2.2** A view of the client of nursing.

Nurses encounter clients in their practice who are represented by their humanity and problems for nursing that are circumscribed by their biographies and current conditions, and who are located within specific local and general environmental contexts. For nurses to understand, assess, and provide services and care to clients, it is necessary to view clients in this complexity, which determines, influences, and shows off not only in the ways they experience health, illness, and suffering, but also how they act toward others and interact in health care situations. Nursing practice relies on how accurately, comprehensively, and justifiably nurses understand their clients. Nurses' understanding of clients is always the starting point, the pivot with which their practice with clients is shaped and carried out. Therefore, it is critical for nurses to establish and possess a framework to obtain the understanding of clients for the production of good practice.

- What is your personal philosophy and model of human beings that influence your views of clients? How would you describe your clients in a general way?
- The author offers a model of human living as a general framework to view clients. How closely is this model in alignment with nursing's general concepts about clients? Is this a useful model for nursing? If not, what is lacking in the model?
- What do you encounter in your practice concerning the environmental implications, both at micro and macro levels, on clients' health and your nursing practice?

## CHAPTER 3

# The Nursing Perspective for Practice

THE PERSPECTIVE FOR NURSING PRACTICE IS the fundamental base upon which the characteristics of nursing practice are shaped, as it is the base with which nurses view, perceive, understand, and interpret clinical situations of nursing practice and formulate their "nursing" approaches to clinical situations. There are several terms that are used in the literature and in nursing practice to refer to this foundation, such as perspective, orientation, posture, vision, and frame. These terms, in a general sense, share a common meaning in that they refer to the base that guides the relevance structuring of what we encounter and how we act as humans. Relevance structuring means selecting those elements in reality that have "relevancy" in the context of the encounter, as it is practically impossible to consider all elements and aspects of reality to construct meanings that allow us to respond to the reality. It is selecting essentially meaningful features of the reality by applying a specific filter. If we do not use this relevance structuring, we would be frozen with data overload. These terms are thus boundary-making devices by which the content and meanings of situations are extracted, selected, and organized to provide specific meanings. As we encounter situations, we selectively view and perceive both the "wholes" and the elements within them to provide us with specific understandings and meanings. We base such selectivity and meaning-making on the posture we have about the world in which we find ourselves. We as humans have general perspectives that are the bases for primary ways of looking at the world, and at the same time we also have specific perspectives according to our roles, positions, and activities in specific situations. At the most general level, a person may view the world as harmonious while another person may view it as competitive and struggling, depending on the person's worldviews and perspectives.

On a more specific level, a person may have a conservative or a liberal perspective with which he or she formulates ideas about political situations. Similarly, nurses as professional practitioners hold perspectives that are the bases for their understandings and interpretations of nursing care situations. For example, the situation of a patient lying on a hospital bed after cardiac surgery is factually the same for all individuals who encounter it, including nurses, physicians, dieticians, family members, and nursing assistants. However, how each person sees, perceives, understands, and interprets this situation would differ entirely depending upon the perspective with which each one of them encounters it. Although each individual nurse has a specific nursing perspective that may vary from other nurses, there is a nursing perspective that is generally shared by all members of professional nursing, which is termed "the nursing perspective." The nursing perspective is derived from the general philosophical and definitional ideas about nursing, and represents the basic beliefs about what the nature of nursing practice should be like. Hence, the term is used to represent the shared, foundational ideas regarding nursing practice.

This use of the term is different from the way "nursing perspective" is used in the literature. For example, a MEDLINE search from 1960 to the middle of 2011 with a key phrase "nursing perspective" gave more than 600 citations. In these publications, "nursing perspective" is used in four different ways:

1. Referring to specific commitments to philosophy, theoretical framework, or beliefs such as "holistic nursing perspective," "transcultural nursing perspective," "caring nursing perspective," or "patient-centered nursing perspective"
2. Defining nursing-specific orientations regarding different types of health care such as nursing perspectives for primary health care, mental health care, women's health, rural health, hospice care, gerontology, or intensive care unit (ICU) care differentiating nursing orientations especially from medical ones
3. Delimiting nursing-specific ways of providing care to patients with different diseases such as nursing perspectives for stroke, cardiac surgery, postoperative care, epilepsy, AIDS, or cancer
4. Specifying specific perspectives with which phenomena in clients or special practice issues are viewed such as nursing perspectives of suffering, healing, spirituality, or childhood, and nursing perspectives of empathy, communication, or bioethics

In these uses, multiple perspectives existing at different levels are mostly used to delineate the characteristics of nursing in the referred contexts, rather than to address the foundational perspective of nursing. Meleis (2011) suggests that the disciplinary perspective of nursing is shaped by four defining characteristics: (a) nursing as a human science; (b) nursing as a practice-oriented discipline; (c) nursing as a caring discipline; and (d) nursing as a health-oriented discipline. This means that the nursing perspective providing the fundamental orientation for nursing practice is determined by the definition of nursing. Determination of the nursing perspective can begin with generic definitions offered by the American Nurses Association (ANA) and the International Council of Nurses (ICN) that state:

> *Nursing is the protection, promotion, and optimization of health and abilities, prevention of illness and injury, alleviation of suffering through the diagnosis and treatment of human response, and advocacy in the care of individuals, families, communities, and populations. (ANA, 2003)*

> *Nursing encompasses autonomous and collaborative care of individuals of all ages, families, groups and communities, sick or well and in all settings. Nursing includes the promotion of health, prevention of illness, and the care of ill, disabled and dying people. Advocacy, promotion of a safe environment, research, participation in shaping health policy and in patient and health systems management, and education are also key nursing roles. (ICN, 2014)*

These definitions provide a perspective of viewing humans and a perspective of "doing in nursing," pointing to the two-dimensional perspective of nursing practice. The nursing perspective based on these definitions (or any other acceptable definitions, for example, the one offered in Chapter 1) provides the foci with which nursing must view the situation of its practice—one focusing on clients with their related clinical situations and the other focusing on what nursing should do for clients. The nursing perspective with the focus on clients specifies the frame that contains health, functioning, illness, disability, dying, and suffering in the context of individual, family, and community; and the nursing perspective with the focus on doing specifies the additional orientation for promotion of health, prevention of illness and injury, caring of the sick, dying, and disabled, and alleviation of suffering. This two-dimensional nursing perspective indicates that when a nurse encounters a clinical situation, he or she not only frames what *exists* in the situation, especially in the client, based on the perspective, but also frames what would be required to respond to the situation "nursingly." In the nursing perspective, the focus on client and clinical situation is the *foreground perspective* as it determines the way the reality of the clinical situation is grasped by nurses in practice, while the focus on what are expected as nursing responses is the *background perspective* as it determines the direction with which nursing practice has to move forward in responding to clients' needs and clinical situations.

The nursing perspective as the foundational way of perceiving and understanding for nursing practice thus differs characteristically from the medical perspective, the social work perspective, the pharmacy perspective, or the perspective of physical therapy because the differences among these health care professions are in their specific foci regarding health and illness, especially in terms of what different professions do in health care. The nursing perspective points to the idea, for example, that nurses' primary focus in a client would not be the enlarged liver, ulcerative lesion in the stomach, or elevated creatinine level, but would be how well the client is maintaining an ideal weight, whether the client is able to follow the medication schedule, or in what ways the client is managing his or her daily life with diabetes. This means that the nursing perspective is the basis for configuring clinical situations to have nursing-specific meanings. The nursing perspective of the *foreground* is based on the beliefs and philosophies that have been established in the nursing culture throughout its development regarding clients and clinical situations, which in general encompass the following key values.

- Clients have unique histories and individuality, but at the same time share common human features including human dignity.
- Clients live and experience their lives as selves and in contexts.
- Clients make meanings about their own experiences as well as about situations, objects, others, and others' experiences that become the bases for their experiences.
- Clients have capacity for self-determination.
- Clients are constantly engaged in environment and contexts that have both fixed and changing features.
- Nursing clients have needs related to healthful living.
- Clinical nursing situations center around clients defined by health and illness matters, and are those requiring nursing attention.

The nursing perspective of the foreground then orients nurses to view and understand their clients in a general nursing way. On the other hand, the nursing perspective of the *background* regarding what nursing is responsible for in relation to clients and clinical situations orients nurses to establish their responsibilities to their clients and clinical situations. The nursing perspective of the background therefore consists of the following values based on the generally held beliefs and philosophies regarding nursing practice.

- Nursing is aimed at helping clients to have healthful living through the maintenance and promotion of health, and prevention of illness and injury.

- Nursing provides care and services for the sick, dying, and disabled in order to achieve the highest possible quality of living.
- Nursing is aimed at alleviating suffering in the context of health and illness.
- Nursing practice involves caring relationships with clients.

These two sets of key values make up the nursing perspective in general, and orient nurses to frame their practice accordingly at the fundamental level. The nursing perspective delineated in this way is a generic perspective of nursing regardless of specific orientations in ontology, epistemology, or theory. Because the discipline of nursing has developed its knowledge for practice from the pluralistic tradition throughout the past several decades, there are different ideas among the scholars and practitioners regarding whether or not the nursing perspective is or needs to be universal or unitary especially in relation to theoretical orientations. The past three decades have brought about tremendous changes in the ways nursing is practiced in relation to the changes in societies and health care systems in general, and the changes in the requirements for health care, science and technology, culture and ideology, and people's everyday lives in particular. Along with such changes, nursing practice also has gone through changes in the perspectives that frame and configure the nature of nursing practice. The frames as the guiding value structures for nursing practice are not fixed but are somewhat fluid, responding to not only the larger structures such as culture, society, and ideology but also to the changes in the profession itself and how it sees its position within the larger contexts.

However, there are certain value systems in nursing that are viewed generally as unifying ideologies regarding nursing practice in the contemporary scene. In this sense, there are four key ideologies that undergird the nursing perspective: the ideologies of *holism*, *health orientation*, *person-centeredness*, and *caring* (Figure 3.1).

The frames for practice configured by these ideologies provide the baseline by which the intricacies of nursing practice are and need to be formulated. These ideologies constituting the nursing perspective are integrated into the perspective of both the foreground and the background, becoming the base both for nursing conceptualizations of clients and for nursing approaches to clients. The ideologies of holism and health orientation are primarily oriented to the perspective of the foreground, while the ideologies of person-centeredness and caring are primarily oriented to the perspective of the background. However, all four ideologies constitute the nursing perspective as a unified frame. This set of four ideologies is different from the Core Professional Nursing Values advanced by the Association of American Colleges of Nursing (AACN, 2008),

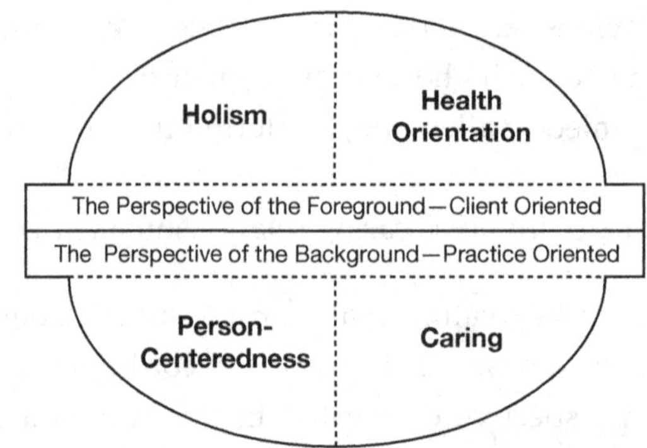


**FIGURE 3.1** Configuration of the nursing perspectives for practice.

as the values specified in this set, which include altruism, autonomy, human dignity, integrity, and social justice, are the ethical, moral values for practice. From this perspective, nurses are advocates, resource providers, educators, carers, helpers, therapists for health-related problems, care managers for clients and families, and coordinators of health care as shown in Figure 3.2.

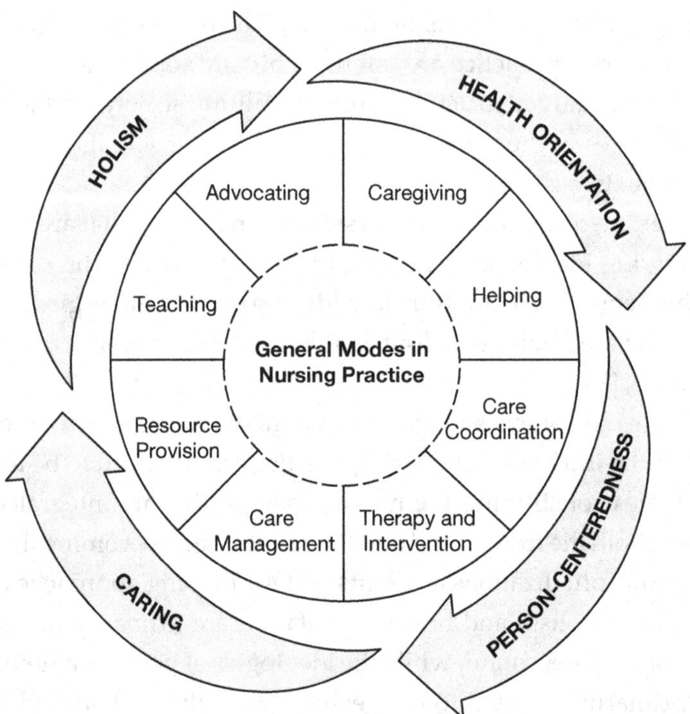


**FIGURE 3.2** The nursing perspective in relation to the general modes in nursing practice.

## HOLISM

Holism as an ideology has been suggested by many as the appropriate unifying nursing perspective. However, holism as a concept has been adopted in nursing at several different levels ranging from the philosophical level to the practice level. More specifically, holism has been upheld as an ontology and has become the base for conceptual and theoretical developments in nursing with specific epistemological postures during the past several decades. However, holism as a value structure that forms the perspective for nursing practice refers to upholding holism as a philosophy for practice against particularistic and reductionistic approaches to viewing humans.

The philosophy of holism especially regarding humans has been hailed as the basic foundation for nursing by many scholars and practitioners (Cowling, Chinn, & Hagedorn, 2000; Donaldson & Crowley, 1978; Roy, 2007; Stevenson & Woods, 1986). It has been identified as the foundation for nursing in order to move away from biomedical and reductionistic orientations, emphasizing nursing's concerns with human experiences as interpenetrating and unitary rather than particularistic and separate. Holism and holistic care have been the most enduring and sustaining value for nursing, although several different terms, such as whole-person approach, total patient care, comprehensive nursing, have been used to connote the same value. Holism as the approach applied in nursing practice can be traced to Florence Nightingale who advocated holistic principles to be applied to the care of the whole patient (Shealy, 1985). The whole-person approach emphasizes the need to consider the patient in terms of body, mind, and spirit, and in the person's "wholistic" relations to environment. Holistic nursing in the form of comprehensive nursing care became the dominant philosophy for nursing practice beginning in the 1950s and 1960s as a way to differentiate nursing from medicine. The holistic nursing philosophy encompassing comprehensive nursing care was a position developed to orient nursing to focus on all aspects of the patient, including physical, psychological, social, and spiritual, in providing care (Kim, 2006c, p. 90).

Holism as an ideology that has roots in the "whole-person" approach in nursing is not in complete alignment with the epistemological movements in nursing for holistic theory developments that began in the 1970s. This occurred in line with the suggestion by Donaldson and Crowley (1978) that nursing should uphold holism as the guiding principle for the discipline's substantive structure. While theoretical holism in nursing has diverse commitments to various tenets of holism, the ideology of holism of the "whole-person" approach is oriented to the nonreductionistic view of clients. It refers to incorporating comprehensive understanding of patients and their problems and integrating such understanding in providing nursing care. It therefore does not necessarily reject knowledge from particularistic or reductionistic theories but puts integration of knowledge as the key to nursing practice. On the other hand, holism in theory development in nursing advocates for holistic theories as the basis for nursing practice. Thus, this notion of theoretical holism can be considered one particular articulation of the holism of the "whole-person" ideology.

## HEALTH ORIENTATION

The ideology of health moves nursing away from diseases and directs nursing's attention to what is involved in healthful living. Chinn (2007) emphasizes the mandate for nursing to affirm its commitment to health and quality of life, especially for all. This was considered a way to dissociate nursing from the biomedical, reductionistic view of human's health problems with the focus on diseases. The initial movement to differentiate nursing from medicine occurred in the 1960s with the textbook by Harmer and Henderson first published in 1955 that identified 14 areas of basic human needs as the major areas of nursing responsibilities. This was followed by Abdellah, Beland, Martin, and Matheney (1960) who proposed a typology of 21 nursing problems for the areas of nursing care in patient-centered nursing, and by Levin (1966) who introduced the concept of adaptation as the basis for understanding and assessing patients' problems (Kim, 2010, p. 5).

The ideology of health orientation is also embedded in the general concept of health adopted by nursing as *the physical, psychological, social, and spiritual well-being.* This ideology focuses on promoting and maintaining health and healthful living (health promotion), actively seeking the maintenance of health (health protection and illness prevention), and supporting the recovery and maintenance of optimal health (health restoration).

## PERSON-CENTEREDNESS

Person-centeredness is an ideology that has emerged during the past two decades in a specific form from the values of emancipation, self-determination, and autonomy, which were the prevailing philosophical undercurrents in the second half of the 20th century. This ideology has arisen out of the postmodern awakening against "controlling" that has become the prevailing approach in health care especially in medicine in modern times. "Controlling" embedded in addressing diseases was beginning to be viewed against the values of human dignity and self-determination, and collaboration between health care providers and clients has become increasingly the preferred mode of addressing problems of health in more recent decades. The Institute of Medicine (IOM) in its report on improving health care for people (IOM, 2001a) defines "patient-centered care" as care that is respectful of and responsive to individual patient preferences, needs, and values, and ensures that patient values guide all clinical decision. It also identified patient-centered care as one of the six quality dimensions for health care, and identified rules for patient-centered care that include: (a) customization based on patient needs and values, (b) the patient as the source of control, (c) shared knowledge and the free flow of information, (d) the need for transparency, and (e) anticipation of needs (IOM, 2001a, p. 8). Mead and Bower (2000) identify five dimensions of person-centered care as: (a) the biopsychosocial perspective, (b) the patient-as-person, (c) sharing power and responsibility, (d) the therapeutic alliance, and (e) the doctor-as-person.

The concept of individualization that has been integrated into the philosophy of nursing practice from the 1950s has sometimes been viewed as connoting the same concept as person-centeredness. However, person-centeredness, although encompassing individualization as one of its attributes (Morgan & Yoder, 2012), goes beyond by focusing on an individual's active role in decision making regarding the affairs of one's own life, including health care. Person-centeredness is an ideology that is based on the concept of singularity of persons and the values of autonomy and self-determination. McCormack (2003) defined person-centered care as "the form of a therapeutic narrative between professional and patient that is built on mutual trust, understanding and a sharing of collective knowledge" (p. 203). The focus of person-centeredness as an ideology is collaboration, sharing, and mutuality in order for nursing practice to uphold individuality and individual's autonomy and integrity from the patient's perspective. Therefore, person-centeredness as an ideology of nursing practice focuses on collaborative client–nurse relationships in which clients' needs, wants, and preferences are actively sought out in decision making, and emphasizes client–nurse partnerships in the delivery of nursing care.

## CARING

The ideology of caring, genealogically, has its beginning in nursing as women's practice of caring and is often viewed to be the traditional roots of nursing. It began with the primary identification with duty and sacrifice. However, the perspective of caring from this orientation has gone through various changes throughout the times, with debates within the profession and in societies at large regarding the concepts of gender roles, dependency, and power (Brilowski & Wendler, 2005; Condon, 1992; Olson, 1993). The focus on caring in recent decades as one of the key mandates for nursing came about with the health orientation and the differentiation of nursing from medicine, which is viewed to focus on cure. Caring has been upheld as the way to focus on persons rather than on "diseases," on person-oriented relationships rather than on working with objectified states of being (i.e., diseases), and on the whole person rather than on particular aspects of a person. Dunlop (1994), however, notes that with the adoption of caring as a specific orientation, nursing translated "love" into the public domain, that is, into the "caring" of the public domain. In addition, "caring" has been transformed into theoretical ideas in nursing during the past several decades, with various developments viewing it either as a specific concept or as a general framework for nursing practice, such as by Benner and Wrubel (1989), Eriksson (1987) and Martinsen (2006) in the Scandinavian countries, Swanson (1991), and Watson (2012) among many others.

The perspective of caring embedded within the nursing perspective, despite the current anxiety regarding the difficulties in coalescing diverse sets of conceptual and theoretical specifications of caring in nursing, endorses the primacy of the humanity of persons, as caring is interpersonal rather than a process of object-to-subject relations (Chinn, 2007; Gadow, 1996; Watson, 2012). The AACN adopted the position that the concept of caring in professional nursing practice encompasses "the nurse's empathy for, connection to, and being with the patient, as well as the ability to translate these affective characteristics into compassionate, sensitive, and patient-centered care" (AACN, 2008, p. 26). The nursing perspective of caring thus emphasizes the view of clients that upholds human dignity and individuality as the primary focus. Caring as an ideology for nursing practice is directly tied to the philosophy of humanism in which human dignity, freedom, equality, and autonomy are the key values (Fagermoen, 2006). It upholds these values in human-to-human relations, therefore integrating the value of altruism (AACN, 2008; Fagermoen, 2006). Caring as an ideology transcends various notions about the concept from conceptual and theoretical perspectives, and refers to the primacy of being concerned for others (clients) as human persons in their totality, with their uniqueness over any other particular persons and regardless of specific concerns.

In addition, these ideologies that configure into the nursing perspective have been further emphasized by the core professional values for nursing suggested by the AACN to be incorporated into nursing education. These core values for nursing include human dignity, autonomy, integrity, altruism, and social justice (AACN, 2008). Human dignity and autonomy are in line with the ideologies of holism and health orientation identified earlier for the foreground nursing perspective referring to the inherent qualities of humans, while integrity, altruism, and social justice are values for how nursing practice should be framed, making up the ideologies of person-centeredness and caring of the background nursing perspective. Social justice for nursing is based on the postmodern awakening regarding nursing's role in promoting and providing for health for all. For example, Kagan, Smith, Cowling, and Chinn (2009) in their discussion of the "Nursing Manifesto" published by Cowling et al. (2000) endorse the value of social justice as the critical foundation for nursing, and propose that holistic, humanistic, and emancipatory values that endorse and enhance social justice are also necessary for nursing practice. Nursing, in recent decades, has embraced the postmodern and postcolonial sensitivity regarding the positions of the vulnerable, and has come to advocate social justice as one of its values. In many ways this is natural, as perspectives are evolutionary and developmental, reflecting the dominant ideologies of the time. Although the basic essence may be retained throughout the years and centuries, the nursing perspective has and will change to reflect the prevailing definition of nursing and ideologies for nursing practice.

## NURSING GAZE AS OPERATIONALIZATION OF THE NURSING PERSPECTIVE

The concept of nursing gaze is somewhat new, and refers to a specific process by which the nursing perspective is operationalized in nursing practice. While confronting clinical situations, nurses in practice develop specific ways of seeing, knowing, telling, and describing them. Lawler (2003) states that the metaphor of gaze indicates a particular stance toward the world, shaped by specific ways of knowing and perceiving. As the concept of clinical gaze has been mostly discussed in the context of medicine, the following introduction to the concept of medical gaze gives us the starting point for discussion regarding nursing gaze.

Clinical gaze and other similar concepts such as clinical eye and clinical mentality have been used to describe the mind-set of physicians by various authors. Atkinson (1995) states that "the production and reproduction of clinical knowledge or opinion are grounded in characteristic modes of perception and legitimization" (p. 47), and advances the idea of "clinical eye and rhetoric" in medicine as the modes by which physicians engage in clinical situations. Furthermore, Good (1994) suggests that medical gaze is acquired by medical students through their learning and socialization processes in the course of medical studies. On the other hand, Foucault (1973a) describes the emergence of the modern form of the clinical gaze during the enlightenment to become intrinsically attached to the objectivation of the patient and the supremacy of medical control. Shapiro (2002) categorizes the medical gaze into three types—the voyeuristic gaze that is oriented to gratifying the physician's curiosity and craving, the avoidant gaze that may characterize a doctor who does not want to engage personally in the patient's suffering, and the scientific gaze as described by Foucault's analyses of clinical gaze that focuses on diseases in terms of signs and symptoms devoid of patient subjectivity. These concepts of clinical gaze, specifically identified for medicine, represent the formation and content of medical perspectives that are the bases for medical practice, especially at the initial stage of medical encounters in which diagnosis is the primary goal. While there is a general consensus regarding the characteristics of medical gaze (or clinical gaze in general) of the modern times to focus on diseases and the treatment of diseases rather than the person, the rise of patient-centered practice (Coulter, 2002) in medicine in recent years is forging a shift in medical gaze to incorporate humanity. At the same time, Bleakley and Bligh (2009) point to the "inhumanizing" method of medical education, with the use of simulation as a possible source for further dehumanizing the clinical gaze of objectivation specified by Foucault. These discussions regarding clinical gaze in medicine view it in relation to formulating or arriving at medical diagnoses. Thus, the clinical gaze is not only the frame by which physicians "investigate" patients in clinical encounters but also the frame used to apply various diagnostic technologies including imaging and tests, and to interpret findings. Several nursing authors raise concerns regarding the impingement of the medical gaze into nursing. Lees, Richman, Salauroo, and Warden (1987) suggest that the nursing gaze became encapsulated into the medical gaze in the advent of quality assurance programs in health care, while Liaschenko (1994) argues in her analysis of home care that the gaze of medicine follows the patient and changes the landscape of the home, making nurses adopt the medical gaze for their practice.

Chater (1999) from the gerontological nursing context suggests that nurses' clinical gaze encompasses the culturally constructed notion about aging and is the basis for configuring nurses' basic understanding about the elderly and attitudes toward elderly care. Nortvedt (1998), on the other hand, emphasizing the ethical dimensions of nursing care, suggests that nurses' clinical gaze is oriented to vulnerability in the patient's human condition and consists of concerned observation. However, Henderson (1994) notes that the practice of nurses' recording about patients in the intensive care unit is guided by the "gaze" that objectifies patients' bodies in concert with the dominant clinical gaze of medicine. This is in line with the idea that nursing gaze dictates specific methods of observation, techniques of registration, in this case the recording, and procedures for investigation applied in practice. May (1992) elaborates this trajectory of nursing gaze into the processes of practice further by suggesting that the nursing gaze establishes nurses' knowledge about the patient in two dimensions: the "foreground" knowledge and the "background" knowledge. According to May, nurses' knowledge about the patient that establishes the clinical definition of the body as objectified and reductive is the "foreground" knowledge and is the framework that specifies the site of action and technical control in nursing work, while nurses' knowledge about the patient that establishes the patient as "an idiosyncratic and private subject" is the "background" knowledge and is guided by nurses' commitment to know the patient as an individual and whole obtained through dialogical investigations focusing on social history and normal modes of behavior. While the "foreground" knowledge is the shared product gained through the concerted efforts of health care professionals especially physicians and nurses within institutions of care primarily guided by the clinical gaze of medicine, the "background" knowledge is obtained by nursing's unique orientation to know the patient beyond the body itself. These discussions point to the characteristics of nursing gaze that go beyond the clinical gaze of medicine, incorporating nursing's basic value orientation in personhood. What is critical is that the nursing gaze interpenetrates into various processes in nursing practice such as assessment, history taking, recording, surveillance, and clinical decision making as well as patient–nurse communication and interaction.

Ellefsen, Kim, and Han (2007) specify nursing gaze as the first component in their descriptive model of nursing practice composed of nursing gaze, clinical construction, and clinical engagement. In this model, nursing gaze is the starting point, which is brought into clinical situations and encounters by nurses as a posture or a set of "attitudes" regarding what they are looking for, and comprises the ontology of client and the ontology of practice. These two components refer to actual processes of nursing practice involved in constructing the clinical case and engaging in action processes of practice. In this descriptive, qualitative study of nurses in acute care hospitals in Korea, Norway, and the United States, the nursing gaze emerged as being constituted of two dimensions: one on the ontology of client with two foci—normality and needs—and the other on the ontology of practice regarding clinical expectations. Although there were some variations among the countries in the contents of the nursing gaze, there were more similarities, and the differences were mostly in terms of emphasis. These two-dimensional contents of nursing gaze integrate the dominant nursing philosophy of helping and restoring for optimal health. Nursing gaze in this study was related to both what the nurses were looking for and where they looked, informing that nursing gaze is the framework for guiding and selecting various approaches used in clinical encounters as well as for identifying specific contents. The contents related to the ontology of "client" have two types—normality and needs. The component of normality refers not only to disease and the illness/recovery trajectory but also to physical and emotional responses as well as individual-specific normality framed by the individual's past experiences. Nurses used the nursing gaze of normality to seek out in their clients how "normal" situations would look and how the "presenting" situation differs from the expected, especially on the basis of previous encounters or clients' history. At the same time, the nursing gaze related to needs directed nurses to seek out patients' needs for health care connecting to the need to know the patient. Patients' needs for nursing approaches and medical therapeutics were viewed to be expressed by characteristics, responses, and experiences and were identified in terms of pathophysiological responses and psychosocial experiences. The nursing gaze is integrated with these two components regarding clients to guide the establishment of the picture of the client and clinical situation. In addition to this direction of the gaze to the client, the nursing gaze is also directed to clinical expectations for nursing. Clinical expectation frames what the nurse has to address in clinical encounters in providing nursing care related to medical diagnosis, the patient's clinical condition, and the context of practice. Nursing gaze on the dimension of clinical expectation connects the content derived by the dimension of client to what nurses ought to do in their practice in specific clinical situations. This dimension of nursing gaze coordinates the priorities for nursing attention, and is guided by the philosophy of nursing practice. These two dimensions are thus in alignment with the notion that the nursing perspective consists of the foreground perspective and the background perspective presented in the earlier section. It seems the operationalization of the foreground perspective specifies the contents of the nursing gaze in terms of clients while that of the background perspective establishes the contents of the nursing gaze in terms of clinical expectation.

While there are apprehensions regarding the content of nursing gaze to be closely tied to the medical, clinical gaze that primarily focuses on the objectification of the body, nursing investigations have shown that the nursing gaze is complex and multidimensional. It incorporates the dominant nursing perspective regarding individualized, holistic care and health-enhancement orientation. The nursing gaze as the operationalization of the nursing perspective in practice may be differentially connected to the medical, clinical gaze, depending upon the context of nursing practice. It seems that there may be configurations of coordinates between the body orientation and the person orientation that shape the nursing gaze differently in acute care nursing versus home care nursing or in mental health nursing versus rehabilitation nursing. The dynamics of health care involving different professionals and organizational complexities may be forces from the sidelines that influence the contents of the nursing gaze. The studies also point out that the nursing gaze of specific nurses may be different from the universal nursing perspective, or may be operationalized in various ways in nursing practice. Because the general nursing perspective is a part of this normative model of nursing practice, it is necessary to gain more in-depth knowledge regarding the characteristics of the nursing perspective held by nurses and how these are operationalized in practice in order to know the impact of the nursing perspective on actual practice.

## THE NURSING PERSPECTIVE AND A NURSING PERSPECTIVE

While the nursing perspective is the general posture identified for nursing practice for the profession and articulated as representing the essential values and philosophies of nursing, a *nursing perspective* is one that belongs to an individual nurse or exists in a specific organization identifying the person's or the organization's specific ways of viewing the world of nursing practice and clinical situations. The nursing perspective is a shared perspective that has some continuity in its development within the profession, representing the prevailing ideologies of the time. On the other hand, a nursing perspective is one that has become established within a person or within an organization through various processes of integration, and could be the same as the nursing perspective or different from it. Hence, the establishment of the nursing perspective has to be seen at two levels—at the collective level, such as how it is established within the profession, in societies, and in organizations, and at the individual level for nurses as practitioners.

The nursing perspective incorporating the key ideologies reflects and is generated through the prevailing discourse and practice in the profession and in the larger culture within which the profession occupies a specific position and meaning. The nursing perspective is a symbolic form generated through "formative processes" through which reality is constructed, organized, and responded to in a distinctive "nursing" way as inferred by Cassirer (1955) for science, religion, art, and history and by Good (1994) for medicine. Good applying Cassirer's theory of symbolic forms analyzes how contemporary clinical medicine "constructs persons, patients, bodies, diseases, and human physiology" through formative processes (1994, pp. 66–67). Good suggests that the construction of medical reality is generated through the formative practices of interpretation in confronting, experiencing, and elaborating the reality to have specific "medical" meanings, and shapes how medical practitioners "apprehend and act on reality, and their efficacy in transforming it" (1994, p. 69). In this analysis Good suggests that medical students learn not only the language and knowledge of medicine but also the fundamental practices of specialized ways of "seeing," "writing," and "speaking" through which physicians engage and formulate reality in a specifically "medical" way (1994, p. 71). Such fundamental practices guided by medicine's long-standing commitment to instrumental rationality are ritualistic and sustain what Bourdieu calls *habitus*, which is a structuring mechanism established as "a historically constituted, institutionally grounded, and thus socially variable, generative matrix" (Bourdieu & Wacquant, 1992, p. 19). The medical perspective identified by Good (1994) centers around the concept of disease, with an emphasis on pathophysiological mechanisms, and the concept of patient, with a focus on medical therapeutics, through which the medical construction is established for what the objects of medical attention should be and how clinical activities need to be pursued. This analytical approach regarding medicine as a social institution arrives at a similar conclusion as Foucault whose analysis of clinical gaze for medicine addressed how the modern medical gaze as a disciplinary power became established in the Western culture through discursive practices. Clinical gaze in the Foucaultian analysis based on discursive practices regarding power shares the same content with Good's analysis of medical perspective as a symbolic form based on fundamental practices of interpretation by practitioners. The analytical works by Foucault, Good, and Bourdieu regarding the generation and sustenance of socially grounded perspectives provide us with an insight that the nursing perspective is the shared base with which reality is grasped, constructed, comprehended, and acted upon in a specific "nursing" way, which requires analysis not only for its contents but also for the processes of its generation and sustenance.

The nursing perspective as discussed in the first section of this chapter has to be viewed as the currently valid way of structuring the "nursing" way of grasping, interpreting, constructing, and acting upon the reality of clinical situations by nursing practitioners in general. As suggested by Foucault, Good, and Bourdieu, it is socially constructed and sustained through various symbolic and social processes (i.e., both discursive and interactional). In nursing, such processes are embedded within the discursive practices in professional organizations and its educational systems, and in the political and legal sectors of societies that control and define registration, licensure, and privileges for nursing practice. The processes of generation and integration of the perspective are also through the relational and controlling processes in the practice settings of nursing, such as forms of patient assignment, handover rituals, and routinizing formulas for patient care. The recent introduction of evidence-based practice in nursing threatens, to some degree, to alter the character of the nursing perspective, moving away from person orientation toward problem orientation. At the collective level, such a shift may be slow, preceded by incorporation into individual practitioners' perspectives as nurses respond to the practical demands for change. On the other hand, policy mandates and political philosophies may be critical forces that can introduce changes. Gavin (1997) voices her anxiety regarding the possibility of toppling the basic ideology of nursing by the policy statements within "The Future Healthcare Workforce" report in the United Kingdom for redefining nursing practice to incorporate the function of "generic carer," which semantically seems to be in line with the ideology of nursing but is in fact against it in essence.

At the individual level, a nurse develops his or her perspective through learning and practice. The literature especially in sociology suggests that although individual perspectives are specific to individuals, practitioners of a specific profession or people with a long-term affiliation in the same organization tend to hold perspectives that are fundamentally similar and share affinity in their essential characteristics. Strong commitments to specific philosophies and values and personal experiences certainly function as powerful forces in generating or changing individuals' specific perspectives. However, as long as nurses continue to engage in social processes of interaction in their practice and are exposed to discursive and symbolic practices of the profession, which have sustaining influence, the nursing perspective learned would be the base from which individual variations that are not too deviant would be generated and formulated. As seen in the study by Ellefsen et al. (2007) there were more similarities in the nursing gaze among the American, Korean, and Norwegian nurses than differences. Individual variations were minimal in the study. A nursing perspective of an individual nurse, therefore, is a reflection of the nursing perspective. This calls for attention to the significance of learning and practice in the generation and solidifying of individual nursing perspectives.

## SUMMARY AND QUESTIONS FOR REFLECTION AND FURTHER DELIBERATION

The nursing perspective as the fundamental posture with which nurses practice reflects the essential philosophies and ideologies of nursing. Because it is the overall, general framework that influences the manner in which nursing practice comes to be shaped, it is critical that the nursing perspective in place reflects what nursing aims to accomplish within health care and as a social mandate. The current winds of human culture will certainly go through various transformations influenced by forces that demand rethinking, reformulating, and revisioning our attitudes and approaches regarding humanity, human life, and welfare. Multiculturalism, the widening distance between the haves and have-nots, and the different dynamics of change occurring because of technology and distribution of resources are beginning to demand revisions in our belief systems and ideologies, especially in human service practice. Nursing stands at the crossroads of technocentrism versus humanism, of scientism versus aesthetics, and of therapeutic efficiency versus caring. The pendulum that shifts various ideological commitments of nursing may require restructuring of the nursing perspective, which could be revolutionary or evolutionary. Nurses, however, have to be proactive controllers of such pendulum if nursing is to shape the characteristics of its perspective. This means that it is both the collective and individual responsibility of nurses to effect either the stability or changes in the nursing perspective, as any drastic change in the perspective will dictate changes in the total characteristics of nursing practice.

- The chapter presents the nursing perspective as configured by four ideologies—holism, health orientation, person-centeredness, and caring. What are the ideologies and values embedded in your personal nursing perspective? What philosophical orientations are inherent in this perspective? How different or similar is your personal nursing perspective for practice in relation to the general perspective offered in this chapter? How does it influence the way you practice nursing?
- How do you view the nursing perspective influencing nursing practice?
- Do you believe it critical for nursing to have a common set of perspectives guiding nursing practice?
- What are the factors that might influence the shaping of the nursing perspective at the professional level?
- What are the mechanisms through which nursing perspectives become established in nursing practitioners?

# CHAPTER 4

# Nursing Knowledge for Practice

GENERALLY SPEAKING, THE ROLE OF KNOWLEDGE in nursing practice is to guide nursing practice. The assumption is that nursing practice as a human service practice needs to be based on knowledge rather than just intuition, sensitivity, experience, and wisdom, all of which are critical for practice but need to be coalesced with knowledge. In nursing practice, various types of knowledge including the basic ones such as physics, mathematics, biology, psychology, and so on, which are applied in most of general human actions, and the knowledge specific to the discipline of nursing are applied. From the perspective of nursing practice specified in this model, the essential knowledge for nursing practice is "nursing knowledge," which is developed with nursing's specific disciplinary orientation. Nursing knowledge for practice is circumscribed by the nursing perspective for its boundary, is driven by the three philosophies of nursing practice for its content, is the grounds for determining the characteristics of the five dimensions of practice, and is the foundation upon which the processes of nursing practice must occur. This means that knowledge for nursing practice is both arising from these structures of nursing practice and influencing the characteristic variations in these structures as nursing is practiced by individual nurses and in specific clinical situations.

Nursing knowledge in the context of nursing practice is constituted by knowledge type and knowledge content. The type of knowledge for nursing practice is considered *nursing epistemology*, and the content of knowledge for nursing practice is considered in terms of the *knowledge domains for nursing*. The knowledge types necessary for practice are determined by the cognitive (i.e., "knowing") needs that are embedded in practice. This means that different cognitive needs are inherently present in practice, to be fulfilled by knowledge

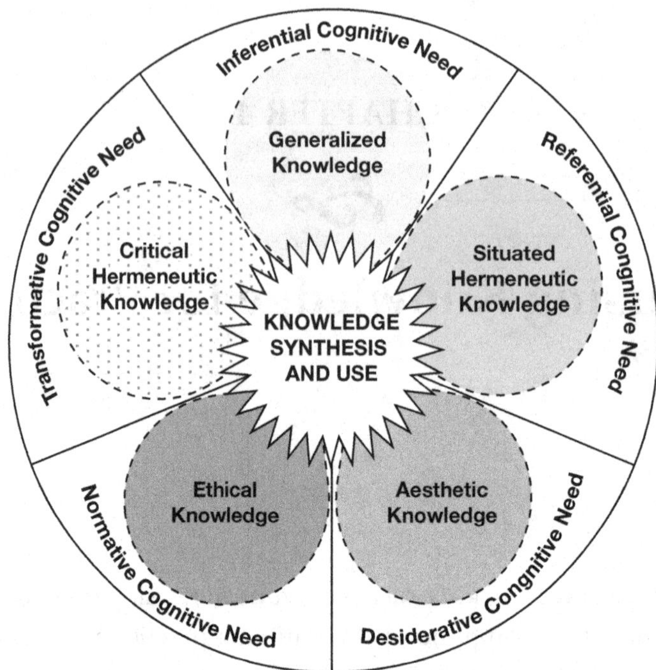


**FIGURE 4.1** The configuration of nursing epistemology.

in order for nurses to be fully guided by the knowledge. The essential contents of nursing knowledge can be specified by the conceptual distribution in the four domains—client, client–nurse, practice, and environment domains.

## NURSING EPISTEMOLOGY

I proposed a nursing epistemology[1] as a way of specifying the types of knowledge necessary for nursing practice (Kim, 2010). The knowledge types for nursing practice are delineated by five specific *cognitive needs* based on a set of ontological commitments necessary for nursing practice regarding human nature, human living, human agency, and nursing practice. There are five types of cognitive needs for nursing practice: (a) *inferential*, (b) *referential*, (c) *transformative*, (d) *normative*, and (e) *desiderative*. These cognitive needs point to five different types of knowledge: (a) generalized knowledge, (b) situated hermeneutic knowledge, (c) critical hermeneutic knowledge, (d) ethical knowledge, and (e) aesthetic knowledge (Figure 4.1).

This model of nursing epistemology is based on a *critical normative epistemology* (Kim, 1997, 2007a, 2007b). This philosophy is an integrated view coming from epistemological realism, emancipatory pragmatism, and normative perspective of human practice. This is based on the sentiments expressed by Good for anthropology and Bhaskar for the social sciences. Byron Good stated for medical anthropology that "[d]isease and human suffering cannot be comprehended from a single perspective. Science and its objects, the demands of therapeutic practice, and personal and social threats of illness cannot be comprehended from a unified or singular perspective. A multiplicity of tongues are [sic] needed to engage the objects of our discipline and to fashion an anthropological, scientific, political, moral, aesthetic, or philosophical response" (Good, 1994, p. 62). The statement Bhaskar makes is that "any social science must incorporate a historically situated hermeneutics; while the condition that the social sciences are part of their own field of enquiry means that they must be self-reflexive, critical, and totalizing in a way in which the natural sciences typically are not. But there is neither antinomy nor unbridgeable chasm nor the possibility of mutual exclusion between the sciences of nature and of (wo)man" (Bhaskar, 1986, p. 101). It is furthermore based on the notion that nursing is a human practice discipline, and that nursing knowledge must provide the foundation from which the practice is shaped for the discipline and for individual practitioners. Nursing knowledge for a human practice discipline with a specific focus on people's health must be for the understanding and explanation of human phenomena of interest to nursing, both those of clients and those of nursing practice itself. In addition, this epistemology is based on several assumptions regarding human nature, knowledge, and practice.

- Human beings, ontologically, are complex, in that humans are natural, physical beings existing concretely as individuals, in concert with others, and contextually engaged in their environment. However, at the same time, humans are also symbolic entities constructed by selves and others, and constrained by history and circumstance, capable of free will, intentions, and self-propelled activities. Hence, there are aspects of humans that are among nursing's epistemic concerns that are (a) knowable objectively and are based on generalizable features, and (b) only knowable by experiencing selves and through interpretations as contextually embedded phenomena.
- It is not possible for one to know (i.e., understand and explain) human beings all at once in a unified, comprehensive fashion. We must tease out aspects of humans based on different ontological foci for proper understanding. This requires specific nursing ontology of humans that can direct us to adopt appropriately different epistemological modes of knowledge generation.

- Nursing practice as a form of human practice requires mutuality that upholds emancipation of involved human agents. Human agents engaged in practice (both clients and nurses) must coordinate their freedom, meanings, and desires as a means of gaining emancipation, mutuality, and goal attainment.
- Nursing practice is founded on a normative, moral, and aesthetic grounding that is formulated through historical, social, and personal processes that go beyond the way scientific knowledge is produced.
- Although knowledge needs to be developed partially and selectively within the given ontological and epistemological foci appropriate for nursing, such knowledge must be considered complementary and inclusive rather than competitive and exclusive.
- The ultimate endpoint for any systematized nursing knowledge is the knowledge of synthesis as it is used in actual practice, and can be revealed and known only by accessing the practice.

These assumptions are supported further by four ontological commitments: (a) ontology of *human nature,* (b) ontology of *human living,* (c) ontology of *human agency,* and (d) ontology of *practice.* The ontology of human nature bespeaks a commitment to the assumption that human nature encompasses humans' species-specific and group-specific features, characteristics, and conditions that exist and are possible as patterns and systematic differences influenced by innate and contextual as well as experiential forces. For example, both human genetics and human socialization play important roles in determining conditions, behaviors, and trajectories of experiences in humans. The ontology of human living, on the other hand, points to a commitment to the understanding of human living as experienced, interpreted, and managed from the totality of the living self, the individual that is conscious, meaning making, historically and contextually embedded, and reflexive all at once. This means that human living is both individually unique and at the same time contextually connected to the culture (i.e., history, language, customs, habits, etc.) in which the living takes place. The ontology of human agency commits to the assumption that humans are agents who are engaged in both independent and coordinated actions in search of certain goals. Thus, human agents are both free and constrained in seeking and moving toward their goals. The paradox of freedom and constraints is the essential feature of human agency, and thus points to the need for coordination regarding meanings, means, and goals. The ontology of practice is based on the assumption that human practice is a service of one human person (the provider or the professional) to another (the patient, the client, the service user) in which the goal is specified for the recipient (the patient), thus requiring ethical, moral, and aesthetic guidelines for practice. This ontology also commits to the notion that practice is not simply scientific, technological problem solving, but is guided by a priori and overarching principles and desiderata.

These four sets of ontological commitments suggest that there are different types of knowledge that will satisfy them and address the specific features of the ontologies. These ontological commitments also mean that the phenomena of interest to nursing are centrally located in humans as both clients and nurses, which will need to be understood, examined, and explained from four different angles if we are to get comprehensive knowledge in nursing. The reason why these ontological commitments connote distinct types of knowledge is that fundamental features of human phenomena have to be abstracted differently from the perspectives of these four ontological commitments. Nursing knowledge has an integrative, synthesizing set of cognitive interests that must embrace four ontological commitments for knowledge content, and that this integrative, synthesizing set of cognitive interests encompassing five types of cognitive needs must be identified as the central aspect of nursing epistemology. This model of nursing epistemology thus is an organized view of what types of knowledge are necessary to carry out nursing practice that indeed is based on knowledge in a systematic way. Furthermore, it can be the starting point at which a nurse in practice raises questions about what types of knowledge are needed in a specific clinical situation to fulfill the goals of nursing practice.

The *inferential cognitive need* is the need for knowing the characteristics and processes of patterned ways in which the reality occurs in nature, and seeks to understand, explain, and predict occurrences in the reality by resorting to the generalized knowledge of the reality. The inferential cognitive need is grounded in the ontology of human nature with the assumptions that (a) some aspects of reality for humans exist in patterned ways (i.e., regularities and systematic differences), (b) it is possible to develop theories that explain how such patterns exist, and (c) it is possible to understand, explain, or predict (not factually but theoretically) individual occurrences by drawing inferences from theories. The knowledge type identified by the inferential cognitive need is the *generalized* knowledge. The generalized knowledge focuses on regularities (patterns) in human conditions, processes, mechanisms, changes, and experiences relevant to nursing and is aimed for general understandings and systematic explanations through objective validation. It is used to make inferences about specific occurrences by making inferences about the specifics to general types, patterns, and processes. In general, the notion of empirical scientific knowledge is in the form of the generalized knowledge referred in this nursing epistemology. For example, a nurse's understanding about a specific patient's postoperative pain is derived inferentially from the general theories of pain that are developed with varying scopes of generalization.

The *referential cognitive need* is based on the ontology of human living, which is entrenched in uniqueness, situatedness, meanings, and contextuality. The referential cognitive need is for deep understanding of human living through knowing about similarities, differences, commonalities, and uniqueness in human living experiences posed against various backgrounds. Although each human experience can be viewed as unique, humans also share certain affinities that can be used for referential understanding. It is, as Taylor (1987) suggests, that understanding is never closed and is open in a hermeneutic circle for restatement and reinterpretation. Through the referential cognitive needs, the unexpected and the unique as well as the similarities and commonalities can be illuminated, and one's insights into individual occurrences expanded. The type of knowledge identified by the referential cognitive need is the *situated hermeneutic* knowledge. This type of knowledge refers to the knowledge of enlightenment, understanding, illumination, elaboration, and appreciation regarding human experience as it is lived in subjective, meaning-making, and situation-bound fashion. The focus is on humans' subjective, experiencing, living selves in situations and their meanings to them, which are ideographically etched and reveal private ways of being and experiencing. The situated hermeneutic knowledge provides knowledge to nurses for an enriched understanding that is necessary to individualize nursing practice.

The *transformative cognitive need* is grounded in the ontology of human agency that is unshakably intertwined with the socially coordinated nature of living. Human agency is associated with the conditions of human engagement with other humans and in social situations framed within the concept of human freedom. This cognitive need is similar to Habermas's (1986) critical cognitive rationality by which he proposes emancipation and mutual understanding as the goals of critical knowledge. It is for acknowledging, understanding, and developing transformations of constraints, distortions, dominations, and misunderstandings in social life in order to attain mutuality with freedom. As nursing practice is a social practice involving people, there is a need to understand problems of social engagement and interaction in nursing practice and health care as well as in general social life in order to free not only nurses, but also other participants in nursing practice, including clients, from systematic constraints and misunderstandings. Such constraints affect (often unknowingly, sometimes consciously) all aspects of human living; for example, how we determine health and illness, how we express our needs for care, or how we view others as well as ourselves regarding competence. The type of knowledge identified by the transformative cognitive need is the *critical hermeneutic* knowledge. This type of knowledge refers to the knowledge of interpretation, critique, and emancipation that is embedded in human living in contexts and with others. Humans' lives in general and more specifically in the context of health and nursing care are intertwined with and interpenetrated in history, context, and others. The focus is on coordinated living between people, including clients and nurses. It includes knowledge about mutual understanding through interpretation, hermeneutic understanding through fusion of horizons in an interactive sense, and emancipatory projects oriented toward "autonomy and responsibility" and the removal of distortions and domination in human living. This knowledge type is *dialogical* and *transformative* and depends on the use of language. In nursing, it gives us the base from which coordinated work of practice, of getting well, and of living together are formulated.

The *normative cognitive need* is grounded in the ontological commitment regarding what constitutes human practice in general and nursing practice in particular. It refers to the need to know what is expected and required in making right and good choices in nursing practice. Ontologically, nursing practice is guided by normative ideals, ethical principles, and value orientations regarding what is right and good for recipients of nursing care (Holmes & Warelow, 2000). Nursing as a human practice discipline is firmly established with goals that are for clients, and requires its practitioners to engage in a practice that ensures the maximum, the best, and the right outcomes for each client. For this to happen, nurses have to rely on the knowledge of normative expectations and ethical guidelines for conduct and decision making and values regarding effectiveness, efficiency, and quality related to goal attainments. The type of knowledge identified by the normative cognitive need is the *ethical* knowledge. It refers to knowledge that is necessary for nursing to determine what is normatively expected and aspired to in its practice. It refers to the knowledge regarding the general and specific normative standards of nursing practice, value orientations embedded in the discipline of nursing and practice, and the grounds for ethical practice. It provides the grounds for making connections between "what is known" in other spheres of knowledge in nursing practice and "what must be" in nursing practice. The focus is disciplinary. The ethical knowledge addresses what are the nature of ethical frameworks for practice, how these frameworks get established, generated, or changed, and their relationships to the larger culture and context.

The *desiderative cognitive need* is grounded in the ontology of practice as a form of self-presentation and self-expression. It refers to the need to know what is desirable in the form of nursing practice to encompass harmony, beauty, and creativity, resulting in individualized, unique caring. This sort of ontological commitment regarding practice has been expressed by Holmes (1992), advancing the notion of nursing practice as aesthetic praxis. This separates the aesthetic ground of nursing practice from the moral ground of nursing practice and signifies the desiderative cognitive need to be oriented to the aspect of goodness associated with desirability rather than necessity. The type of knowledge identified by the desiderative cognitive need is the *aesthetic* knowledge. This type of knowledge provides the basis for grounding nursing practice in the values of goodness, harmony, and individuation. Knowledge in this sphere addresses various modes of self-presentation and self-expression necessary to create aesthetic practice, and different aesthetic frameworks for practice in relation to events, situational context, society, and culture.

These five types of knowledge based on four areas of ontological commitments and five different types of cognitive needs make up the knowledge that is necessary for nursing practice. Knowledge synthesis drawing from these five types of knowledge has to occur as the process through which knowledge is used in nursing practice. The fulfillment of the five cognitive needs by drawing knowledge from the five types of knowledge in nursing practice involves both an individual process of knowledge use by nurses in practice and a disciplinary process of knowledge development in nursing. First, nurses must know that their practice has to synthesize knowledge from these five spheres in order to fulfill their cognitive needs for practice. Moreover, the discipline of nursing must seek to enrich its knowledge base by addressing all of these cognitive needs, which are to be satisfied in practice.

## NURSING'S SUBSTANTIVE KNOWLEDGE DOMAINS

While the model of nursing epistemology provides a way of organizing a set of cognitive needs that points to five types of knowledge necessary for nursing practice, nursing knowledge also has to be specified in terms of content. The substantive characteristics of nursing knowledge are oriented to four different domains[2], each of the domains having a specific "locational" focus. The four domain specified in the model of nursing domains are: (a) the *client* domain, (b) the *client–nurse* domain, (c) the *practice* domain, and (d) the *environment* domain (Figure 4.2).

The substantive knowledge of the client domain is concerned with the phenomena pertaining to clients of nursing both as humans and as the recipients of nursing care. The knowledge in the client domain is for understanding, describing, explaining, and/or predicting phenomena in the client. Phenomena of interest to nursing pertaining to clients are always circumscribed

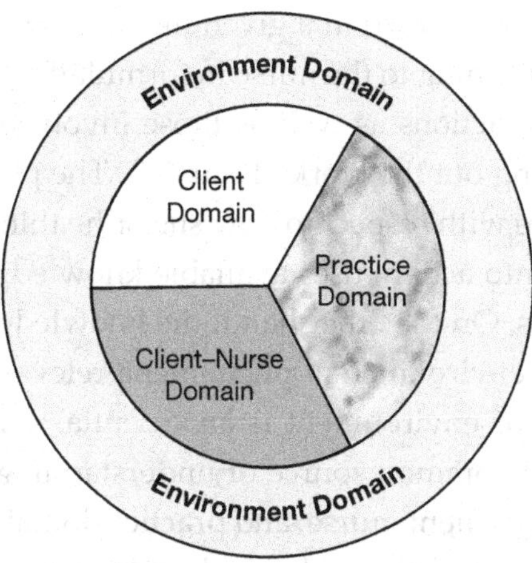


**FIGURE 4.2** The substantive knowledge domains of nursing.

by nursing's focus on health and human living. The knowledge of the client domain developed with the nursing perspective is the base for nurses in practice to appreciate, understand, explain, and predict clients' phenomena, as well as prescribe for clients' needs and problems. The knowledge of the client domain, whether it is about the fundamental features of human life relevant to nursing or about particular issues, problems, and concerns existing in clients that are critical for nursing practice, is necessary for nurses to make client assessments and clinical decisions and to carry out nursing activities for clients.

The knowledge in the *client–nurse* domain is for understanding, describing, explaining, and/or predicting phenomena that exist or can exist when a nurse and a client (or clients, or clients and families) are together as experiencing humans. As nursing practice involves human-to-human engagements and services, the knowledge regarding the many facets of relations between client and nurse in the process of providing nursing care is critical for nursing practice. The knowledge in this domain is concerned with various modes of contact, including spatial, physical, communicative, emotional, and interactive modes, in client–nurse engagement.

The knowledge in the *practice* domain is for understanding, describing, explaining, and/or predicting phenomena of nursing practice. This domain encompasses phenomena and concepts related to what nurses do "in the name of nursing." It includes phenomena particular to the nurse who is engaged in nursing work. The concept of practice adopted for the delineation of knowledge for this domain refers to the cognitive, behavioral, and social aspects of professional actions taken by a nurse in addressing clients' needs and problems and in fulfilling the role of nurse in a given nursing care situation. It encompasses phenomena pertaining to the nurse in formulating, thinking about, and contemplating nursing actions as well as those involved in the nurse doing nursing, that is, carrying out the work of nursing. The phenomena of concern are located in the nurse with respect to how she or he thinks, makes decisions, transfers knowledge into action, uses available knowledge in actual practice, or takes certain actions. On the other hand, the knowledge in the *environment* domain is for specific environmental phenomena relevant to health care and nursing. The domain of environment is an essential component of nursing knowledge, as it is the common source of understanding and explaining the phenomena in the client, client–nurse, and practice domains. The environment is thought to be composed of physical, social, and symbolic components, varying in temporal and spatial contexts. *Environment* refers to the external world that surrounds the client and also forms the context in which client–nurse interchanges and nursing practice take place.

The four domains as the substantive knowledge areas represent ways of organizing the contents of knowledge necessary for nursing practice. This structure of knowledge domains for nursing and the nursing epistemology identifying the critical cognitive needs and their attendant knowledge types specify what sorts of knowledge in terms of types and contents necessary for nursing practice. Nursing knowledge organized in these two matrices gives direction to both nurses in practice to extract out knowledge specifically required in given clinical situations and to the discipline in developing the knowledge base necessary for nursing practice.

## SUMMARY AND QUESTIONS FOR REFLECTION AND FURTHER DELIBERATION

Nursing knowledge, organized by the five types of cognitive needs in the four domains, is the comprehensive, unifying base from which nurses must draw knowledge that is applicable and useful in singular, unique clinical situations (Figure 4.3). Knowledge development in each of the domains in terms of the five cognitive needs will add to the comprehensive knowledge base necessary for nursing practice. So far, there has been active knowledge development for the inferential cognitive need in the client domain, whereas knowledge development in other sectors of this configuration has been somewhat lacking. There has to be an ongoing assessment of knowledge development in all of the sectors of nursing's knowledge base if nursing is truly to be a knowledge-based practice.

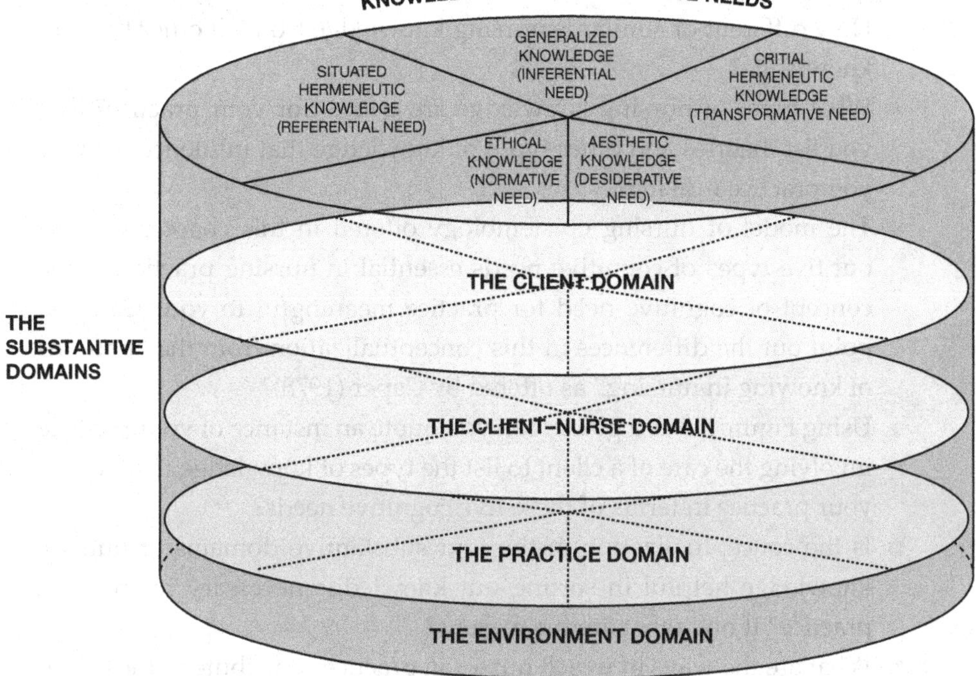


**FIGURE 4.3** Knowledge types and the substantive knowledge domains of nursing. Adapted from Kim (2010, p. 271).

While nursing's knowledge development is usually pursued by researchers, theoreticians, and scholars, the ultimate synthesizer and knowledge generator is the nurse in practice. Practicing nurses must be able to identify the critical aspects of their clients, situations, and their own practice by alternately dissecting and gaining understanding of specific types of knowledge and at the same time layering and knitting together the multiple types of knowledge to produce "the practice." Synthesis of knowledge in practice involves *how* (i.e., method) nurses bring forth knowledge that exists in many different sectors (such as in the public domain, in themselves, in clients and families, and in situations) to bear relevance in specific situations, and what (i.e., content specifiable in the five knowledge types in the four domains) types of knowledge become incorporated into nursing work that is carried out in specific situations. Knowledge synthesis is carried out by nurses in practice by eliciting nurses' personal knowledge, drawing upon situation-specific knowing, and accessing public knowledge. The process of knowledge application in practice is discussed in detail in Chapter 10.

- What do you consider to be the critical features of nursing knowledge? How different or similar is nursing knowledge from all other types of knowledge?
- What types of nursing knowledge are critical for your practice? Can you list theories and other types of knowledge that influence the way you practice nursing?
- The model of nursing epistemology offered in this chapter extracts out five types of cognitive needs essential in nursing practice. Is the concept of cognitive need for practice meaningful to you? Can you point out the differences in this conceptualization from the "patterns of knowing in nursing" as offered by Caper (1978)?
- Using Figure 4.3 as a guide, can you quote an instance of your practice involving the care of a client to list the types of knowledge that go into your practice in terms of these five cognitive needs?
- Is the conceptualization of the four substantive domains of nursing knowledge helpful in sorting out knowledge necessary for nursing practice? If not, what are the reasons?
- What are the ways in which nurses in practice contribute to the development of nursing knowledge for practice?

## NOTES

1. This section has been adapted extensively from Kim (2010).
2. This section has been adapted extensively from Kim (2010, pp. 59–89). This book provides an in-depth study of the four domains in Chapters 4 through 8.

# CHAPTER 5

# Three Philosophies of Nursing Practice: Philosophies of Care, Therapy, and Professional Work

NURSING PRACTICE GUIDED AT THE FIRST level by the nursing perspective is further guided by the philosophies of care, therapy, and professional work identified at the third general level in the model of nursing practice. Philosophies of nursing practice are the orientations that determine the nature of work (i.e., being and acting) that nurses have to accomplish for their clients. The philosophies of nursing practice are determined primarily by the assumptions regarding the nature of nursing practice delineated out in the definition of nursing practice. The concept of nursing practice for the consideration of its philosophical underpinnings begins with Aristotelian notions regarding human activity. Aristotle in his *Nicomachean Ethics* Book VI differentiates three forms of human activity as *theoria, poiesis,* and *praxis,* which are guided by different forms of knowledge (wisdom)—*theoria* by *episteme* (theoretical wisdom), *praxis* by *phronesis* (practical wisdom), and *poiesis* by *technē* (technical knowledge; Lobkowicz, 1967). While the goal of *theoria* is truth and that of *poiesis* is the end product, the goal of *praxis* is in the action itself as being good, just, and noble. Therefore, the criteria for judgment regarding the value of these forms of human activity are different, in that for *theoria* the criterion is whether or not it is truth seeking, for *poiesis* it is the worthiness (or usefulness) of products, and for *praxis* it is virtuous action for human flourishing. These ideas have been interpreted variedly by many philosophers and social scientists during the past two centuries. Most notable are the interpretations of the term *praxis* by Marx as the philosophy of praxis, turning the focus of philosophy on human action rather than on metaphysics, and by Arendt (1998), who specified the meaning of *praxis* as the highest form of human action, which is most closely identified in terms of political life differentiating it from labor and work. From the perspective of critical philosophy, Habermas (1983/1990) defined his concept of communicative action in terms of *praxis* differentiating it from instrumental action in social forms of life, while Freire (1970/1992) advanced the concept of *praxis* to encompass both reflection and action oriented to transformation. From the interpretive perspective, Bernstein (1983) advanced the concept of *praxis* and *phronesis* within ontological hermeneutics following Gadamer's linking of the notion of "application" as *praxis* among the three forms of hermeneutic experiences (i.e., understanding, interpretation, and application) to formulate practical philosophy.

There are semantic difficulties associated with both translating *praxis* into English as "practice," which has various meanings, and interpreting it in relation to human action in general or to specific sorts of human actions such as political, economic, and professional actions. Because of these differences, its use in the context of nursing as well as in various human practice disciplines has been somewhat confusing. This is especially evident in the nursing literature because nursing is a "practice"; thus, the term *praxis* is sometimes used in place of "practice" without referring to its philosophical roots, and is also used to align with specific philosophical interpretations of the term. The use of the term "practice" in nursing in the same sense as "nursing caring" to differentiate nursing from medicine, which is viewed in terms of "curing," also has added to this confusion. In nursing, there are several different adoptions of the concept of *praxis* to articulate the nature of nursing practice and of nursing knowledge (Connor, 2004). At one extreme are the proponents who insist that nursing is or should be solely *praxis*. This position focuses on the idea that *praxis* is "doing (acting)" rather than "making" with a particular orientation of doing guided by *phronesis*, which is the capacity to act with regard to human goodness and human flourishing grounded in moral virtue (Flaming, 2001; Lauder, 1994). This position is akin to the position taken by Carr and Kemmis (1986) and Dunne (1993, 2003) among others for the discipline of education in which teaching is viewed as *praxis*, with *phronesis* as the basic ingredient for its practice (Kristjánsson, 2005). At the extreme of this position is a complete rejection of systematic, established knowledge (mostly identified as scientific knowledge) as the basis for nursing practice, embracing *phronesis* as the only viable base. Nursing practice also has been viewed as *praxis* in the tradition of Freire (1970/1992) and Schön (1983), emphasizing reflection and action as the key aspects that can move a practice to be good (e.g., Clarke, 1986; Rolfe, 1997b, 2006). In the reflection-oriented *praxis* for nursing practice, the emphasis is on using, developing, and refining knowledge coming from practice itself. On the other hand, the notion of *praxis* in line with the critical postmodern perspective has been adopted in nursing to focus on social change and emancipation as the key mandates for nursing (Henderson, 1994; Kendall, 1992). Nursing *praxis* in the postmodern, critical perspective is a project for emancipation of theory and action and for correcting social practices. Finally, there is a *praxis* orientation in nursing that focuses on the Aristotelian emphasis of *praxis* on particulars and the way it has been embraced within the philosophy of hermeneutics. In this interpretation, nursing as *praxis* is a situationally particularistic human experience that can only be understood and experienced in that particular situation (Cowling, 2000). These conceptualizations of nursing practice solely focusing on the notion of *praxis* in the Aristotelian sense are limiting and do not embrace the complex nature of nursing practice as a specific human service practice. Nursing practice in its complexity can be viewed to encompass all three forms of human activity including *theoria*, *poieia*, and *praxis* by which the three teleos of "truth" for nursing knowledge generation in practice (i.e., for *theoria*), "product" for obtaining specific outcome states of well-being in clients (i.e., for *poiesis*), and "goodness" for acting with clients for their humanity (i.e., for *praxis*) are upheld.

An articulation of a philosophy of professional service practice can begin with a philosophy of human action, action defined as intentional one. Moya (1990) proposes the concept of human agency as the central figure in intentional action, having three required characteristics: (a) commitment to normativity, (b) reflective thinking, and (c) subjectivity. Professional practice as a specialized form of human action is then enacted by human agents (i.e., professionals) who are reflective of their desires and values in relation to selves with commitments to act normatively that is specific in the professional context. The structure of norms for professional practice determines the essences undergirding a philosophy of professional practice. Thus, it encompasses how nurses in practice need to accomplish their work in order to meet the social mandates of the practice, and it provides the philosophical guidelines for the practice. The structure of norms for nursing practice is configured on its service to clients and its service as professional work, both as the core aspects of nursing responsibilities.

Nursing practice as a human service practice (as teaching, social work, medicine, etc.) has to be viewed with the primacy of goal directedness with goals residing in clients, which means nursing practice is to produce outcomes in clients. The goal of producing clients' outcomes that are fundamentally tied to human flourishing in the context of health and healthful living is processed in nursing through caring and therapeutic actions occurring in the health care context. This is in contrast to viewing nursing only as "caring," pitting it against medicine as "curing," of which dichotomizing is simplistic and erroneous. Scholars such as Watson who consider nursing solely as caring tend to stretch the concept of caring to embrace all aspects of nursing's responsibilities. However, such approaches have not been successful in depicting nursing in all of its complexity. Gadow's (1995) clinical epistemology for nursing suggests that nursing as a relational narrative encompasses responsibilities for the immediate vulnerability of the client as well as for treating and governing the client's diseases. This means that nursing practice is oriented to both caring for the client's vulnerability and to curing (i.e., therapy) problems stemming from diseases and illness experiences. Nursing practice is an integrated set of human actions that are enacted both in direct contact with clients as well as away from clients in order to address goals specifically established for clients. It is carried out for and with clients as wholistic entities and as having specific clinical problems in order to fulfill nursing's professional responsibilities.

This idea points to three modes of "attending" in nursing practice as: (a) attending to clients as persons, (b) attending to clients in terms of clinical problems, and (c) attending as work. Nursing practice is configured by these three modes of attending, which need to be guided by specific philosophies of practice. Goals of nursing practice are determined by its responsibilities primarily to clients and their problems. Nursing practice requires its attention to clients in two ways: (a) clients as persons with individuality and vulnerability, and (b) clients with clinical problems. Nursing practice involves attending to clients as persons via "caring," that is, helping, and attending to clients' clinical problems by instituting nursing therapeutics and problem-oriented approaches at the same time. This means that nursing practice must coordinate these two aspects of "attending" guided by two philosophies of practice related to its attendance to clients: (a) the *philosophy of care* focusing on clients as human persons in their totality, and (b) the *philosophy of therapy* focusing on clients' problems for resolution or improvement. At the same time, because nursing practice is a form of professional work, it is also guided by the norms regarding how nurses work as professional, social agents of health care provision to individuals and groups in health care organizations. This then requires the *philosophy of professional work* as the third set of philosophies of nursing practice. These three philosophies of nursing practice specified for three different modes of attending in nursing practice constitute the system of over arching, foundational value constructs, providing guidelines for how nurses are to "be" and "act" in their practice. It is critical to accept that nursing practice is *not* caring, therapy, or professional work at different times or different situations separately, but consists of actions (in a broad sense) coordinated, integrated to reflect, and guided by the philosophies of care, therapy, and professional work in totality at all times and in all situations. While the philosophy of care for nursing practice has a relationship orientation, the philosophy of therapy for nursing practice has an instrumental orientation, and the philosophy of professional work for nursing practice has a social orientation. Together, these three philosophies guide the nature of nursing practice to be human service for the betterment of clients in the context of health and illness. These three philosophies are specified by a set of principles specific to each of the philosophies, which are thought to be critical in expressing the essential elements of the philosophies. None of the principles stand alone to represent the referred philosophy, as the intention is to identify a set of principles that together represent each philosophy.

## THE PHILOSOPHY OF CARE

Nursing practice in its relational character sees clients as human persons who are viewed to be individuals with unique biographical and experiential histories, and focuses specifically on persons' experiencing, living, and suffering. Thus, nursing practice in the relational sense, in general, involves engagements of nurses with their clients as humans sharing, interacting, and connecting in their humanity, which is referred to here as "care." A great deal of controversy exists in the literature regarding whether the caring in nursing is unique with special characteristics or is fundamentally the same as in an ordinary sense that is possible to all humans (Warelow, 1996). The concepts of care and caring that enter into the frame of the philosophy of care within this model of nursing practice are specified from an interactive perspective. Caring is a specific relational construct to be differentiated from such concepts as exchange, communication, and role relationship. As a relational construct, caring involves a carer and a cared-for meeting on an unequal footing. Therefore, although caring is viewed in a relational perspective, it is the relational approach for nurses. Even though clients could be caring, the requirement here is the nurse to be caring in his or her relations with clients, specifying that it is intentional caring. In ordinary human relations, caring among people is not a requirement, although it is desirable and is often present in human relations. Gilligan's work (1982), which differentiates the ethics of care from the ethics of justice to uphold the value of the female mode of moral development, and Noddings's work on care ethics (1984) have generated a great deal of discussion in nursing: Some identify the ethics of care as the primary ethical orientation for nursing, while others suggest nursing to be governed by ethical frames other than the ethics of care

(Edwards, 2009; Nortvedt, 2003, 2011). Austgard (2008) analyzed the writings on nursing caring by Benner and Wrubel, Eriksson, Martinsen, Nissen, and Watson and concluded that the central theme of agreement regarding nursing caring by these authors is that caring is a moral practice characterized by the holistic view of humans and directed toward meeting clients' fundamental needs in the context of their experiences and values. The articulation of the philosophy of care as one of the fundamental orientations for nursing practice goes beyond the concept of the ethics of care coming from Gilligan's work and subsequent derivations (Edwards, 2011; Warelow, 1996). This means that the philosophy of care as a philosophy must transcend various conceptualizations of "care" and "caring" in nursing, although the position taken regarding caring in this model agrees with the general orientation of various caring theories identified by Austgard. It proposes that the philosophy of care must be specified in terms of the principles that can guide nursing practice to embrace care to be the mode of attending to clients as persons.

The mode of attending to clients as persons in nursing practice is preconfigured by three specific positions for clients, that is: (a) clients as the cared-for, (b) clients with vulnerability, and (c) clients being thrown in (i.e., trapped in situations of care). As these three positional characteristics of clients have implications for clients to be dependent and passive in their relations with nurses, the philosophy of care must be oriented to upholding clients' rights and voices in client–nurse relations and, at the same time, aimed at helping clients to move toward higher levels of flourishing and well-being. The focus of this mode of attending is person oriented rather than problem oriented and is for clients to live well in a general sense. The philosophy of care for nursing practice includes the following four principles:

- Individuality
- Autonomy
- Human integrity
- Human flourishing

The philosophy of care with respect to *individuality* specifies that clients are to be viewed and approached as persons having unique biographical and experiential histories, patterned ways of living, specific contextual engagements, and needs and desires. Because nurses also hold individualities with the same characteristics, the key goal in the philosophy of care in terms of individuality is understanding—understanding not in a superficial sense, but deep understanding with an appreciation for the meaning and uniqueness of individuality for clients in health care situations. Thus, this principle for the philosophy of care is for "knowing of clients" in terms of not only their individuality, but also the meanings of individuality to clients themselves.

The philosophy of care with respect to *autonomy* is related to correcting the power imbalance between the nurse and the client in their relations, as stated previously in light of the preconfigured dependent positions for clients in nursing practice situations. Upholding autonomy in clients also means emancipation of clients as well as of nurses from power domination. Upholding the value of autonomy has to be based on genuine trust and respect for individuals' capacity and affinity for self-determination. This also refers to the undesirability of abuse of power by nurses inherent in their relations with clients. Caring without a true commitment to autonomy can be suffocating to clients and controlling, fostering passivity and dependence. Upholding autonomy makes it possible for caring not to be self-centered on the part of the nurse.

The philosophy of care with respect to *human integrity* refers to caring that is oriented to maintaining persons' personhood. Nurses' approaches to and relations with clients are meeting with clients of specific personhoods. Preservation of personhood in human relations in order to uphold human integrity calls for an appreciation of human worthiness as individual beings. Caring has to be oriented to preserving human worthiness in each client of specific personhood, however different or similar the person is from all others.

The philosophy of care with respect to *human flourishing* identifies the generalized orientation for the well-being of clients. This emphasizes nursing responsibility to help clients have better lives and flourish to the extent possible. Caring has a generalized orientation to clients as it is not aimed at specific issues or needs, but is aimed at clients' living that is as positive as possible and is devoid of suffering as much as possible. Human flourishing refers to being able to expand oneself and one's life to the highest level of fulfillment in terms of responsibilities and well-being. This principle thus refers to the wholistic rather than particularistic focus of nursing's attending to clients.

These four principles of the philosophy of care make up the values and normative foundation for the mode of "attending to persons" in nursing practice, laying out the goals of understanding, emancipation, human worthiness, and well-being as one set of the essential orientations in nursing practice. The philosophy of care guides nursing practice to be humane, person-centered, emancipatory, and wholistic by a complementary integration of these four principles. This means that the nursing practice of attending to clients as persons is guided by the philosophy of care articulating all four principles together at all times rather than one or two separately.

## THE PHILOSOPHY OF THERAPY

The mode of attending in nursing practice specific to the philosophy of therapy is "attending to clients in terms of clinical problems." This "attending" is particularistic, goal oriented, and strategic. It is based on the professional mandate for nursing to address, intervene, and solve clients' health-related problems in the realm of nursing responsibilities. Nursing therapy as articulated by McMahon aims to achieve beneficial outcomes for the patient's problems by using interventions applied "with due regard for the goals and individuality of the patient" (1998, p. 10). Kitson (1997) endorses that one of the ways nursing can influence health outcomes in clients is through the provision of individual interventions. The requirement is that nurses are to identify clients' problems for attention, deliberate ways of dealing with identified problems, and institute ways of dealing with problems for the best outcome possible. Clients' problems are targets (i.e., the objects of nursing attention) requiring therapeutic actions, interventions, or strategies. The focus on clients' problems as human conditions requires a complex set of principles as the base for the philosophy. Nursing therapeutics attending to clients' clinical problems are never just *poiesis* in the Aristotelian sense, although Aristotle attributes the work of medicine to *poiesis*, because nursing therapeutics are very seldom carried out without the engagement of clients in the process and also because clinical problems have to be understood and attended to in the context of the person who experiences them. Clinical problems are never independent of the person, and have to be "treated" in the context of the person experiencing them. In addition, nurses often act to facilitate or enhance therapeutic effects rather than directly produce the effects; in such situations, it is the client who is directly engaged in the therapy. In this sense, nursing's therapeutic actions are coordinated actions to address clients' problems. Although the final goal of therapy or problem solution is the outcome through "technical" control, the philosophy of therapy cannot be limited to outcomes only, but has to be extended to cover all aspects of nursing practice in this "attending." There are four principles that are essential features of the philosophy of therapy:

- Effectiveness
- Efficiency
- Individualization
- Openness to choice

The philosophy of therapy in terms of the principle of *effectiveness* focuses on outcomes of nursing's therapeutic actions with the goal in beneficence not only in relation to clinical problems, but also more critically in terms of the client as a whole. What a nurse does for clients with regard to their problems has to result in outcomes that are beneficent to clients and effective in solving problems. The effectiveness principle in nursing therapy is based on three assumptions: (a) clinical problems are of clients as persons, and are to be attended for solutions in the context of the person; (b) the basis for therapy is rationality connecting actions to outcomes, providing foresights for the predictability of outcomes; and (c) the reality of therapeutic paradox exists for therapies for human conditions, requiring consideration in instituting therapeutic actions. This means that the principle of effectiveness in nursing practice is configured by the balancing of beneficence for the person and solving clinical problems, complicated by the degree of predictability, and circumscribed by therapeutic paradox.

The philosophy of therapy in terms of the principle of *efficiency* focuses on the manner with which therapy is instituted with the goal in finesse. Efficiency in therapy is important because it is the criterion that ensures timeliness, fluidity, and fidelity. While the principle of effectiveness is oriented to outcomes (i.e., results of therapy), the principle of efficiency is oriented to processes of actions involved in therapy to ensure the value of finesse in action. This principle calls for nurses to take into account the use of resources including time and procedural requirements in therapeutic actions.

Although when solving problems effectiveness and efficiency are of critical importance, individualization in therapy is necessary to attain effectiveness and efficiency. The philosophy of therapy has to be specified in terms of the principle of *individualization* because therapy without individualization is technical and mechanistic, thus, unfitting to solve human problems. Therapy in nursing practice has to be instituted with full consideration of clients as individuals and in light of the context in which clinical problems are experienced. Ontologically, clinical problems do not exist outside of the person, and are intrinsically of the person. Individualization is required because not only clinical problems and therapeutic actions are experienced individually, but also responses to therapeutic actions are individual specific. The goal of individualization is harmony among clinical problems, therapy, and outcomes framed in individuals' singularities, experiences, and contexts. Individualization of therapy ensures fittingness of therapeutic choices and actions to the individuality of clients.

Therapies for and approaches to human conditions, especially those related to health and illness, for which nursing is responsible, are developed from various philosophical and theoretical perspectives especially dependent upon conceptualizations of clinical problems. While there are nursing scholars and practitioners who advocate nursing practice to be framed within a specific perspective (e.g., adaptation, holism, and existentialism), the position taken here is that although such commitment to a perspective is for the nurse, it is critical that clients have the right to choices available in various therapeutic perspectives and therapies. This means that, for the nurse, the philosophy of therapy has to encompass the principle of *openness to choice* regarding therapy in order to ensure a possibility of choice in clients. Openness to choice in nursing means having the mindset that allows clients' preferences and choices regarding therapies. The goal in this principle is thus selectivity for clients with regard to therapeutic choices. This principle is especially connected to the perspective of person-centeredness.

The philosophy of therapy is represented by the principles of effectiveness, efficiency, individualization, and openness to choice, which guide nursing practice in attending to clients in terms of their clinical problems to ensure beneficence, finesse, harmony, and selectivity. These principles ensure that nursing therapy is to be selected, designed, and instituted as a part of nursing practice to fulfill its goal to solve clients' problems and as a human service practice for health.

## THE PHILOSOPHY OF PROFESSIONAL WORK

Professional work involves carrying out responsibilities assigned to the role in specific institutional contexts. Professional work responsibilities are defined by the professional role in relation to its practice to clients delineating the scope and type of service it has to render. The manner with which professional work has to be accomplished is guided by a set of standards established by the profession itself and by social and legal mandates that determine the profession's practice. Professional work of nursing is guided primarily by the legal mandates for nursing practice as nursing is a licensed profession, and is further delineated by the standards of practice established by national and international nursing organizations. For example, the American Nurses Association's standards of professional nursing practice (2010b) include: (a) the Standards of Care that specify the general requirements for care processes within the frame of the nursing process in terms of assessment, diagnosis, outcome identification, planning, implementation, and evaluation; and (b) the Standards of Professional Performance that specify the requirements regarding nurses' performance in relation to quality of care, education, collegiality, ethics, collaboration, research, and resource utilization. While the first set of standards is oriented to how nursing care is to be provided to clients, the second set is in relation to nurses' professional role performance. Although such legal mandates and professional standards provide guidelines for nursing practice specifying the scope, components, and criteria, these tend to be at the level of operationalizing the values for the practice of nursing. There is a need to specify the philosophy of nursing practice in relation to professional work in order to round out the overall philosophical base for nursing practice at a more general level than what is articulated in such standards of practice. Professional work defined by the mode of "attending in nursing practice" as to *work*, differentiated from attending to clients as persons and to clients in terms of clinical problems, refers to nurses' responsibilities within institutions of practice, in terms of nurses' own practice, and in relation to others involved in health care. Therefore, the philosophy of professional work is configured by three principles:

- Distributive justice
- Competence
- Collaboration

The principle of *distributive justice* in the professional work of nursing is related to nurses' responsibilities required by their positions in institutions of health care. Nursing practice occurs in health care settings for particular clients and at the same time for a group of clients. Nurses' attending to clients, both as persons and in terms of clinical problems, singularly and particularly have to be juxtaposed with nurses' attending to work with organizational responsibilities that involve distribution of services and prioritization. Although there are various conceptualizations of distributive justice, the criterion of accountability is most critical in guiding nursing practice, as it has to maintain its primary focus on individual clients while at the same time ensuring the best care to all clients whose care is the responsibility of the nurse. Distributive justice that involves prioritization and selective attention has to be based on accountability for each and all clients. Therefore, the goal with this principle is accountability. Nortvedt, Hem, and Skirbekk (2011) contend that the ethics of care has to be the guide to ensure individualized, relational practice of nursing even in dealing with role obligations inherent in institutional nursing. They propose that balancing between the values of relational obligations and instrumental obligations in nursing practice has to be achieved based on the considerations for vulnerability and contextual needs. The key to this proposal is accountability in individualized care.

The principle of *competence* refers to the requirement that nursing practice maintains the quality of competence both in its processes and outcomes so that the goals of nursing practice are successfully achieved in the individualized care role, institutional role, and professional role. The goal for this principle is excellence achieved through competence that is gained through education, experience, and reflection. The term *competence in nursing* has been used with various meanings, as suggested by the review of the literature, ranging from its reference to behavioral capacity focusing on performance in a role, the ability to perform tasks and roles to the expected standard of a particular job, an individualized set of personal capabilities or characteristics, and a set of characteristics or attributes that underlie competent performance in an occupation (Cowan, Norman, & Coopamah, 2005). This term is used here in a generic sense rather than in the connotation attributed to competence in the work of Benner (1984, 2009) who positioned it in the middle of the ladder for expertise development in practice. As the principle has been extracted for the philosophy of professional work, competence has a general reference to the professional role in nursing practice, and refers to the capacity to function effectively in providing nursing care in various situations of practice. The concept of competence as a principle for the philosophy of practice is critical in order for the practice not to be entrenched within ineffective routinization, an indifference to situational variations and differing complexity in practice, and a self-sealing tendency in learning in practice. The concepts of competence, expertise, and quality of practice are addressed in detail in Chapter 11.

The principle of *collaboration* has been extracted as a critical component for the philosophy of professional work because coordination is necessary in providing health care to people. Health care is a complex service provided by various health care professionals and various health care settings among which collaboration is required in order to move toward meeting the unified goal of helping clients to attain health and good living and to minimize suffering. The goal of collaboration is coordination among services and service providers including family and the social network involved in clients' care. Collaboration is based on mutual understanding, sharing, and complementarity, and is possible through communicative action (Habermas, 1986). Collaborative practice is addressed in Chapter 9.

## SUMMARY AND QUESTIONS FOR REFLECTION AND FURTHER DELIBERATION

The philosophy of nursing practice consisting of the philosophies of care, therapy, and professional work is the fundamental guide for nursing practice. The elements identified for the three philosophies of practice, which orient nurses to practice in appropriate, benevolent, and effective ways, are summarized in Table 5.1.

**TABLE 5.1 Elements in the Extrication of the Philosophies of Nursing Practice**

| PHILOSOPHY OF NURSING PRACTICE | MODE OF ATTENDING IN NURSING PRACTICE | ORIENTATION | PRINCIPLES | GOALS |
|---|---|---|---|---|
| **Philosophy of Care** | Attending to clients as persons | Relational | Individuality<br>Autonomy<br>Human integrity<br>Human flourishing | Understanding<br>Emancipation<br>Human worthiness<br>Well-being |
| **Philosophy of Therapy** | Attending to clients in terms of clinical problems | Instrumental | Effectiveness<br>Efficiency<br>Individualization<br>Openness to choice | Beneficence<br>Finesse<br>Harmony<br>Selectivity |
| **Philosophy of Professional Work** | Attending to work | Role | Distributive justice<br>Competence<br>Collaboration | Accountability<br>Excellence<br>Coordination |

The philosophy of nursing practice consisting of the philosophies of care, therapy, and professional work is the foundation that directs how nursing is to be practiced in patient care situations. Integration of these philosophies in practice, especially in the processes of practice, is necessary for nursing practice to fulfill its legal, professional, and social mandates. The philosophy as a whole has to be the guide in selecting, designing, and instituting nursing care for clients. Nursing practice has to encompass all three philosophies in all situations for it to be truly and comprehensively professional and service oriented.

- What is your philosophy of nursing practice? Can you characterize your philosophy of practice in terms of the three philosophies of practice identified in this chapter?
- How has this chapter helped you to think (or rethink) about the philosophy of nursing practice?
- Is the philosophy of nursing practice a critical component affecting the nature of nursing practice? If so, in what ways is it critical?
- How is the philosophy of nursing practice related to the definition of nursing practice and the nursing perspective?
- How do nurses develop their philosophies of nursing practice?

# CHAPTER 6

# Five Dimensions of Nursing Practice

## CHARACTERIZATION OF NURSING PRACTICE

NURSING PRACTICE AS A FORM OF human practice takes up specific characteristics that reveal how the practice is configured as the practice occurs. Thus, individual nurses' practices can assume varying sorts of characteristics as the practices are carried out in clinical situations. From an analytic stance, nursing practice is viewed to encompass five distinct dimensional qualities—scientific, technical, ethical, aesthetic, and existential—that are integrated together to characterize the practice of "being," "thinking," and "doing" in nursing. This is based on the assumption that all human practice is encompassed by these five dimensions. The distinctive characteristics of nursing practice in these five dimensions that set nursing practice apart from ordinary human practice are in the goals and meaning structure of nursing practice. Nursing practice is normative, goal oriented, and intentional work for clients to better their health. Therefore, these five dimensions commit nursing practice to specific sorts of principles, knowledge, and modus operandi at the normative level. These dimensions are organized by five distinct types of rationalities that govern nursing actions in terms of the principles, knowledge, and modus operandi inherent in the dimensional orientations. The term "rationality" is used in the sense Rescher defined it: "[...] a matter of seeking optional (best available) resolutions to the problems we face in life" (1987, p. 29). Rationality defined in this way is concerned with the manner with which human problems are resolved, and refers to methodology in applying general principles required in arriving at the "best" available resolutions. It also means making choices based on specific justifications. Thus, rationality involves evaluation against a set of standards for action, providing reasons for action. Hence, rational human practice is based on justifications for practice evaluated as the best in the situation. Rationality has to be the base that characterizes nursing practice because nursing practice is a goal-oriented human service; that is, it is intrinsically normative. The assumption in this model of nursing practice is that there are five distinct rationalities that guide in seeking the best available resolutions for actions in clinical situations, which are designated as scientific rationality, technical rationality, moral rationality, aesthetic rationality, and practical rationality. Each of these rationalities is organized about a set of specific general principles, which are the values for each dimension and that, through their application in practice, characterize the essential features of nursing practice from a specific dimensional perspective. Each type of rationality defines the "best" available resolution for problems and specifies a dimensional character of nursing practice—scientific rationality for the scientific dimension, technical rationality for the technical dimension, moral rationality for the ethical dimension, aesthetic rationality for the aesthetic dimension, and existential rationality for the existential dimension. Because rationality is the base for actions in nursing practice, we can conceptualize that the quality of nursing practice is determined by how well all five types of rationalities are applied in guiding actions in nursing practice. Thus, the dimensional characteristics of nursing practice result from the application of these five types of rationalities in practice (Figure 6.1).

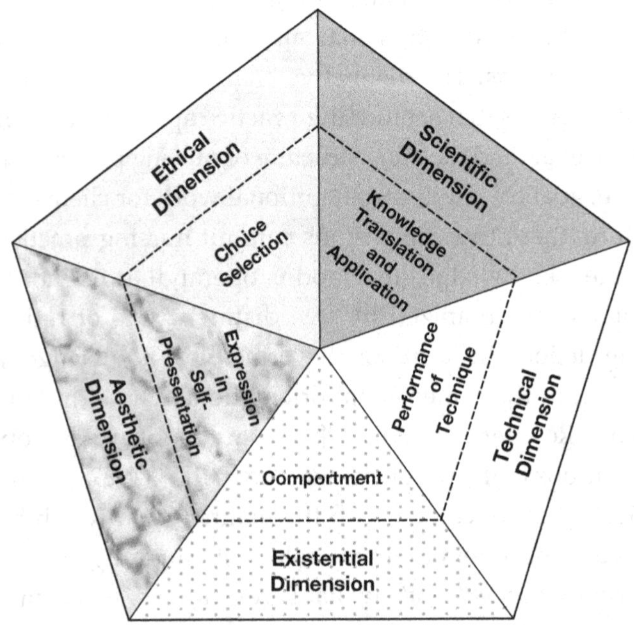


**FIGURE 6.1** The characteristic dimensions of nursing practice.

This conceptualization of dimensions in the model of nursing practice is different from Carper's (1978) specification of four patterns of knowing in nursing (empirics, aesthetics, ethics, and personal knowledge), which focuses on the ways of knowing necessary for practice rather than the characteristic dimensions of practice itself shaped by how value systems (principles), knowledge, and modus operandi are weaved into practice. This characterization of nursing practice focuses on nursing practice itself rather than on the discipline of nursing as a knowledge system, and therefore also differs from the proposal by Donaldson and Crowley (1978) who suggest that the syntax of nursing discipline is composed of two sets of value systems, those of science and professional ethics. This characterization of nursing practice in terms of five dimensions also differs from the idea embedded in the evidence-based practice in nursing, which adheres to the notion that health care practice is "... the integration of best research evidence with clinical expertise and patient values" (Sackett, Straus, & Richardson, 2000, p. 1), depicting only two dimensions of practice. These ideas do not fully articulate the characteristics of nursing practice. The five dimensions specified for this level in the model of nursing practice are not simply regarding the types of knowledge or the value systems suggested by Carper (1978) and Donaldson and Crowley (1978), but refer to the characteristics of nursing practice represented by different rationalities determining the application of value systems, knowledge, and modus operandi in practice. The five different dimensions represent the characteristics of nursing practice, because nursing practice is viewed to be a special type of human actions guided by the perspective, the knowledge, and the philosophies, and also because it is believed that a system of human actions for goal orientation is shaped by rationalities that determine how different types of value systems, knowledge, and special modus operandi are applied in practice.

The characteristics of nursing practice have to be viewed from a holistic rather than a particularistic stance, because each independent human action (such as a thought, a decision, a movement, an utterance, a behavior, or a technique), however specialized it is, is not nursing practice by itself. Nursing practice is a stream of human actions as a set carried out for goals in a client in a specific nursing care situation. So, "practice" is composed of human actions, but is not a simple sum of various human actions, and has a meaning of its own as a whole. Therefore, the dimensions refer to the specific characteristic orientations of nursing practice *not* in order to separate out nursing practice into five types (i.e., *not* as scientific practice, technical practice, ethical practice, aesthetic practice, and existential practice), but to show how five different sets of characteristics meld into and make up nursing practice. Nursing practice is a goal-oriented system of human actions, which have to be designed by various guidelines for problem solving, caring, and service. These various guidelines have been identified as rationalities, with an assumption that although rationality is a construct based on human reasoning, each type of rationality applies a specific set of general principles as the value system for reasoning. When we talk about principles, principles are conceived to hold variability. This means that humans do not articulate these rationalities in a uniform, universal manner, but exhibit in their actions, behaviors, and thoughts varying levels of articulation of the principles embedded in the rationalities. This means that the characteristics of nursing practice in this dimensional sense vary from one nurse to another and from one clinical situation to another. However, nursing practice involves a synthesis of all five types of rationalities, which are oriented to producing the best possible outcomes in clients. The best practice then would be one that reflects the articulation of the principles identified for the five dimensions of nursing practice at the highest, optimal level.

## THE SCIENTIFIC DIMENSION

The scientific dimension has become the central aspect of nursing practice, resulting from the development of nursing's knowledge system and its professionalization in modern times. To suggest that nursing practice has a scientific dimension specified by scientific rationality means that nurses are to follow the general principles of scientific rationality in carrying out nursing actions and base their actions on knowledge developed through the application of scientific methodology. Although there is a certain level of debate and an objection for nursing to be identified purely as a scientific discipline, that nursing practice should rely on scientific knowledge is a generally accepted and prevailing notion. This also means that even the extremists who advocate for the turn to "nursing as an art" or "nursing as experiential praxis" would not negate the necessity for scientific knowledge as the base for nursing practice, even if the contribution is not thought of as primary. Specifying the scientific dimension as one of the five dimensions of nursing practice also means that nursing practice is *not* solely "scientific" but has a scientific "side" as one of its characteristics.

One of the critical challenges nursing has faced during the past several decades is associated with the turn in the views regarding the nature of science and scientific knowledge development. The long tradition of science and scientific rationality based on empiricism and positivism, dating back to the 17th century and continuing on into the middle of the 20th century, has undergone a dramatic turmoil and shift during the past several decades, especially since the

1970s, with debates coming from relativism, historicism, and postmodernism. Although there is a certain level of unrest and disagreement within the field of philosophy of science regarding how science should develop and what constitutes the essential nature of science, there seems to be general consensus in various scientific disciplines that scientific knowledge provides us with the necessary knowledge to improve human life.

The key scientific value that needs to be upheld in this consideration of the scientific dimension in nursing practice is "heuristic power." While there has been a great deal of discussion and controversy regarding what should be considered the key scientific values, such as truth, objectivity, verisimilitude, consensus, for our purpose in describing the scientific character of nursing practice "heuristic power" establishes the orientation by which all matters of science for practice need to be considered. With this value as the pivotal center for the scientific dimension, the following starting assumptions regarding knowledge in general and scientific knowledge in particular provide the baseline for the dimensional proposal in this model.

- Human knowing and knowledge development are embedded within the human culture, including language and history, in such a way that pure objectivity in scientific knowledge development is untenable, and that all knowledge is context dependent.
- However, this does not mean that it is impossible to attain a level of consensus regarding scientific rationality and validity in science. Various forms of human discourse make a general consensus possible for acceptance of validity claims of different types of scientific theories.
- The empiricist ontology has been replaced by an ontology on which the nature and the world appear both essential and constructed, thus requiring description, understanding, and explanation from a web of critical investigations.
- Scientific rationality encompasses (a) logic as the basic method of derivation and inference, (b) reliance on the explanatory power of theories to understand the nature, and (c) grounding of knowledge in experiences.

Thus, the general principles undergirding scientific rationality are *logic, explanatory power*, and *experiential grounding*. The principle of *logic* in scientific rationality links the nature of phenomena nurses encounter (the particularities) to general and known cases having references to theories for understanding, description, and explanation. The principle of logic is applied to make sense of special, singular cases (i.e., specific clients and clinical situations) referring back to general and known cases and to gain understanding about encountered cases. This is based on the assumption that, however unique a clinical situation is, every case can be considered a kind of general type and has a reference to a class of known cases. This principle is necessary, as scientific knowledge, especially in terms of scientific theories, is for generality (not necessarily as universal generalizations) and for referentiality. This means that the scientific character of nursing practice has to be based on how well the principle of logic is applied to gain as comprehensive as possible understandings about specific clinical situations extracted out of the general and referential scientific knowledge.

The principle of *explanatory power* in scientific rationality, specifically oriented to the value of heuristic power, calls for an attainment of best possible descriptions and explanations regarding phenomena encountered. Scientific rigor and application of appropriate scientific methodology to develop theories are the prerequisites for establishing the base for strong explanatory power. Scientific rationality in this regard is oriented toward ensuring that the knowledge has relevance in providing us the ground for depth understanding. In the culture of evidence-based practice, nurses are required to seek out the best available explanatory frameworks that can give the fullest possible scientific answers to problems encountered in practice. However, the principle of reliance on explanatory power does not mean simply to adhere to "the power" of theories for explanation in a statistical sense, but to coalesce, integrate, and select out knowledge (and theories) that give the fullest understanding and explanation about phenomena. Thus, theories need to be developed with various aims such as for understanding, description, interpretation, explanation, and prediction following different methods and approaches. One of the critical issues pertaining to the principle of explanatory power in relation to nursing practice is the quality and availability of knowledge for practice. In order to rely on a fullest possible explanatory power to understand clinical situations and carry out nursing actions, it is necessary to have a comprehensive knowledge base.

On the other hand, the principle of *experiential grounding* refers to the necessity for knowledge to be grounded in experiences of the nature, making it scientific. Scientific knowledge has to be about experiences of the nature in which experiences refer to various ways of reality. The scientific dimension of nursing practice is concerned with phenomena in clinical situations of nursing care. This principle thus identifies nursing's concerns with theories that are grounded in experiences. This neutral version of scientific rationality embraces the changing landscape of science within which the nature of scientific theories and scientific methodology is evolving to integrate the context dependency, coherence in explanatory fidelity, and the immutable angst in the dichotomy of object–subject relations in knowledge development. In the present context of scientific knowledge development in general and within the realm of nursing in particular, upholding this principle of experiential grounding regarding scientific knowledge means to acknowledge many different ways of developing knowledge about the experiential reality. The validity claim about knowledge must be in relation to the knowledge's reference to experiences of the nature.

The scientific dimension of nursing practice is therefore characterized by how these three principles are applied in practice. It reflects choices and applications made by nurses in their practice through scientific rationality with a specific value system involving the principles of logic, explanatory power, and experiential base. These principles are applied in reasoning, in selecting, and in applying scientific knowledge for practice. However, for scientific rationality to work well, the discipline has to have an enriched scientific knowledge base. Nursing's scientific knowledge base has to be well developed to address key questions of nursing care as a precondition.

The essential modus operandi for the scientific dimension of nursing practice is knowledge translation and application. Nurses should know the existing scientific knowledge relevant to nursing practice, be able to translate the meanings of the knowledge in the context of specific nursing care situation, and select and apply the best available knowledge to address clinical nursing questions. Nurses in practice should translate existing knowledge's meanings and values in relation to specific clinical situations, and apply appropriate knowledge in order to arrive at understandings and explanations as well as to formulate individual-specific nursing care approaches. The scientific knowledge selected by applying the principles of logic, explanatory power, and experiential base thus guides what the nurse does in practice scientifically.

## THE TECHNICAL DIMENSION

The technical dimension of nursing practice refers to the performance of techniques in nursing practice, and is guided by technical rationality. Nursing practice involves actions carried out with specific goals, and such actions have technical dimension in terms of how they are performed. The focus is on "techniques" in nursing practice, which are in various action forms, including communicative and discursive such as those used in teaching, guiding, or caring; behavioral such as in instituting comfort measures, giving medication, or being present; and mechanical in the sense of using tools such as in changing dressings, cleaning tracheostomy tubes, or working with vital monitoring systems. The technical dimension is framed by technical rationality defined in a narrow sense. Technical rationality in a broader sense has been articulated in the literature in association with scientific rationality, and is often referred to within the formulation of scientific–technical rationality. The use in this model is narrower, as scientific rationality has been identified to encompass this broader sense. Its use in this model is also narrower than the concept specified by Schön (1983) in his work on reflective practice in which he identified technical rationality in the heritage of positivism. Technical rationality in a narrow sense only refers to the rationality in relation to the performance of techniques. In this narrow sense, it is in line with "procedural rationality" that focuses on the methods of technical application, and it refers to the rational process to determine and deliver the most appropriate means (i.e., techniques) to achieve a predetermined end. Techniques in nursing practice, which are components of nursing approaches derived from theories for caring, problem solving, and role playing, therefore are guided by scientific knowledge, and have the special characteristics of being applied to human beings. As techniques of nursing practice are performed for human clients, the technical rationality that governs them has to take into consideration the humanistic and interactive nature of technical application. Techniques of nursing practice are experiential, in that they are performed by nurses with clients, and thus are intricately interwoven with humanity and human interaction. These techniques include, for example, such techniques as selecting a specific word or phrase in conversations with clients, delivering a teaching program, and caring for a tracheal tube.

The general principles of technical rationality in this narrow sense and specifically applied in nursing practice as the value system for the technical dimension are *optimization, coordination, contextualization,* and *flexibility*. These principles of technical rationality are oriented to efficiency and effectiveness of technical delivery. Technical rationality based on these principles makes it possible for nursing practice to be efficiently and effectively delivered to solve clients' problems and attend to their needs.

The principle of *optimization* focuses on the need to have applied techniques to produce outcomes according to the plan. In order for techniques to be optimal, techniques should be delivered as close as possible to what the theories have specified. This means that the aspects of technique, such as design, the method of delivery, and timing, should adhere to the theories from which the techniques have been derived. Optimization calls for consistency and coherence in relation to design and skillfulness in delivery. For example, when a nurse carries out a diabetic teaching program, the scientific dimension of it is related to whether or not the content and method of a teaching program is based on the best science currently available as determined by the scientific rationality of logic, explanatory power, and experiential base. The technical dimension in relation to the principle of optimization is related to how well the teaching program is designed and delivered to produce the desired outcomes in the clients, given its scientific base. It refers to the manner with which nursing actions are performed to optimize their intended goals.

The second principle of technical rationality is *coordination*. The principle of coordination is related to the way a given technique is delivered in coordination of various aspects of human actions, such as the use of resources, the involvement of environmental elements, and combining with concurrently happening activities. The use of resources involves coordinating available resources present in the self, others, and environment, while coordinating the involvement of environmental elements and combining with concurrently happening activities into nursing practice means to manage whatever coexists in the situation of practice to align with the practice actions. In delivering a diabetic teaching program, for example, the nurse has to coordinate the presentation of the teaching material with his or her verbal actions, elicit the client's participation to try out the testing of equipment at appropriate times, cue in with various stimuli in teaching, and coordinate the participation of a family member.

The third principle of technical rationality is *contextualization*. The principle of contextualization means making adaptations of techniques to fit into the context of a specific client and the situation of nursing practice. The context of a specific client includes the uniqueness of individuality such as age, gender, family and cultural background, language, personal history, and life experiences. Techniques should be designed and delivered by preconfiguring to fit with the client's individuality in these respects, making "procedural" adjustments and adaptations. In addition, contextualization also means making a predetermination of adjustment made in relation to the situation of nursing practice. The situation of nursing practice includes various social and environmental components of practice that may affect the delivery of techniques. Contextualization means foreseeing what needs to be adjusted in design and delivery of techniques of nursing practice, maintaining the need for effectiveness in the outcomes.

The fourth principle of technical rationality is *flexibility*. While the principle of contextualization is oriented to the need to foresee what adjustments should be made in relation to client individuality and situational specificity, the principle of flexibility is a requirement for the need for adjustments at the moment of delivery. Flexibility is in responding to constantly changing and emerging situational configurations at the time of delivering techniques. This is critical in human practice in which the delivery of techniques involves clients who respond and interact. Bourdieu describes such adjustments as "on the spot," "in the twinkling of an eye," "in the heat of the moment" in practice (1990, p. 80). For a nurse to insist on adhering to techniques as designed without being able to adjust to situational changes is to be inflexible. Such inflexibility will result in adverse reactions in clients, probably producing ineffectual outcomes. Flexibility means to respond to "on the spot" needs by making adjustments in the delivery of techniques.

The technical dimension of nursing practice guided by the technical rationality undergirded by these four principles thus refers to how techniques of nursing practice are designed and delivered to be in line with scientific rationality and at the same time to have the characteristics of optimization, coordination, contextualization, and flexibility in their designs and delivery. While the value system for the technical dimension is configured by the four principles of technical rationality for nursing practice, the knowledge base for technical dimension is based on designs of techniques. Because designs of techniques involve integration of various scientific knowledge including theories both about phenomena and about delivery of techniques, this knowledge base is often referred to as "applied science." For example, the technique of teaching a diabetic patient has to be designed to incorporate at least the theories regarding diabetic illness experiences, of compliance, of teaching and learning, and of communication, which are to be reflected in the scientific dimension. At the same time, the essential modus operandus for the technical dimension in nursing practice is performance of techniques, referring to actual behaviors in nursing practice. The characteristics of nursing practice in terms of the technical dimension thus are represented by the degree and appropriateness of optimization, coordination, contextualization, and flexibility inherent in the performance of techniques in nursing care.

## THE ETHICAL DIMENSION

The ethical aspect has been considered critical for nursing practice dating back to the premodern period of nursing even before its emergence as a profession. Nursing as a human service profession is based on and informed by a set of moral values, and nursing practice is guided by ethical standards established upon such moral values. Nursing's professional organizations have been involved in establishing sets of ethical standards for nursing to be used as the guides for ethical nursing practice. For example, the International Council of Nurses (ICN) has published the *ICN Code of Ethics for Nurses* since 1953, with the most recent statements made in 2006. The *ICN Code of Ethics for Nurses* encompasses four principal elements of ethical conduct, including (a) nurses and people,

(b) nurses and practice, (c) nurses and the profession, and (d) nurses and coworkers (ICN, 2006). The major moral values undergirding this code of ethics are related to upholding and respecting (a) individual human rights, values, customs, and beliefs; (b) informed choice; (c) confidentiality; (d) social responsibility for health of the public and for maintaining a healthful environment; (e) professional accountability; (f) self-respect; (g) human dignity; and (h) professional role accountability. The American Nurses Association (ANA) also has developed and updated the *ANA Code of Ethics for Nurses*. The *ANA Code of Ethics for Nurses* published in 2015 includes nine statements regarding (a) compassion and respect for individual dignity, worth, and uniqueness; (b) the nurse's primary commitment to the patient; (c) promotion and advocacy for the patient's health, safety, and rights; (d) individual responsibility and accountability in one's own practice; (e) responsibility for self-growth and competence; (f) responsibility for the provision of quality health care; (g) responsibility for the advancement of the profession; (h) participation in collaborative practice; and (i) the role of the professional organization and its members in determining the matters of the nursing profession (ANA, 2015).

Moral values are embedded within these statements as presented in the ANA's interpretive statements (2015), which include (a) respect for human dignity, (b) the right of self-determination, (c) primacy of the patient's interest, (d) patient rights, (e) practice accountability, (f) self-respect, (g) social accountability, and (h) professional accountability. The moral values reflected in these statements of ethics for nurses are related to how nurses should view, work with, and provide care to clients and what should guide the ways nurses perform their responsibilities in relation to individual clients, to clients in general, and to society. As these ethical statements cover not only nursing practice but also the nurse's role as a professional person, there is a need to delineate more specific moral principles that undergird nursing practice to characterize it in terms of ethical dimension.

Nursing practice, because it works with goals in clients, requires an ethical base upon which actions and choices are made for and on behalf of "the other" (i.e., the client). There has been a great deal of controversy regarding appropriateness and validity of various ethical frameworks and theoretical paradigms in nursing practice (Beauchamp & Childress, 2012; Edwards, 1996; Gadow, 1999; McCarthy, 2006; Varcoe et al., 2004; Volker, 2003). While such debates are central to the bases upon which ethical issues that arise in nursing practice should be addressed both theoretically and practically, the validity of the ethical dimension in nursing practice is not an issue in this debate. The ethical character of nursing practice is established by the nature of nursing practice, which is framed by service obligation to clients and is concerned with client vulnerability.

The ethical characteristics of nursing practice refer to choices made on behalf of clients in nursing practice related to the universally accepted ethical values in the context of client vulnerability. Client vulnerability in nursing practice can be specified in two ways—one related to client's health status and the other in terms of social position of clients in the health care environment and in relation to health care professionals. Because clients often have to rely on decisions made for them regarding treatment and care by nurses (as well as by other health care professionals), their vulnerability is enhanced by such dependency. It is only through the moral agency of the nurse and the reliance on decision making guided by both the ethical values and the contextuality of client vulnerability that it is possible to attain a high ethical character in the practice. The ethical values of autonomy, beneficence/nonmaleficence, justice, fidelity, and care (Beauchamp & Childress, 2012) are in general accepted as representing the values for nursing practice. Rodney and colleagues (2009) found that there is a general consensus regarding the features of "moral horizon" for nursing practice such as relief of suffering, preservation of human dignity, the fostering of choice, physical and psychological safety, the prevention and minimization of harm, and patient/family well-being. Even if there is a debate regarding the stability and universality of these ethical values for nursing practice, the structure of ethical values and related moral horizon for nursing practice are the base from which ethical, moral issues need to be resolved in practice. As nursing practice is an occurrence in specific clinical situations, ethically oriented decision making in practice requires a specific rationality for evaluations to uphold these ethical values. What is required in nursing practice in relation to upholding these ethical values is the application of moral rationality in specific nursing care situations, bringing in both specific client vulnerability and the contextual nature of the situation into value judgments. This is the base by which moral sensibility is established for deliberations requiring nurses to deal with what Taylor calls "the diversity of goods" (1985b).

Moral rationality is defined as "doing the *intelligent* thing in matters of belief, action, and evaluation in order to do the *right* thing in regard to actions affecting the interest of others" (Rescher, 1987, p. 36). Moral rationality specifically delineated for nursing practice goes beyond the general moral rationality, which is oriented to "others" in a general sense, with a presupposition that morality has to be bounded both by self-interest and other interest (Moshman, 1995). More specifically, moral rationality in nursing practice is oriented to the moral responsibility regarding "specific others" who are patients with vulnerability. A commitment to the universal ethical values, to the contextual humanity, and to the intersubjective nature of decision making is critical for the moral agency in nursing practice and in applying moral rationality in practice. The moral rationality to characterize the ethical dimension of nursing practice is therefore specified by the principles necessary to apply the ethical values and at the same time to contextualize situations of decision making. The principles for moral rationality in nursing practice are the guidelines in how nurses can reason, deliberate, and fulfill responsibilities with *right* actions regarding the goals in patients' health and well-being. The nature of *right* actions are preconfigured by the ethical values for nursing practice, and the principles are the means by which decisions regarding *right* actions are made. The moral rationality consists of four principles as the guiding structure for decision making in relation to upholding the ethical values of nursing practice: *holistic understanding*, *contextuality*, *truthfulness*, and *compassion*. Application of the moral rationality specified by these four principles in nursing practice makes it possible to arrive at decisions on the basis of ethical values rather than on nurses' personal needs, interests, wishes, and desires or on contextual pressures.

The first principle, *holistic understanding*, refers to the need to rely on the holistic understanding of clients and clinical situations in making choices for and with clients related to their health and well-being. Holistic understanding of clients and clinical situations means to grasp a whole picture that results from coalescing and integrating various aspects of clients and clinical situations, including the history, background, and current status and event. It is opposite to discrete, segmented, and event-specific understandings, which could be sincere and in-depth, but without being integrated into the whole. The principle of holistic understanding for moral rationality is based on the assumption that any aspect of human lives is intrinsically embedded within the unitary nature of human lives. This means that any deliberation regarding ethical decision making has to rely on holistic understanding of the person, the situation, and the event. This principle is in line with the ways holistic ethics is advocated for applied ethics (Lantz, 2000).

The second principle, *contextuality*, refers to the contextual nature of human lives as well as situations of practice involving clients and clinical situations. The principle of contextuality emphasizes the critical ways context, in terms of history, time, culture, and environment, determine the characteristics and meanings of individuals themselves, their experiences, and events involving people. Contextuality is a critical principle in making ethical choices because each person, each clinical situation, or each event is circumscribed by contextual features, making each to be what it is. Contextual uniqueness of each person, each clinical situation, and each event brings about the particularistic character and meanings of each, requiring attention to the uniqueness in making ethical decisions.

The third principle, *truthfulness*, means approaching ethical decisions with an attitude of openness, sincerity, and honesty. While the principles of holistic understanding and contextuality require ethical understanding, the principles of truthfulness and compassion are attitudinal principles.

The principle of truthfulness prevents deceit and hidden agendas from influencing ethical decisions by requiring openness with one's biases and self-interest and making practitioners deal with ambivalence and conflicts with an open, sincere posture. This is a critical principle for moral rationality in nursing practice as well as in all human service practices, since the consequences of ethical decisions affect clients and their families more directly than practitioners. This is also because truthfulness can be distressful, tiresome, and troublesome in conflicting situations, as sometimes practitioners have to face the impossibility of making decisions if truthful.

The fourth principle, *compassion*, refers to an attitude of what Marcel (1964) called "human fraternity." The principle of compassion is a relational attitude to other humans as in "disponibilité" (availability), which means being available to the other with one's resources at hand to offer (Marcel, 1964). Compassion as fraternity puts a person on par with another in a noncompetitive plane, assuming the spontaneous responsibility for the other. Compassion is a humanistic attitude in a relational sense, and is the base for sharing the mutual, intersubjective humanity so that there is a genuine offering of sharing. As the principle for moral rationality, it is the base for making ethical decisions involving sharing and helping.

Holistic understanding, contextuality, truthfulness, and compassion together as the principles for moral rationality are the base upon which ethical decision making is processed for ethical values critical for nursing practice. The key modus operandus for the ethical dimension is choice selection for the benefit of clients and their families and for positive health outcomes. Choices are made through moral rationality by applying the principles of holistic understanding, contextuality, truthfulness, and compassion together in each given situation of nursing practice. Because the outcomes of choice are in clients and their families, moral rationality guided by these principles is critical in ensuring the best possible outcomes. The knowledge necessary for the ethical dimension has two bases: the knowledge regarding ethical standards for professional nursing practice that provide the guidelines for ethical practice, and the knowledge regarding various processes involved in ethical decision making including ethical theories, processes of ethical decision making, and various philosophical positions regarding applied ethics.

## THE AESTHETIC DIMENSION

The aesthetic dimension of nursing practice has been a controversial issue especially with the debate that characterizes nursing either as a science or as an art. In this model of nursing practice, this debate is viewed to be without merit, because the notions that consider nursing solely as either science or art are viewed as untenable and inappropriate. As a human service practice, nursing practice is represented as an integrated form that can be depicted with a scientific character and an aesthetic character along with technical, ethical, and existential characters. It is also a non sequitur to specify one or another of these dimensions to represent the essential characteristics of nursing practice, because nursing practice is represented by all five dimensions, together and integrated, in its characteristics. The terms "art" and "aesthetic" represent a rather controversial usage in the literature. While there are definite differences between these two terms from a strictly philosophical sense, and three distinctive camps exist on the use of these terms in the nursing literature (Kim, 2010, pp. 212–214), in this exposition "art and aesthetic" are used interchangeably to refer to the expressive nature of nursing practice.

When we speak of the aesthetic dimension of nursing practice, the concept of art used in this context is not in line entirely with the conventional notion of art in which artwork and its meaning and appreciation are the central focus for understanding and analysis. Nursing practice is not viewed to be artwork in a strict sense of production, but is viewed to encompass an artistic character in the expressions embedded in practice. Therefore, philosophies and theories regarding the production and appreciation of artwork have to be reinterpreted in the perspective of viewing nursing practice as having an artful character.

Nursing practice involves presentation of self—the nurse—to clients/families and in clinical situations. Self-presentations in practice, in this sense, are expressions made by nurses through physical, behavioral, and discursive actions in their relationships with clients and in specific clinical situations. Thus, nursing practice has an aesthetic aspect, in the same sense that Freire (1970/1992) considers education as art. The aesthetic aspect of nursing practice indicates that nurses are artists with their artistic products in the form of self-presentation in relationships with clients and in clinical situations. This means that what nurses do with clients (i.e., discursive, behavioral, and physical "doings") have the artistic character, and needs to be guided by specific principles, knowledge, and modus operandi in order for nursing practice to be expressive and creative in an artistic sense. The artistic dimension of nursing practice refers to the creative presentation of the self in consideration of what is desired, meaningful, and beautiful in relation to the client and the world in which nursing is practiced (Kim, 2010). It is relational in its character as all art is relational. That is, art involves an expression, an exposition, or a product for which there is a receiver, a reviewer, or a responder who experiences it in a distinctively personal way. However, nursing practice as art is different from the ordinary notion of art as an object of appreciation, in which there is no personal and immediate involvement of producers of the art with recipients of art. In nursing practice, nurses' self-presentations in relation to clients and clinical situations are expressions of values and ideals of nursing (Holmes, 1992), and involve creativity to attain situational harmony in personal, situational, and immediate engagements of specific clients and nurses (Kim, 2010).

As the art of nursing practice is relational and situational, the focus for the aesthetic dimension is more on the process of nursing practice than the outcomes of nursing practice. Certainly the outcomes of nursing practice would be enhanced by "good" art, but the focus is on the "good" art itself that is experienced together with clients as nursing practice unfolds. Hence, the ultimate goal of the aesthetic dimension of nursing practice is in making the relational experiences of nursing practice to be harmonious, beautiful, pleasing, and sublime. This also means that since all nursing practice has the aesthetic dimension, some nursing practice would be "bad" art in these terms, making the experience to be less than satisfactory both for clients and nurses. Scruton states that "we are *presenting* ourselves, *making ourselves present*, and the act of presentation is one in which appearances mediate between self and other, and between self and self. Aesthetic choices are signs of what we want to be *for* others, and also *for* ourselves" (2011, p. 311). In "doings" in nursing practice, not only through discursive acts but also through various forms of actions, nurses are applying aesthetic judgment to coordinate their "self-presentations" in practice with clients, nurses themselves, and with context. Freire (1970/1992) suggests that for education such coordination brings about the fundamental rupture of the student–teacher dichotomy in which all participants in dialogues are simultaneously teachers and students. In nursing practice, it would also mean that the rupture of dichotomy between the giver (the nurse) and the receiver (the patient) will occur through the aesthetic dimension of the practice. Chinn's nursing art (2001) also aligns with this notion.

From the practice perspective, self-presentation must be guided by aesthetic rationality that seeks to optimize the most satisfactory, pleasing, and fulfilling senses in nurse–client and nurse–situation relations. Aesthetic rationality is framed by the contextuality of self-presentation. That is, self-presentations and relational experiences from the aesthetic perspective are contextually bound. Therefore, aesthetic rationality for nursing practice has to be based on the principles that are oriented to the relational and expressive aspects of actions. The principles for aesthetic rationality in nursing practice are therefore identified as *unity*, *harmony*, and *finesse*. Application of the aesthetic rationality specified by these three principles in nursing practice makes it possible to arrive at self-presentations in nursing practice on the basis of aesthetic values in terms of nursing's relational aspects of practice. Aesthetic values specific to nursing practice are viewed to include beauty, sublimity, empathy, and sensibility, because the aesthetic character of nursing practice is inherently in nurses' relationships with clients and clinical situations requiring "pleasure" and "enjoyment" to be relational rather than the practice simply as the production of art. These three principles of the aesthetic rationality are the guiding structure for determining how nurses present themselves in practice situations in order for their practice to be enhancing of other characteristics of practice as well as to produce aesthetic character of the highest level.

The first principle of *unity* refers to the need for streams of nursing actions to be unified as a whole by which self-presenting expressions are continuously integrated to bring about empathy and mutual sensibility. The concept of unity advanced by Dewey (1934/1987) refers to the way for discrete parts of an experience to flow together without seams, continuously merging and integrating so that "the experience" becomes aesthetic experience that is distinctively unified to stand out as vital, noteworthy, or memorable. The unity in an experience as an "integrated complete experience" to Dewey (1934/1987, p. 43) yields the enjoyment characteristic of aesthetic perception, thus making it aesthetic experience. For nursing practice, the aesthetic character is revealed through the unity of nurses' discrete forms of self-presentation that are integrated and merged as a whole to express empathy and sensibility toward clients. This means that aesthetic character in nursing practice is not in each specific expression but in the final form of integration and unity resulting from continuously stringing and integrating various expressions (such as physical, behavioral, and discursive) together to reveal nurses' attitudes of sensibility toward specific clients or specific clinical situations. This means that a single, discrete expression is neutral in its characteristics from the aesthetic perspective (such as the color yellow is neutral until it is used in a painting), and that only when a stream of expressions is merged into a unity, it will reveal certain aesthetic characteristics. This idea is in line with Chinn's definition of nursing art as "the nurse's synchronous arrangement of narrative and movement into a form that transforms experiences into a realm that would not otherwise be possible" (2001, p. 291). For example, a statement "you are suffering" by itself is a proposition regarding a state; however, when it is combined in a stream of expressions that includes a concerned facial expression, gentle grasping of a hand, and a combination of other sayings, it as a unity becomes a practice of comfort with aesthetic character.

The second principle of *harmony* refers to the fittingness of human actions in a relational sense. It is specifically contextually oriented, and focuses on the need for nursing practice to be harmonious with client singularity and specificity of clinical situations. Harmony means blending together of different elements, parts, and aspects without confliction and competition, while retaining distinctive identities or characters of those parts that are brought together. Harmony is akin to the concept of fittingness that is viewed by Zaibert (2006) as "aesthetic normativity that is intrinsically good and beautiful." Harmony in art in the formal sense means bringing together different elements to produce a sense of beauty and sublimity in artistic products. Harmony is achieved usually by putting together different elements such as color, shape, feel, tone, and pitch in artistic work to produce beauty and sublimity. However, the principle of harmony applied to nursing practice in a relational sense goes beyond the fittingness of different elements with each other and as a whole. The principle of harmony is applied in nursing practice in relation to how nurses' expressions (actions) are harmonious with specific clients and specific clinical situations. To be harmonious with a client means to make the nurse's self-presentations to be specifically designed to fit with the specific client's characteristics and needs, and to be harmonious with a clinical situation means to make the nurse's self-presentations to be in alignment with what is going on in the clinical situation. Therefore, for general artistic products, the principle of harmony is oriented to beauty and sublimity, whereas the principle of harmony in nursing practice from the aesthetic perspective is additionally oriented to empathy and sensibility. Ways of speech, of body movements, of behaving with clients have to be fitted to client singularity in order for nurses' self-presentations to encompass the sense of beauty, sublimity, empathy, and sensibility.

The third principle of *finesse* refers to the design of artistic work to reveal artistry. Finesse is revealed in artistic work that is seamless, thoughtful, natural, and pleasing, and refers to the quality of artistic work. Finesse often refers to refinement, delicacy of performance, execution of artisanship, and skillful, subtle handling of a situation. In nursing practice, finesse from the aesthetic perspective is revealed in expressive acts that flow seamlessly, exhibit authenticity, and are pleasing to the nurse as well as to the client in a specific situation. The principle of finesse is therefore oriented to the values of beauty and sublimity, and is specifically upheld through the application of creativity and a habit of exercise aimed at refinement. To have finesse in nursing practice means to have expressions of excellence, especially in relation to beauty and sublimity, in nurses' self-presentations with clients and in clinical situations. Self-presentations in nursing practice therefore are enacted through thoughtfulness and authenticity applying creativity and resulting from continuous efforts for refinement.

Unity, harmony, and finesse as the principles for aesthetic rationality are the base upon which self-presentations in nursing practice attain the highest values of beauty, sublimity, empathy, and sensibility. The aesthetic dimension of nursing practice guided by the aesthetic rationality framed by these three principles thus refers to how nurses' self-presentations as expressions are made to be artful in nurses' relations with clients and in clinical situations. The knowledge necessary for the aesthetic dimension has three bases: the knowledge regarding the nature of various self-presentations in nursing practice and different forms of aesthetic self-presentations especially in terms of relational expressions, the knowledge regarding how creativity is cultivated and applied in human practice, and the knowledge of design in relation to producing beauty, sublimity, empathy, and sensibility in self-presentations of nursing practice. The key modus operandus for the aesthetic dimension is expression in self-presentations, which result through aesthetic rationality in applying the principles of unity, harmony, and finesse together in each given situation of nursing practice. Because the outcomes of expressions as aesthetic ones are in clients, as well as in nurses, as feeling states, the aesthetic dimension of nursing practice elevates the quality of nursing practice to a higher level.

## THE EXISTENTIAL DIMENSION

The existential dimension is an unavoidable aspect of human "doing" as a presence since human presence involves the "person" as an existential being located in particular contexts and at specific times of human living. Existentially, humans reveal and make themselves known in situations by projecting their meanings of themselves and engaging with the world as particular selves of particular times. The existential person therefore is a unique, acting being, with a set of specific history, memory, corporeal as well as mental and spiritual identity, and with a specific attitude and understanding about himself or herself and the world. This notion is rooted in the tenets of existentialism (Barrett, 1962; Dreyfus & Wrathall, 2008; Fackenheim, 1961), and is also akin to Heidegger's phenomenology, which considers human existence as "being-in-the-world" (Heidegger, 1927/1962). However, in this model it is framed as one dimension of nursing practice rather than the whole of human practice, because it is believed that nursing practice as a form of human practice is a special type because it is goal oriented, social, and deliberative, necessitating it to encompass five dimensions analytically. When existentialism is upheld as a philosophy, it is a way of seeing human life with a focus on human existence, and when phenomenology is upheld as a philosophy, it is an approach to understand and analyze human existence. However, in the view of nursing practice, it is necessary to consider "existence" of humans as one of several dimensions of human life in this analytical view of nursing practice as a way of characterizing nursing practice. This stance may be debatable from the perspectives of the existential and phenomenological philosophies as these philosophies view human existence as an unpartitionable phenomenon. However, although it is possible to view nursing practice as a form of human existence in this regard, it is believed that it has to be viewed as one dimension of the totality of nursing practice in an analytical sense. Thus, the existential dimension of nursing practice refers to the ways of existing of nurses in relation to particular patients and specific clinical situations as "selves." It is the engagement (i.e., comportment) of a nurse as a unique self in a particular clinical situation (most of the time involving a specific client) with one's own "endowments," commitments, choices, habits, history, and vulnerability but transcending these with choices and decisions so that self-identity is revealed in his or her existence. The existential dimension of nursing practice refers to how nurses engage with the world and comport themselves in clinical situations projecting their identities and meanings of selves, and revealing habits of their beings. Thus, it is what is present in such comportments that characterizes the existential dimension. Existentially, nursing practice could be caring, understanding, self-centered, winning oriented, disguised, appropriate, alienating, habitual, aloof, knowing, and so forth. Each instance of a nurse's existential presence is unique in itself, has particular meanings, and involves the nurse as an entirety, but always in relation to a particular client or a particular clinical situation.

From the practice perspective, the existential dimension is guided by the existential rationality in order to align with the tenets of nursing practice, especially in terms of goal orientation in clients' well-being. Because existence is "self-making-in-a-situation" (Fackenheim, 1961, p. 37), self-making of nurses in clinical situations has specific meanings in relation to why nurses are in clinical situations, more critically why an individual nurse is in a particular clinical situation at a particular time. Human existence, thus, is contextually, temporally, and individually meaningful. Therefore, existential rationality for nursing practice has to be based on the principles that uphold commitment, freedom, and choice oriented to enhancing the purposes of nursing practice through the engagement of the nurse as an agent of "doing" of nursing in a particular clinical situation. The principles for the existential rationality in relation to nursing practice are identified as *authenticity*, *particularism*, and *understanding*. Application of the existential rationality specified by these three principles in nursing practice makes it possible for nurses to be "present" in clinical situations of nursing practice as genuine, particularized, and prudent comporting of selves. These three principles of the existential rationality are the governing structure for determining how nurses engage and comport with their self-identities in practice situations in order for their practice to be human encounters of highest quality.

The first principle of *authenticity* comes from the philosophy of existentialism, in which self-making in existence involves a burden of choice requiring one to be true to oneself (by proper coordination between transcendence and facticity) and to take full responsibility of choices that one makes (Sartre, 1958). Authenticity in existence refers to being true to oneself and true to situations in one's "doings," and means making choices that are framed by freedom and one's being. Since one's being is a complex of facticity and at the same time a transcended entirety, "doings" reflecting choices are governed by how authentic one is in coordinating this "being." Authentic existence with the burden of its inherent responsibility also reflects commitment to oneself. Nursing existence as nursing comportment governed by authenticity, therefore, means a genuine commitment of the nurse in being an individually responsible presence with the client and in the clinical situation, projecting the responsibility of being "the nurse" in the situation. In this sense, the nurse is *not* any nurse, but a particular nurse at a particular time in relation to a particular client and in a particular clinical situation. The existential character of nursing practice revealed in nursing comportment governed by authenticity is in the genuine "caring" of the nurse-self and of the client, and in opposition to simply fulfilling the required nursing role.

The second principle of *particularism* is oriented to the need for antiroutinization of human practice, especially in terms of professional services such as nursing practice. Humans develop standard approaches in "doings" mostly through experiences and repeated exposures to similar life situations. While routinization and standardization in human practice offer various advantages in carrying out services in an expedient, streamlined fashion, it tends to overlook specific characteristics of presenting situations. Particularism, in the existential sense, refers to the position that takes every situation as a particular instance with unique characteristics and presenting conditions. It is associated with the principle of authenticity, but goes beyond to address the need to the particularity of each "doing" or comporting in existence. Human encounters with others as well as in situations present unique features and meanings in their physical, social, and psychological occurrences, which at the same time are also interpreted in the human's mode of understanding the world in the framework of class identity. Grasping our world in the framework of class identity is a shortcut way of dealing with complex features of the life world. In so doing, we also develop ways of acting and "doing" in our encounters in the world that respond primarily to our class-identity interpretations. This means that human existence is entrenched with pulls for standardized choices as well as for particularized choices. When human existence is fully entrenched with standardization, it represents alienation and dehumanization, while when it is fully represented with particularization paying attention to the particular characters of a particular situation, it represents a genuine concern for the other. In nursing practice, particularism leads to nurses' comportments that fit with a particular client or with a particular clinical situation. A nurse who comports with all patients in a same kind fashion would be known as "the kind nurse" but would seldom be referred as "my nurse."

The third principle of *understanding* does not refer to cognitive, epistemic understanding, but refers to "the grasping" of meanings of oneself and a situation in a wholistic fashion. Such understanding is based on the concept of human agency advanced by Taylor (1985a, 1985b). Taylor states that a crucial feature of human agency is the capacity for "strong evaluation" with which responsibility for our "doings" becomes central to our beings and that is articulated through self-reflection (Taylor, 1985a, pp. 15–44). The key feature in this notion of human agency is insightfulness regarding choices one must make through articulations that are based on reflections examining "different possible modes of being of the agent" (Taylor, 1985a, p. 25). Further elaboration of this conception of human agency in the context of human existence points to the necessity of a person's understanding of the self and the situation in a wholistic, integrated fashion. Such understanding is "articulated" in the choices of "doings" in existence one makes in a specific situation, reflecting the significance of the situation to the self. Understanding as a principle for this existential dimension refers to the need to grasp the meanings of clinical situations and of the self in clinical situations in order for nurses being in clinical situations to have specific meanings. Understanding is critical for nurses in their posturing in clinical situations as the meanings of such situations are grasped by nurses in relation to their beings and their self-identities. In clinical situations nurses' beings and self-identities are intrinsically and unavoidably configured by them being nurses. Therefore, such understanding is nursing oriented and projects toward grasping the meanings from the nursing orientation.

Authenticity, particularism, and understanding as the principles for the existential rationality are the base upon which comportment in nursing practice attains the highest values of commitment, freedom, and choice in order for the nursing presence to have clinically significant meanings. The existential dimension of nursing practice guided by the existential rationality framed by these three principles thus refers to how nurses' comportments are made to be meaningful and have significance as nursing situations.

The knowledge necessary for the existential dimension can be specified in terms of self-knowledge and phronesis. Self-knowledge is a form of knowledge that is possible only through self-reflection, and is critical both for authenticity and understanding. On the other hand, phronesis in the sense that Aristotle (*Nicomachean Ethics,* Book VI) articulated refers to the insightful knowledge regarding what "doings" should be to bring about goodness and rightness in situations. Phronesis as knowledge is embedded intrinsically and integrally within persons, is oriented to the knowledge of attending to situations wholistically, and is experiential. Phronesis in the context of nursing practice then would refer to the insightfulness regarding clinical situations and nurses' approaches to clinical situations. The key modus operandus for the existential dimension is comportment. Nurses' comportments result from the existential rationality, with the articulation of the principles of authenticity, particularism, and understanding together in each given situation of nursing practice. Nursing comportments thus project qualities regarding genuineness, closeness/alienation, and satisfaction.

## SUMMARY AND QUESTIONS FOR REFLECTION AND FURTHER DELIBERATION

Characterization of nursing practice as it occurs in clinical situations is depicted in this dimensional specification. This is a way of describing what characteristics become evident in nursing practice by identifying five different aspects specified as the scientific, technical, ethical, aesthetic, and existential dimensions. When we talk about the characteristics of nursing practice, we refer to the qualitative differences and significances, as nursing practice is enacted in clinical situations with particular appearances, activities/actions/behaviors, meanings, and hidden processes. The five dimensional characteristics of nursing practice are viewed to be governed by the specific rationalities for the dimensions, and the principles specific to the rationalities. Table 6.1 shows the components for the dimensions of nursing practice.

As stated earlier, this dimensional configuration is not oriented to specifying nursing practice by different types, but refers to the aspects of nursing practice that bring about specific characterizations that result in a holistic view of nursing practice. Nursing practice is characterized by these five dimensions that are integrated to represent effectiveness, efficiency, goodness, sublimity, and commitment. Nursing practice represented by the qualitative variations in these dimensions can thus be examined to determine its quality in terms of both each characteristic dimension and its integrated nature.

**TABLE 6.1 Five Dimensions of Nursing Practice and Their Specifications**

| DIMENSION | VALUES | PRINCIPLES FOR THE RATIONALITY | KNOWLEDGE | MODUS OPERANDI |
|---|---|---|---|---|
| **Scientific Dimension** | Heuristic power | Scientific Rationality<br>Logic<br>Explanatory power<br>Experiential grounding | Scientific knowledge | Knowledge translation and application |
| **Technical Dimension** | Effectiveness<br>Efficiency<br>Craftsmanship | Technical Rationality<br>Optimization<br>Coordination<br>Contextualization<br>Flexibility | Designs of techniques | Performance of techniques |
| **Ethical Dimension** | Autonomy<br>Beneficence/ nonmaleficence<br>Justice<br>Fidelity | Ethical Rationality<br>Holistic understanding<br>Contextuality<br>Truthfulness<br>Compassion | Ethical knowledge | Choice selection |
| **Aesthetic Dimension** | Beauty<br>Sublimity<br>Empathy<br>Sensibility | Aesthetic Rationality<br>Unity<br>Harmony<br>Finesse | Knowledge of creativity<br>Knowledge of self-presentation | Expression in self-presentation |
| **Existential Dimension** | Commitment<br>Freedom<br>Choice | Existential Rationality<br>Authenticity<br>Particularism<br>Understanding | Self-knowledge<br>Phronesis | Comportment |

- Can you describe your practice in the five dimensions that characterize nursing practice by thinking about a recent case of nursing practice? Are you able to differentiate the characterizations according to these five dimensions? If not, why do you think it is not possible? Can you relate these five dimensions to your own practice?
- These five dimensions of nursing practice are viewed to characterize nursing practice analytically. Can you relate this analytical view to a descriptive view of the characterization of nursing practice?
- What are some of the tools necessary to analyze characterizations of nursing practice in these five dimensions?
- How is this dimensional level in the model related to other general levels—the perspective, the nursing knowledge, and the philosophy of nursing practice?

CHAPTER 7

# The Process of Nursing Practice

NURSING PRACTICE CONCEPTUALIZED IN THIS NORMATIVE model has the focal structure of processes as central to how "practice activities" are brought into actuality. The processes of nursing practice are the workings of how certain mental and/or behavioral activities in practice are produced. Although what occurs in specific situations of nursing practice may vary according to goals and contexts, it is actualized through the processes of deliberation and enactment that are the major human processes for practice. In this sense, while the three structures of nursing practice, that is, the perspective, the knowledge, and the philosophy, are the foundational groundings providing directions, orientations, and commitments for nursing practice in relation to *how* it should occur, the structure of processes refers to actual workings for *what* occurs in practice. The resulting nature of nursing practice, that is, "what occurs in practice," is reflected in the five dimensional characteristics. Nursing practice encompasses "activities" that are carried out by nurses either without or with the physical presence of a client. Yet, the goals of such "activities" are always oriented to the client. These "activities" in practice refer to intellectual or cognitive as well as behavioral ones involved in providing nursing care to clients.

The conceptualization of nursing practice with the focus on the processes of deliberation and enactment adopted in this model can be viewed vis-à-vis the general conceptualization of action in philosophy and the conceptualization of practice as in "praxeology" in sociology in order to specify the undergirding assumptions regarding human action in this model. Philosophy of action, since Aristotle in his *Nicomachean Ethics,* has addressed how human actions come about, distinguishes "intentional" action from mere happenings, and invokes human agency as central to the production of human action, based on the assumption that human agency is central to linking one's *desires*, *beliefs*, and *goals* and the production of actions. To Aristotle (Aristotle/Ross, 1980), human action is rational and based on a choice one makes through deliberation in the context of desires. Davidson (1982) asserted that an action, in some basic sense, is something an agent does that was "intentional under some description." Moya (1990) notes that the core of human agency is "an ability to commit oneself to do things in the future…" and that "the ability to commit oneself to act goes hand in hand with the ability to make one's own desires and other sorts of reasons objects of reflection and evaluation" (pp. 167, 168–169). Moya further considers agents as "having a subjective point of view of the world and acting according to it" with attributions of "beliefs, desires, hopes, intentions, values, and so on," and states that such states can be "falsely attributed when we shift to a perspective other than the agent's," that is, mental concepts "introduce intentional contexts" and "intentional states are subject to overall normative constraints of coherence and are holistically attributed" (1990, p. 71). Therefore, intentionality, reflection, and choice framed by desires, norms, and the agent's subjectivity are tied to actions not as mere happenings, but as committed ways of acting. This philosophy of action thus is the fundamental view in conceptualizing nursing practice as a special class of human actions.

The concepts of practice advanced in sociology lead these basic notions about human action further from the interpretive perspective, by explicating the concept of human agency and rationality in the social context. Taylor proposes that the human agent is "not only as partly responsible for what he does, for the degree to which he acts in line with his evaluations, but also as responsible in some sense for these evaluations" (1985a, p. 28). He further proposes the concept of human agency as having the capacity for evaluating desires to include the features of "strong evaluation" involving reflective articulation of one's preferences in which one applies evaluative language and self-interpretations that are shaped by experiences (Taylor, 1985a).

The basic assumptions regarding the processes of nursing practice are related to the definition of nursing practice, especially in terms of its goal-directed nature, specifically of its orientation to the well-being of clients in relation to healthful living. It is also based on the assumption that nursing practice is a form of human practice in which there is a complex interplay of mental/cognitive and behavioral activities. Nurses in practice are situated in continuously changing clinical situations that include clients, and are required to respond to and act upon the requirements inherent in such clinical situations in a responsible, goal-directed, and outcome-foreseeing manner. It means the practice involves the continuous workings of the processes that inhere specific actions. Let us consider a clinical situation in order to point out specific analytical issues related to the processes.

> *Edward Baxter, 69 years old, was admitted to the stroke unit 24 hours ago with a diagnosis of acute ischemic stroke. He was found slumped on the floor having fallen off the chair by the dining table by his wife on her return from grocery shopping. He was conscious, but his speech was incoherent, and he was not able to move his right arm and right leg. He was taken to an emergency unit where it was determined that he did not meet the criteria for thrombolytic treatment having passed the 3-hour time window of stroke event. The initial imaging of the brain revealed evidence of neither hemorrhage nor early ischemic changes. His initial NIHSS [National Institutes of Health Stroke Scale] score was 14. He was admitted to the unit for acute post-stroke treatment and care. He has a history of hypertension, ischemic heart disease, and diabetes. Alice Jones, RN, is the nurse for the care of Mr. Baxter on his second day of hospitalization. His vital signs are within the normal limits with a blood pressure of 158/92 mmHg. Other general signs and symptoms he is exhibiting presently are: dysarthria with slurred speech, moderate paresis, and severe weakness of the right side, a score of 93 on MMASA (Modified Mann Assessment of Swallowing Ability) assessed in the morning of the second day, and right-sided sensory loss. He has been sleeping on and off, and is withdrawn even from his interactions with family members. The nurse's assessments of depression and fatigue indicate mild to moderate levels. A plan of care has been established that involves intensive therapy and care by the nursing staff, speech-language therapist, physical therapist, and social worker, and a psychiatric consult has been requested. A plan of care has also been established to maintain diabetes control as well. Ms. Jones has started to assemble information for a discharge plan, and has consulted with Mr. Baxter's wife regarding the home situation. She has instructed the patient and his wife regarding position for eating, pace of eating, and diet to prevent aspiration. Observation and monitoring for any signs of infection and difficulties associated with possible incontinence are being carried out.*

Nursing practice by Ms. Jones for this patient on this shift consists of various activities involving the integration of deliberation and enactment. The following activities that culminate into the care of this patient can be gleaned:

- Systematic assessment activities—for problems associated with post-stroke status especially concerning dysarthria, paresis, muscle weakness, dysphagia, sensory loss, depression, fatigue, and mood changes

- Surveilling and monitoring activities—regarding potential aspiration, urinary continence, movement, moods, and further stroke activities
- Institution of nursing therapies—positioning, mobility assistance, diabetic control, fatigue management, nutritional balancing, comforting, oral care, and safety measures
- Teaching and counseling of the patient and family—regarding post-stroke experiences, eating and possibilities of aspiration, mobility, and speech
- Discharge planning—information gathering and assessment of the home situation, family preferences and capacities, discharge destination options, and rehabilitation needs
- Coordination with other health care professionals—consultations and collaboration with the physicians, speech-language therapist, physical therapist, and social worker

These activities (both mental and behavioral) are carried out with the integration of (a) the information, situation, and preferences of Mr. Baxter and his family; (b) Ms. Jones's knowledge, experiences, and attitudes regarding nursing practice and care of this patient; and (c) the contextual aspects of nursing practice including the medical care plans. In making decisions and carrying out specific actions, Ms. Jones integrates her nursing perspective, her survey of key knowledge, and her commitment in the philosophies of care, therapy, and professional work to bring about the best possible care for Mr. Baxter. The nursing practice of Ms. Jones for the shift in the care of Mr. Baxter is seamless, but organized, and is oriented to the highest possible well-being of the patient at the present with a view and plan toward the health-related well-being of the future. Ms. Jones's moment-to-moment activities involve moving between deliberations and enactments in relation to these sets of activities of nursing care for Mr. Baxter. At one moment, Ms. Jones may deliberate about what Mr. Baxter's "withdrawn" posture means, which may be followed by her asking the patient how he is feeling, and about what he is concerned, oriented to a careful assessment of depression and fatigue responses; and at another time, she may consider possible barriers to successful rehabilitation for Mr. Baxter, then confers with Mrs. Baxter regarding their home situation, her husband's life history, and his modes of dealing with difficult situations. She may also observe that he is having difficulty consuming his meals, and deliberate about how eating can be improved for him.

Nursing care as depicted in this scenario indicates that the practitioner is involved in a set of actions—deliberative activities that are purely mental and enactment activities that often involve both mental and behavioral

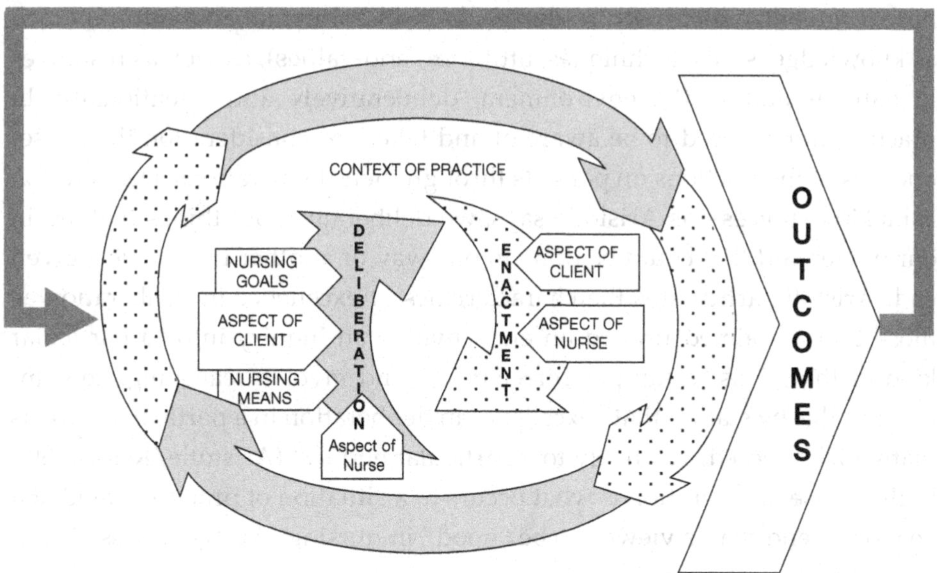


**FIGURE 7.1** The processes in nursing practice.

activities in a specific situation of practice encompassing aspects that pertain to (a) the client, (b) the context, (c) the agent-self, and (d) the nursing frames. Nursing practice is a complex series of actions that can be partitioned into two processes—deliberation and enactment (as shown in Figure 7.1)—as the basic processes that can be analytically partitioned for a full understanding of how nursing practice is actualized in clinical situations.

Although these two processes are conceptualized as analytically separate, the occurrence of these processes is neither linear nor are they independent of each other, and the two processes are connected intricately and interactively in actual practice situations. This means that a nurse may be engaged in a sequence of activities in a given clinical situation, in which the activities are all deliberative, deliberative and enactive, or a series of enactments. Deliberation and enactment may be viewed in the context of "events" in clinical situations that require specific nursing attention as well as in the context of the delivery of nursing care for a specific client.

## THE PROCESS OF DELIBERATION[1]

Nursing practice is deliberative in that it is designed and intended to address the goals for patients. Deliberation is a special type of mental activity that requires an intentional attention by the actor. It requires nurses to know how to mobilize their own resources, both instrumental and cultural (such as knowledge, skills, techniques, attitudes, and values), as well as resources in patients and in the environment, deliberatively and intentionally. In practice, nurses need to be aware of and take into consideration the consequences of their actions on patients through their deliberations. Deliberation is making choices—as Aristotle says, we deliberate about things that are in our power and that could be done in one way or another to achieve a given end. Aristotle articulates the characteristics of excellence in deliberation as those that are aimed toward an end, involve an inquiry into "a particular kind of thing," as "a kind of correctness," and involve reasoning; he summarizes this by stating that "excellence in deliberation in a particular sense is that which succeeds relatively to a particular end ..." (Aristotle/Ross, 1980). In this sense, deliberation is what occurs in a situation of practice aimed at a goal or an end that is viewed to be "good" in nursing, the "goodness" being located in the outcomes in patients.

Deliberation in nursing practice refers to phenomena in the nurse-agent as she or he is mentally and intellectually addressing the clinical situation in anticipation of actual delivery of nursing services. Aristotle presents the meaning of deliberation in relation to practical wisdom (prudence or *phronesis*) in *Nicomachean Ethics* Book VI as making choices to bring about human good through actions involving reason for figuring out the means to attain an end with a view for what is a "good" end (Aristotle/Barnes, 1984). Hence, deliberation is connected to action and is oriented to a result. The nurse in the process of deliberation: (a) considers the meaning and nature of information, (b) processes a given set of information vis-à-vis existing relevant structures, (c) surveys and draws on both the public and personal knowledge arenas, (d) contemplates future courses of action and establishes intentions, and (e) makes judgments and choices about conceptual and action decisions. The process of deliberation involves the practitioner engaging in mental activities to develop a program of action as analytically separated from the enactment of action. It focuses on the structuring of information the practitioner gains of the situation, the practitioner's judgment about the meanings of information, and the arriving at decisions as to what the nurse should do or needs to do to meet the demands of the situation. This may involve a situation with a specific, single problem to be addressed, or one that is entrenched with coexisting, multiple problems, and issues requiring decisions not only for problem solutions, but also for coordination of judgments and choices. Deliberations are viewed to be analytically connected to a network of five structural units: (a) aspects of client, (b) aspects of nurse-agent, (c) nursing goals, (d) nursing means, and (e) context of nurse-agent.

## The Structure Related to Aspects of the Client

The structure related to aspects of the client is the focal framework upon which the significance of nursing for a client is established situationally, that is, for a given situation or an event, or holistically for that client's nursing care. This structure encompasses those elements that are related to the nature of specific problems confronting the client, that provide the client with meanings and perceptions about the problems and situations, and that are related to personal resources present and available in the client. As shown in Figure 7.2, these elements can be differentiated as general or specific, identified in relation to health problems and health-related experiences, knowledge, capacity, attitudes, motivation and commitment, habits, and personal experiences and history. This structure thus defines the elements that the nurse must bring into a varying focus in deliberating about a program of nursing actions. It is the major frame that provides information to the nurse during this phase. Because what the nurse knows about or becomes exposed to with respect to aspects of the client rather than what "actually" exists within this structure is of significance for deliberation, the critical issue is what information regarding the client the nurse brings into the process of deliberation. The concept of knowing the patient has been discussed in the literature to address processes by which nurses attain comprehensive understanding about the patient, which is brought into deliberation (Jenny & Logan, 1992; Liaschenko, 1997; Radwin, 1996;

| Structure of the Client | | Structure of the Nurse | |
|---|---|---|---|
| **General Aspects** | **Specific Aspects** | **General Aspects** | **Specific Aspects** |
| Health problems and health-related experiences | | Personal frame of reference | |
| Knowledge | | Knowledge | |
| Capacity | | Capacity/competence | |
| Attitudes, motivation, and commitments | | Values, value commitments, and attitudes | |
| Habits | | Motivation and feeling states | |
| Experiential history and contextual grounding | | Experiential history and contextual grounding | |

**FIGURE 7.2** Structures for deliberation: Aspects of the client and of the nurse.

Tanner, Benner, Chesla, & Gordon, 1993; Whittemore, 2000). The concept of "knowing the patient" refers to developing an in-depth understanding of the patient as an individual located in a specific health care situation with a unique background and specific modes of living. This means that the process of deliberation is a continuing process that is used to build up the content of "knowing the patient."

## The Structure of Nurse-Agent

This structure refers to the aspects of variability in the nurse, which are possible for activation in the process of deliberation. As shown in Figure 7.2, it is organized into two aspects of the practitioner (i.e., the general and specific situation-bound) with respect to six categories:

1. The frame of reference the nurse is adopting in providing personal meanings regarding nursing practice in the form of standards, commitments, locus of interest, philosophy, and worldviews
2. Personal knowledge existent in the nurse both as organized and as unorganized entities
3. Personal capacity for practice as resources such as energy, skills, and modes of thinking
4. Value commitments from the ethical and moral perspective that guide the nurse's practice
5. Motivation and feeling states
6. Experiential history both as a nurse and as a human being

The structure of nurse-agent is critical in the process of deliberation because professional practice requires the agent's primary focus on others (i.e., clients) and other-directed actions (i.e., actions for the benefit of clients). The practitioner has to negotiate with himself or herself regarding the paradox that ensues with the coexistence of this other-directedness in orientation and the fundamentally self-centered nature of human actions. It means that the practitioner, in having the goals of practice embedded in the client, engages in the phase of deliberation both with and without the conscious recognition of the extent to which the nurse's own aspects are involved. The elements identified within this structure are what the nurse brings into the nursing practice setting, and are basically attained, accumulated, and transformed through professional socialization and experience. Their mobilization in and impact on the processes of this phase are selective and variable in different clinical situations.

One critical concept in the aspects of the nurse that has received a great deal of attention in the literature is the concept of *phronesis* or practical wisdom as specified by Aristotle, which is viewed to be a necessary quality for deliberative praxis to attain goodness (i.e., human flourishing) in human life. Connor (2004) suggests that phronesis is the key concept that undergirds various praxiological discussions in nursing. Svenaeus (2003) on the other hand proposes hermeneutical phronesis, which is based on interpretation, as the way to know the best thing to do for a particular patient in a particular situation and time. Benner (2000) emphasizes phronesis as the essential feature of nursing practice with which the nurse as an embodied and socially embedded moral agent produces good practice. Flaming (2001) in a similar way proposes phronesis, which involves the combined use of intuitive reasoning from the knowledge of the particular and the knowledge of universals, as the basis for deliberation to arrive at an ethically correct nursing action in a particular nursing situation. Phronesis is viewed vis-à-vis scientific, research-based thinking that is generally oriented to knowledge of universals and generalities, with the conception that phronesis focuses on the knowledge of particulars and situationally embedded understandings with a concern for producing socially and morally good actions (i.e., praxis). While phronesis is viewed to be a quality associated with intuition and morality, it is sometimes viewed as a more critical quality than the possession of scientific knowledge. However, while phronesis refers to a quality of process that becomes an integral part of the process of deliberation, the possession of knowledge for practice refers to the structural property that is invoked in deliberation.

The current culture of evidence-based practice claims the critical importance of both the possession of scientific knowledge and the ability to use the knowledge that exists in the public domain. Certainly, professional practice must be based on the knowledge of the discipline, and the expectation is for the nurse to possess a rich decisional base that can be used in deliberation. Professional practitioners including nurses in contemporary society are confronted with relevant knowledge that is continuously developing, updated, and revised in the public domain; as well, they are engaged in updating and accumulating personal knowledge through their professional experiences. Knowledge invoked in specific nursing practice situations is what is present and available to a nurse at the given moment. How that knowledge is organized, what it encompasses, and how it becomes available to the practitioner in deliberation are critical and will be taken up in Chapter 10.

The variability in the nurse-agent in relation to the six categories specified in this structure influences how deliberation is made, and whether or not a given deliberation is of a highest quality. The frames of reference and value commitments are internalized and reinforced through education and social experiences, while personal knowledge and personal experiences are critically tied and require conscious efforts by practitioners for integration and upgrading. Personal capacity and feeling states are situational, requiring conscious attention by practitioners for their potential influence on the quality of deliberation.

## The Structure of Nursing Goals

As shown in Figure 7.3, this structure encompasses the goals inherent in a clinical situation, both latent and manifest, and is differentiated on two dimensions: scope and orientation. Goals in clinical situations may be general from the nursing perspective, such as promotion of health or attainment of client autonomy, and specific to the situation and problem at hand, such as preventing aspiration or improving feelings regarding a sudden immobility as in Mr. Baxter's situation. In addition, goals may exist differently from the perspectives of the client, the nurse, and others such as family members and other health care professionals. For any given clinical situation in which nursing actions must take place, there exists a set of goals identifiable as a varying combination of the generalized and specific goals for the client, the nurse, and others. There may be alignment or misalignment among these goals, as the client, the nurse, and others (such as family members) could be oriented to primarily different aspects of the client's well-being, different priorities, or

| **Structure of Nursing Goals (Orientation)** | | **Structure of Nursing Means (Availability)** | |
|---|---|---|---|
| **General Goals** | **Specific Goals (Situation or Problem Specific)** | **General Means and Approaches** | **Specific Means and Strategies** |
| Goals defined by client | | Repertoire at large | |
| Goals defined by nurse | | Personal repertoire | |
| Goals defined by others | | Conjectured means and approaches | |

**FIGURE 7.3** Structures for deliberation: Aspects of nursing goals and of nursing means.

different motivational structures. How the nurse becomes cognizant of and puts emphasis on different sets of goals in deliberation is one of the problematic aspects in the process of deliberation.

## The Structure of Nursing Means

In a similar manner to the structure of nursing goals (as shown in Figure 7.3), the structure of nursing "means" is differentiated into two aspects: the scope of application and availability. Nursing means include strategies of nursing applicable in clinical situations to bring about some ends that are relevant to nursing practice. Nursing means, from the view of the scope of application, can be general, in that the target for the application is the client as a human person, or specific to the situation or problem. Nursing means can be available in the public arena, mostly as validated forms of strategies, or privately to individual nurses, attained mostly through personal experience, or as conjectures existing only as tentative ideas. The nurse-agent thus also brings varying combinations of means emerging from this structure into the process of deliberation. The structure of nursing means in the process of deliberation is relevant in making connections between goals and future actions, and is the backboard for drawing possible and necessary nursing actions. The process therefore must involve juxtaposing the elements within this structure with the elements of the structure of nursing goals with a view toward establishing a program of action that makes the practice coherent, meaningful, strategically effective, and sensible.

## The Structure of the Context of Nurse-Agent

The structure of the context is the background upon which the nurse's deliberation is processed and refers to elements in the physical, social, and symbolic spheres of the practice environment. Deliberation takes place in the context of a practice situation that contains not only the environmental entities, but also the meanings of such entities. The examples of the elements within this structure that impinge on the deliberation process are noise, conflicting demands present in the situation, value structure or culture of the situation, an institutionalized form of practice (what Bourdieu [1977, 1990] calls institutional *habitus*), level of institutional integration of roles, a lack of staff, and being assigned to several complex clients. One major aspect of the context is medical plans and activities, especially in clinical situations in which clients are primarily medically managed, such as in hospitals. Medical management formulates critical contextual background for nursing as it specifies particular activities for clients in regard to medical diagnosis and treatment.

Deliberations involving these five structures are not only oriented to making choices for actions to be pursued, but also in doing so that the present situation of deliberation is contiguously linked to the future in association with the chosen actions. Normatively, it is expected that a practitioner be engaged in the deliberation phase with a commitment to achieving fidelity of strategy, competent delivery, timeliness and relevancy of program, and efficacy of outcomes. This view points to the idea that the process of deliberation necessarily needs to be rational and prescriptive; however, the phenomena as they exist in actual practice may be more haphazardly or intuitively organized than programmatic or intentional.

Clinical decision making, clinical judgment and diagnosing, information processing, priority setting, and nursing care planning are examples of phenomena in this process.

## THE PROCESS OF ENACTMENT[2]

The process of enactment refers to the phase at which the nurse performs activities in nursing. The phenomena of enactment in nursing are conceptualized as human action being carried out and performed behaviorally by a nurse-agent in the context of nursing care. If one believes that the reality of enactment has a direct and complete causal relation with intention, and intention is a sufficient explanation of an enactment, then it would not be necessary to consider this phase separately from the phase of deliberation. However, I believe this view is not tenable from the theoretical considerations, as this belief is too simplistic and unidimensional contrary to our experiences. The conceptualization of human action within the disciplines of human service practice requires us to consider human action in a much more complex way. Enactment in human service practice is not only realized by the nurse-agent, but also invariably involves another human being (the client) who is also an engaged, enacting agent. In addition, certain aspects of nursing practice require deliberation as separate activities of the nurse. Furthermore, the connections between deliberation and enactment are not uniform and linear, and can take various forms according to differences in the nature of practice setting. For example, a critical care situation often requires on-the-spot, immediate action responses, whereas in a home-care setting, enactment of nursing actions may be separated from deliberation by a prolonged time lag. Alternatively, a nurse may do a deliberation, whereas the enactment needs to be done by a third person through delegation of actions.

Facts of enactment are nonetheless time-bound, possibly have multiple meanings, and are fleeting, as depicted by Bourdieu in describing game playing as an example of practice. Game playing per Bourdieu involves on-the-spot adjustments with what one encounters in the instance of playing, but also with what are foreseen as impending in the immediate future in the continuity of time (Bourdieu, 1990). An enactment is connected to deliberation, but integrates on-the-spot adjustments that connect what exists at the time of enactment to the immediate future. We feel the urgency of human enactment, as it is bound to the present and future at the same time, which becomes a thing of the past instantaneously. We also feel the urgency of human action in the human agent's engagement, as well as the finalization of an action once it is enacted. Action science proposed by Argyris, Putnam, and Smith (1985) and the notion of reflective practice advanced by Schön (1983) examine the reasons for practitioners' failure to achieve intended consequences in their practice and the reasons for the possible disparity that exists between what practitioners believe they are doing and what they actually do.

Nursing practice as *doing* and *acting* occurs as nurses are engaged in actions such as assessing patients, observing, carrying out treatments, caring, teaching, or counseling. And such *doings* require doing them correctly and skillfully, doing them at the right moments, doing them in concert with other things happening at the same time, doing them with foresight, and doing them while valuing patients' identities, worth, wants, and humanness. Nursing practice as *doing* is *praxis* in the sense that was originally articulated by Aristotle, who differentiates *praxis* as *doing* and acting, guided by a moral disposition to act truly and rightly with a commitment to human well-being, from *poiesis* as making of something or producing (*Nicomachean Ethics*, Book VI, Chapter IV; see also Lobkowicz, 1967, pp. 9–15). *Praxis* to Freire (1992) means "reflection and action upon the world in order to transform it" and refers to "the dialectic relation between the subjective and the objective in which men engage and confront reality by critical intervention for transformation of it" (pp. 36–37). Along the same lines, Holmes and Warelow (2000) proposed nursing "as a form of praxis" in which it is "seen as a standard of excellence, an ideal ethical goal for which to strive; it is also what Marxists would describe as an attempt to make an irrational world more rational, or a way of making useable sense of one's practice world" (p. 175). Nursing practice as doing in this sense transcends mere acting or performing and is elevated to the realm of morally committed human actions of nurses.

The process of enactment of doing is analytically separated from the process of deliberation, and involves acting and behaving in a specific practice situation involving the practitioner, the client as a recipient of service as well as a responding human "other," and the contextual frames within which the actions take place. In this process, nursing action is analytically conditioned by three structural units: (a) the client, (b) the nurse-agent, and (c) the context of nursing action. Enactment is bound by time, space, and physical locality in relation to the acting agent, that is, the practitioner. Although it is conceptualized to be analytically separated from the process of deliberation, it does not mean that the process of enactment does not have mental elements, as human actions cannot be considered devoid of mental contents. Separating this process from the deliberation process allows us to examine nursing practice for what is actually done and accomplished concretely in clinical situations.

As an enactor in this process, the nurse brings into the situation of enactment the agent-self with all of his or her capabilities and limitations, desires and hesitancies, sensibility and hardiness, habits and quirks, history and background, and beliefs and knowledge. Such aspects of the nurse accommodate how actions become actualized, by making them good or bad, skillful or cumbersome, with passion or without, coordinated or disjointed, organized or disorganized, efficient or inefficient, ethical or unethical, and artful or mundane.

The client—often as a coengager in the enactment of nursing actions—brings into the situation all aspects that makes the client a specific individual, also engaged in his or her life of the specific situation that is ongoing for him or her. Through the client's responses, behaviors, and presence, enactment is also accommodated to fit with the aspects of the client as it is performed in clinical situations. This is especially critical in situations of enactment that require active participation by the client, such as in teaching, dialogue, and so forth.

The contextual aspects of the situation of the enactment are the physical, social, and symbolic aspects of the environment that are bound to the enactment in a spatiotemporal sense, both immediately and remotely, but significantly. The context of enactment both confines and allows forms of nursing actions that are possible. As an immediate "situ" of practice, the context exerts forces that are both stable and changing. Both the stability and changeability are associated with physical, social, and symbolic aspects of the environment of practice. Stability of the context allows nurses to assume predictability, while the continuously changing nature of the context requires nurses' enactment to be flexible, accommodating, and revisional. Nurses, regardless of their deliberation, need to adapt actual performance of nursing actions to situational contingencies that exist in an immediate environment. For example, a nurse may "end up" delegating a specific action to a health care assistant even though her or his intention was to do it herself or himself, and a nurse may need to stop teaching a patient about diabetic self-care, as she or he is paged for immediate attention to another client.

The context of practice is not only a physical and social situation of a given moment of practice, but also a structured social field that has an established condition of social patterning, both of which aspects exert manifest and latent influences on one's practice. One way of viewing the "context" of practice is to borrow the concept of *field* from Bourdieu (1990). Bourdieu's work (1990) on *practice* focuses on three concepts—*habitus, field,* and *capital.* Human practice to Bourdieu is interplay of *habitus* and *field* in relation to *capital* both as resources for use and gain, in which mediation between "socialized" subjectivity (habitus) and structured objectivity (field) occurs. Habitus is viewed as "the durable and transposable systems of schemata of perception, appreciation, and action that result from the institution of the social in the body (or in biological individuals)" (Bourdieu & Wacquant, 1992, pp. 126–127). On the other hand, field refers to a specific complex of social relations established as a network of objective relations between positions that "are objectively defined in their existence and in the determinations they impose upon their occupants, agent or institutions, by their present and potential situation (situ) in the structure of the distribution of species of power (or capital) whose possession commands access to specific profits that are at stake in the field, as well as by their objective relation to other positions (domination, subordination, homology, etc.)" (Bourdieu & Wacquant, 1992, p. 97). Capital represents power over a field, distributed over positions in a field. Both habitus and field are social, in that the field structures the habitus, and the habitus contributes to constituting the field, that is, the habitus is "the product of the embodiment of the immanent necessity of a field" and the field is constituted by sets of specific dispositions human agents possess giving the field its meanings. To Bourdieu, human agents are engaged in their everyday practice in relatively autonomous fields of modern life, such as economy, arts, science, or education, each of which consists of a specific complex of social relations, and is the site of a logic and a necessity that are *specific and irreducible* to those that regulate other fields. It means for nursing practice that nurses are engaged in their practice in the field of health care, which is composed of a specific complex of social relations constituted by the logic of healing and service with players distributed in different positions of clients, families, health care professionals, and managers. In this theoretical orientation, a nurse's enactment of practice or a system of a nurse's practice can only be analytically viewed to reflect the habitus mediated within a field of practice.

Technical competence, nursing aesthetics, delegation behavior, nursing documentation and nursing description, ritualized practice, caring, ethical practice, nurse talk, and tailoring nursing actions are examples of phenomena in the practice domain with a focus on the enactment process.

## THE PERSPECTIVE, THE KNOWLEDGE, AND THE PHILOSOPHY OF PRACTICE IN THE PROCESSES

These two processes of nursing practice are "workings" that produce the contents of nursing practice. As these are processes involving human's mental/cognitive– and behavioral/action–oriented activities, they are guided specifically by those background elements that make them specifically "nursing." These background elements are conceptualized in this model as the perspective, the knowledge, and the philosophies. The perspective of nursing practice orients nurses' activities to be committed to the welfare of clients and to the views regarding humans in the context of nursing care and nursing as a specific form of human practice. Nurses' commitments to the perspective of nursing frame their practice to be a meaningful social practice oriented to human health and service. Holism, health orientation, person-centered practice, and caring as the key elements of the nursing perspective are integrated into the processes as the guiding frames in viewing goals for clients, ways of accomplishing the goals, and finding specific modes of delivering nursing care. Furthermore, the nursing perspective provides the frames of reference with which nurses consider their clients, clients' problems, and "nursing" ways of providing health care both in the processes of deliberation and of enactment.

Nursing practice in its processes incorporates and utilizes various forms, types, and contents of knowledge in order to make it a knowledge-based practice. Nursing knowledge is the specialized knowledge for nursing practice, and when applied in practice, makes the nature of nursing activities to be *nursing*, differentiated from ordinary human activities and other professional activities. However, knowledge applied/used in nursing practice includes both nursing knowledge as well as other relevant knowledge for general human practice, requiring nurses to hold both types of knowledge. The view advanced in this model regarding nursing knowledge in terms of the five types of cognitive needs for practice proposes that in every nursing practice instance, nurses need to consider inferential, referential, transformative, normative, and desiderative cognitive needs. The understanding and knowledge that undergird practice cannot be of one cognitive type, but need to be comprehensive so that the complex nature of humans and of practice is addressed in delivering care. Table 7.1 lists the most essential theories and knowledge applicable in the nursing practice, using Mr. Baxter as an illustration in addressing five different types of cognitive needs for nursing practice. This list is not exhaustive or complete. The knowledge illustrated in this table has to be available either within the stock of private knowledge of the nurse or in the public domain for extraction by the nurse.

**TABLE 7.1 A List of Theories for the Nursing Care of Mr. Baxter: An Illustration**

| TYPES OF COGNITIVE NEEDS | | | | |
|---|---|---|---|---|
| **INFERENTIAL NEEDS** | **REFERENTIAL NEEDS** | **TRANSFORMATIVE NEEDS** | **NORMATIVE NEEDS** | **DESIDERATIVE NEEDS** |
| Biobehavioral theories of stroke and its process<br>Theories of stroke symptoms and symptom trajectories<br>Theories of pain, fatigue, depression, and sleep<br>Theories of physical and psychological functioning<br>Theories of stroke therapy<br>Theories of recovery<br>Theories of speech<br>Theories of communication<br>Theories of comfort and safety<br>Theories of social interaction<br>Theories of self-identify and self-image<br>Theories of learning<br>Theories of support | Stories of stroke experiences<br>Variations in individual responses to stroke and stressful events<br>Variations in verbalization of stressful experiences<br>Variations in the recovery trajectory from stroke<br>Meanings of stroke experiences and recovery<br>Life stories and stroke experiences | Critical theories regarding disability, dysfunction, and chronic illness<br>Theories regarding marginalization and stigma<br>Critical theories regarding social role and social responsibility<br>Theories of powerlessness and helplessness<br>Theories regarding attribution of responsibility<br>Transformative theories for mutual understanding, power equalization, empowerment, and communication<br>Theories of resource allocation | Ethical theories of caring and advocacy<br>Value theories regarding personhood, integrity, and dignity<br>Standards of care for recovery | Communicative aesthetics<br>Theories of self-presentation<br>Person-centeredness processes<br>Aesthetics of bodily presentation<br>Aesthetics in learning and teaching<br>Environmental aesthetics |

This set of knowledge is applied in the processes of deliberation and of enactment, guiding what sorts of decisions are to be made on behalf of the client and how certain actions by the nurse are to be performed in delivering nursing care. The way such knowledge is integrated into the processes is seamless, sometimes accomplished with little conscious awareness of the integration by the nurse, and other times carried out with conscious efforts by the nurse to apply and integrate specific knowledge. The application of knowledge within these processes is complex, and is addressed in the next chapter.

On the other hand, the philosophies of nursing practice, which are identified as the philosophies of therapy, care, and professional work in this model, are woven into nurses' practice through their commitments to uphold them as an integrated philosophy. It thus means that there is a need for nurses to be committed to these philosophies if practice is to be "nursing." These philosophies as a set are the basis (a) by which nurses seek out what problems there are in clients and how to address and solve problems for their clients, (b) with which nurses approach clients with caring attitudes and caring behaviors, and (c) by which nurses delineate and accomplish their professional responsibilities in providing nursing care to clients. Nurse Jones would be oriented to uphold these philosophies in her deliberations and enactments by adhering to the values embedded in the philosophy of care (i.e., individuality, autonomy, human integrity, and human flourishing), the philosophy of therapy (i.e., effectiveness, efficiency, individualization, and openness to choice), and the philosophy of professional work (i.e., distributive justice, competence, and collaboration). These values as the principles are the guideposts in the deliberations and enactments for nurses being committed to the profession and the values of their practice. Of course, there will be variations in the degrees of nurses' commitments to these philosophies and of their integration into the processes of nursing practice. This variation would be revealed in the quality of nursing practice. While the nursing perspective is the first-layer frame for practice, the philosophies of nursing practice form the second-layer frame for practice to be "nursing" and professional. The perspective, the knowledge, and the philosophy for the processes of nursing practice are the foundation by which the characteristic features and contents of the processes of deliberation and enactment in nursing practice are determined.

## THE DIMENSION OF NURSING PRACTICE AND THE PROCESS

The processes of deliberation and enactment in nursing practice are inherent in the nursing practice activities, and determine the characteristics nursing practice takes on as it is delivered to clients. The dimension and the process in this model of nursing practice have an intrinsic connection via the processes determining the dimensional characteristic variations in practice and, in turn, the dimensions providing the structures for how the processes are to be applied in practice (Figure 7.4). The fashion by which the processes ensue in practice informs the dimensional characteristics in terms of scientific, technical, ethical, aesthetic, and existential aspects; at the same time, the rationalities and principles embedded in the dimensions are guides by which the processes should proceed. In

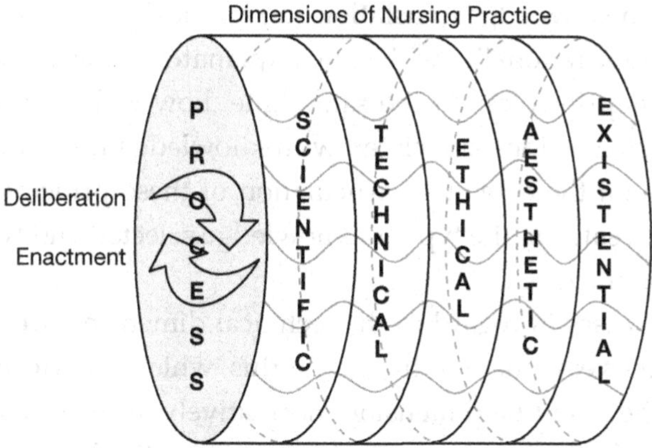


**FIGURE 7.4** Integration of the processes of nursing practice into the five dimensions of practice.

this sense, nursing practice is characteristically represented by the dimensional features as the results of how the processes occur; and at the same time, the processes occur in relation to how the rationalities for the dimensional characteristics become integrated into the practice. Nursing practice thus has two sides that are integrally meshed to reveal its quality, as shown in Figure 7.4.

The quality of nursing practice therefore is determined by how fitting the processes are in practice in relation to the rationalities for the dimensions of nursing practice. The processes of deliberation and enactment have to occur revealing their adherence to:

- The principles of logic, explanatory power, and experiential grounding in the mode of knowledge translation and application in terms of the scientific dimension
- The principles of optimization, coordination, contextuality, and flexibility in the mode of performing of techniques in terms of the technical dimension
- The principles of holistic understanding, contextuality, truthfulness, and compassion in the mode of choice selection in terms of the ethical dimension
- The principles of unity, harmony, and finesse in the mode of expressing in self-presentation in terms of the aesthetic dimension
- The principles of authenticity, particularism, and understanding in the mode of comportment in terms of the existential dimension

The processes of deliberation and enactment in regard to the scientific dimension are involved in the dimension's essential modus operandi, which is knowledge translation and application. Therefore, normatively, nurses' deliberation and enactment in knowledge translation and application in practice have to be guided by scientific rationality with logic, explanatory power, and experiential grounding as its principles. At the same time, how well a nurse deliberates and enacts nursing actions associated with knowledge translation and application depends on the extents of articulation of these principles in practice. This could be revealed in the types of knowledge selected and types of knowledge applied in practice.

These processes in regard to the technical dimension are thus involved in the dimension's essential modus operandus, which is performance of techniques. As in the scientific dimension, normatively, nurses' deliberation and enactment in performing techniques of nursing practice have to be guided by technical rationality with optimization, coordination, contextuality, and flexibility as its principles. Performance of techniques in nursing practice such as carrying out a program of patient teaching or nursing assessment would then have to be based on nurses' deliberations regarding, for example, sequencing or resource-use decisions, and on nurses' actual enactment of such techniques in practice with skillfulness and flexibility. The quality of nursing practice in relation to the performance of technique therefore will depend on how well the principles of the technical rationality are articulated in practice, which can be judged by the degree of effectiveness, efficiency, and craftsmanship.

The processes of deliberation and enactment in regard to the ethical dimension are associated with the dimension's essential modus, which is making ethical choices for clients. Normatively, therefore, nurses' deliberative and enactment processes have to be guided by the moral rationality with holistic understanding, contextuality, truthfulness, and compassion as its principles. Nurses in their encounters of decision situations involving clients, which are oriented to ensuring clients' well-being and ability to flourish, have to deliberate about and act on decisions articulating these principles in order to ensure autonomy, beneficence, justice, and fidelity for clients.

The processes of deliberation and enactment in regard to the aesthetic dimension are associated with the dimension's essential modus operandus, which is expression in self-presentation of the nurse in practice. Nurses' deliberations and enactments therefore have to be guided by the aesthetic rationality with unity, harmony, and finesse as its principles. Nurses' self-presentations in discursive and behavioral expressions have to represent the articulation of these principles applied in the processes.

The processes of deliberation and enactment in regard to the existential dimension cannot be thought of in the same analytic sense as they are integrated into the other four dimensions. This is because the existential dimension with comportment as the essential modus operandus is a part of nursing practice simply as "existence." This means that existence is a priori to the analytical processes of deliberation and enactment, and is revealed only through reflection. The processes of deliberation and enactment are latent in comportment. In order to ensure that nurses articulate in their practice the principles of commitment, freedom, and choice of the existential rationality, nurses have to be self-aware and reflective of their existence and their engagements with the world. It is through reflexivity and self-awareness that nursing practice can existentially uphold these principles.

The articulation between the dimensions of nursing practice and the processes of nursing practice is integrative, and is revealed in nurses' quality of practice. How well nurses can translate and apply knowledge, perform techniques of nursing practice, make ethical decisions, present themselves in various expressive modes, and comport existentially will thus depend upon the degree of articulation of the principles associated with the dimensions' rationalities. An example of a nurse carrying out pain management for a patient with malignant cancer shows the complexity associated with this event of nursing practice, as identified in Table 7.2. A nurse may not be as systematic and comprehensive in her or his practice with this event as depicted in this table, but the quality of this practice would be revealed in relation to the five dimensions.

**TABLE 7.2 Deliberation and Enactment Involved in Pain Management in Relation to the Five Dimensions of Nursing Practice: An Illustration**

| DIMENSION | DELIBERATION | ENACTMENT |
|---|---|---|
| **Scientific Dimension** | Assessing one's own stock of knowledge regarding pain management<br>Selecting knowledge to be applied in pain management<br>Evaluating the quality of knowledge selected for their heuristic power<br>Deciding on how the selected knowledge is to be applied in pain management<br>Deciding on a pain management program | Searching for new knowledge in the public domain regarding pain management<br>Carrying out the pain management program applying knowledge selected for the program |
| **Technical Dimension** | Assessing what sorts of techniques are involved in the pain management selected<br>Deciding on timing, sequencing, and resources-needs in relation to the selected pain management<br>Assessing the types of environmental control necessary for the pain management<br>Assessing one's own skillfulness in instituting the pain management | Instituting the pain management program adjusting for individual's needs and preferences, and tailoring to the patient<br>Mobilizing resources in carrying out the pain management program |

(continued)

**TABLE 7.2 Deliberation and Enactment Involved in Pain Management in Relation to the Five Dimensions of Nursing Practice: An Illustration (*continued*)**

| DIMENSION | DELIBERATION | ENACTMENT |
|---|---|---|
| **Ethical Dimension** | Assessing the presence of ethical issues in the pain management (e.g., issues associated with substance abuse, personal preferences, the nature of pain, and social control)<br>Addressing ethical issues and making a choice of approach in collaboration with the patient | Articulating the choices with the patient and family<br>Advocating for the patient and family regarding the decisions |
| **Aesthetic Dimension** | Thinking through various expressive modes necessary in pain management<br>Deliberating about creativity in expressions in pain management | Combining various expressive modes of actions (talking, using gestures, body language, etc.) in the pain management to fit with the patient's needs and preferences<br>Managing the environment creatively to enhance the effects of pain management |
| **Existential Dimension** | Comporting reflexively to ensure authenticity, particularism, and depth of understanding in the situation | |

## SUMMARY AND QUESTIONS FOR REFLECTION AND FURTHER DELIBERATION

The processes of nursing practice are the core of how "doings" occur in nursing practice. Therefore, the processes have to integrate the perspective, the knowledge, and the philosophy of practice, and are to be embedded inherently within the five dimensional characteristics that determine the quality of practice. Elaboration of what structures are involved in the processes points to the complexities involved in the processes. The concept of nursing process that has been integrated into nursing practice during the last several decades points out the logical components in nursing practice rather than the actual processes that occur in "doing" in nursing. The components in nursing process (i.e., assessment, diagnosis, identification of outcomes, planning, implementation, and evaluation) are oriented to identifying specific actions in the components rather than the processes of how such actions must occur. This means that the processes of deliberation and enactment in nursing practice are inherent in each component of the nursing process as the modes of actions. It is how well and competently a nurse engages herself or himself in the processes of deliberation and enactment reflecting the five rationalities for practice, that would produce the qualities in the six steps of the nursing process.

- Think of a recent case of nursing practice involving a client and reflect on how the processes of deliberation and enactment discussed in this chapter were involved in your practice.
- Are there other essential processes besides the processes of deliberation and enactment that describe your practice?
- Discuss how the processes you applied in your practice are related to your perspective, knowledge, and philosophy of practice.
- Can you characterize your practice by reflecting on the integration of the processes with the five dimensions of nursing practice?
- How do the processes of deliberation and enactment get integrated into the general modes of nursing practice, such as care giving, advocating, helping, teaching, therapy/intervention, care coordination, care management, and resource provision?

## NOTES

1. This section has been extended from Kim (2010).
2. This section has been expanded further from the text in Kim (2010).

# CHAPTER 8

# Essential Tools of Nursing Practice

One of the definitions of the term "tool" in the Webster's English Dictionary is "something necessary in the practice of a vocation or a profession." Although this term is used in this chapter in the general sense of this meaning, "something" is translated not as material entities but as human cognitive and behavioral strategies, approaches, and methods. For every profession, there are basic, essential tools with which its practice is configured at the baseline and that are assembled, integrated, and "tweaked" to address its responsibilities in a given situation of practice. In this sense, essential tools of a profession are seen to be applicable across situations and problems. The essential tools of nursing practice are, thus, identified as those cognitive and behavioral strategies applicable across nearly all clinical nursing fields, and are essential and necessary to fulfill nursing responsibilities of patient care.

From the 1980s, nursing has been engaged in developing a language system to identify with what sorts of problems nursing is concerned (nursing diagnosis), what sorts of client outcomes nursing is expected to produce (nursing outcomes), and what sorts of strategies are performed in nursing care situations (nursing interventions). These concerns have been culminated into the development of the North American Nursing Diagnosis Association (NANDA) classification system for nursing diagnosis, the Nursing Outcomes Classification (NOC) system, and the Nursing Interventions Classification (NIC) system for nursing interventions (Bulechek, Butcher, Dochterman, & Wagner, 2013; Herdman, 2009; Moorhead, Johnson, Maas, & Swanson, 2013). The NIC is a comprehensive, research-based, standardized classification of interventions that nurses perform, consisting of 554 interventions in 30 categories within seven domains at its latest revision (Bulechek et al., 2013). It contains interventions performed by nurses on behalf of patients directly or indirectly and independently or collaboratively with other health care professionals in order to enhance client outcomes. While this list represents a vast array of nursing interventions, the interventions are most strictly oriented to specific outcomes in clients, and probably intentionally do not include those nursing activities that are more generic to the general processes in nursing practice. The elucidation of essential tools of nursing practice made in this chapter, therefore, is to fill this gap by examining all essential and critical nursing approaches that are necessary to meet the goals in nursing practice going beyond therapeutic interventions, fulfilling the roles that are embedded within nursing practice. Essential roles in nursing practice are generally understood to encompass the roles of advocate, caregiver, helper, educator, care coordinator, therapist/interventionist, care manager, and resource provider. Nursing practice involves applying the essential tools of nursing practice in these roles and at the same time specialized strategies and interventions for clients' problems, which are integrated together to provide comprehensive nursing care. It means that the orientation of the essential tools is not in relation to specific clinical nursing problems, but in general nursing care. The essential tools of nursing practice are foundational and critical in carrying out responsibilities associated with the domains of nursing practice identified by Benner (1984), which are helping, teaching-coaching, diagnostic and patient monitoring, managing rapidly changing situations effectively, managing patient crises, administering and monitoring therapeutic interventions and regimes, monitoring and ensuring quality of health care practice, and performing organizational and work-related responsibilities. In order for nurses to function effectively in these domains of practice, it is necessary to develop competence in the essential tools and apply these tools in conjunction with more specialized strategies and approaches required in specific clinical situations.

The essential tools of nursing practice are organized into four groups: (a) tools in general practice processes, (b) caring and person-oriented tools, (c) general nursing therapeutics tools, and (d) professional role–related tools, as shown in Table 8.1. Figure 8.1 shows the constitution of nursing approaches applied in nursing practice.

## ESSENTIAL TOOLS IN THE GENERAL PRACTICE PROCESSES

The general practice processes refer to those actions that are involved in providing nursing care to all clients regardless of their health problems and settings of care. Essential tools in the general practice processes include both cognitive and behavioral strategies ranging from clinical decision making,

**TABLE 8.1 List of Essential Tools for Nursing Practice**

| TOOLS IN GENERAL PRACTICE PROCESSES | CARING AND PERSON-ORIENTED TOOLS | GENERAL NURSING THERAPEUTICS | PROFESSIONAL ROLE-RELATED TOOLS |
|---|---|---|---|
| Nursing process<br>Clinical decision making (clinical judgment, clinical problem solving, clinical reasoning)<br>Nursing assessment<br>• General and focused assessment<br>• Knowing the patient<br>• Outcomes monitoring<br>• Surveillance*<br>Nursing vigilance<br>Tailoring<br>Critical path development*<br>Program development*<br>Referral* | Caring<br>Empowerment<br>Presence*<br>Support* (emotional and spiritual)<br>Client advocacy<br>Client–nurse alliance<br>Active listening*<br>Nursing aesthetics | Anticipatory guidance*<br>Supportive counseling<br>Teaching*<br>Cultural brokerage*<br>Comforting and comfort measures<br>Security enhancement*<br>Client safety management<br>Environmental management*<br>Symptom management | Documentation*<br>Information management<br>Handover communication (shift reporting*)<br>Consultation*<br>Delegation*<br>Care management |

*Note:* *The strategy is included in the Nursing Interventions Classification (NIC) list (Bulechek et al., 2013).

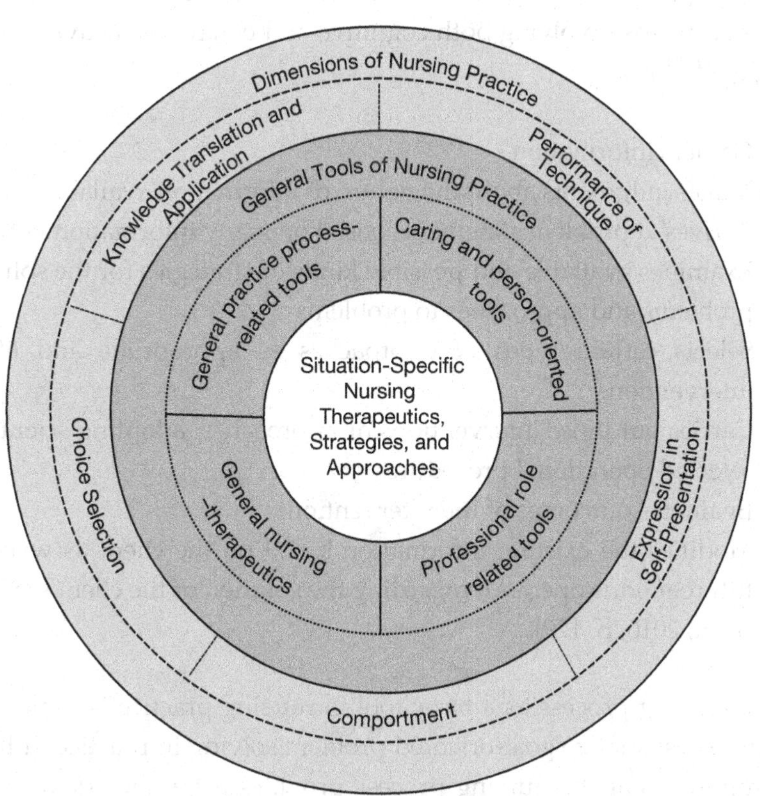


**FIGURE 8.1** Nursing tools, approaches, and strategies in nursing practice.

assessments, care planning, program development, referrals, and transition care. Nurses carry out these actions as routine parts of their practice with clients; these actions are essential for their everyday practice.

## Nursing Process

The nursing process as a tool in nursing practice refers to an organized system of progressing with patient care, and was originally advanced by Orlando (1961), adopted from a problem-solving model. It is a linear system beginning with assessment (information gathering), diagnosing (problem identification), outcomes identification (identification of expected outcomes from nursing approaches and interventions), planning (selection of nursing approaches and interventions regarding identified problems), implementation (actual delivery of planned actions), and evaluation (evaluation of outcomes). The American Nurses Association (ANA) states that the nursing process is "the common thread uniting different types of nurses who work in varied areas" and "the essential core of practice for the registered nurses to deliver holistic, patient-focused care" in the steps of assessment, diagnosis, outcomes identification, planning, implementation, and evaluation (ANA, 2010b).

It is a process involving both cognitive and behavioral activities encompassing the following:

- Gathers information
- Makes judgments about the nature of information available
- Arrives at problem statements based on many information networks
- Examines available and possible kinds of strategies for the solution of problems and approaches to problems
- Selects certain types of approaches as appropriate and effective interventions
- Carries out those interventions or approaches, adopting scientifically selected operational procedures
- Evaluates outcomes of the interventions
- Modifies the existing information based on the client as well as the future modus operandi regarding the solution of the client's problems (Kim, 2010, p. 179)

The nursing process as a basic tool in nursing practice is to be applied as a way to systematize goal-oriented problem solving in practice. It has also been proposed that the nursing process provides a framework with which comprehensive patient care can be carried out in a rational fashion, moving from information gathering, planning, and implementation, to evaluation.

## Clinical Decision Making (Clinical Judgment, Clinical Reasoning, and Clinical Problem Solving)

The term "clinical decision making" embraces the meanings embedded in clinical judgment, clinical reasoning/clinical inferencing, and clinical problem solving, which are often used interchangeably in the literature. These concepts refer to the mental process of decision making in clinical professions, such as nursing and medicine, albeit with subtle differences in their meanings or the outcomes of such process. We take up the concept of clinical decision making as a broad concept that refers to the process of decision making in clinical situations, which ranges from making decisions about the nature of problems presented by patients, such as in making nursing diagnosis, to deciding upon a type of therapeutic action to be taken to address a patient's problem. Invariably, however, clinical decision making involves selecting among alternatives, be they different diagnostic labels or different therapeutic actions. Clinical decision making is used here in the same sense in which Tanner (2006) and Simmons (2010) use the term "clinical reasoning." Clinical reasoning by Tanner "refers to the processes by which nurses and other clinicians make their judgments, and includes both the deliberate process of generating alternatives, weighing them against the evidence, and choosing the most appropriate, and those patterns that might be characterized as engaged, practical reasoning (e.g., recognition of a pattern, an intuitive clinical grasp, a response without evident forethought)" (2006, pp. 204–205). Simmons (2010), in the concept analysis of clinical reasoning, states that clinical reasoning is "a complex cognitive process that uses formal and informal thinking strategies to gather and analyse [sic] patient information, evaluate the significance of this information and weigh alternative actions, and … is dynamic, expansive and recursive, as information, interventions and alternative actions are considered or discarded at multiple cognitive entrance points" (p. 1155). Clinical decision making thus refers to a complex mental process related to information management, interpretation, and choice making in clinical situations with an aim to arrive at decisions that are the basis for nursing actions.

Clinical decision making has been addressed by various theoretical ideas such as cognitive heuristics (Elstein, Shulman, & Sprafka, 1978), information processing (Simon, 1979), expected utility theory (von Neuman & Morgenstern, 1953), and pattern recognition (Dreyfus & Dreyfus, 1986). Recent development in cognitive science suggests that the human brain, as a storehouse and as a processing machine, engages in various shortcutting techniques to bypass elaborate processing of information within the constraints of short-term and long-term memory and the brain's computational capabilities (Pinker, 1997). For example, cognitive heuristics have been identified as shortcuts that people use in making decisions, selecting alternatives, and conceptualizing situations (Kahneman, Tversky, & Slovic, 1982). At the same time, retrieving and selecting knowledge for use in specific instances are influenced by various situational contingencies: (a) the content and structure of a person's private knowledge and specific working knowledge incited in given situations; (b) other personal characteristics such as likes/dislikes, emotional stability, fatigue, and competency level; and (c) contextual factors such as physical, psychological, and social noise in situations, time constraints, available resources, and the presence of social, institutional norms and rules. Not only has the efficiency but also the inadequacy in clinical decision making, as in general decision making, been described and explained by the use of heuristics, the limits in human information processing, calculation errors in expected utility formulas, and the role of experience in pattern recognition. Along this line, Tanner (2006) concluded from the review of the literature on clinical judgment in nursing that clinical judgment is influenced more profoundly by the contextual features in decision making than the actual thinking processes involved, and extracted five key influencing features:

1. What the nurse brings into the situation in terms of knowledge, perspective, and disposition especially toward what is good and right
2. The nurse's personal knowing of the patient including his or her typical patterns of responses and concerns
3. The contextual characteristics of decision-making situations such as nursing units in terms of culture, norms, and routine practice
4. The nurse's initial grasp of the situation, the demands of the situation, and the goals of the practice propelling to adopt a specific reasoning pattern or a combination of reasoning patterns
5. Reflection in and on practice as a critical source for developing clinical knowledge and improving clinical decision making

This means that the competency in clinical decision making is developed through the firm grounding of general perspectives, values, and attitudes as well as developing a stock of personal knowledge in the nurse, and at the same time, the nurse's personal knowing of the patient and the definition of the clinical situation at hand. The nurse as the decision maker is the major variable in this sense. The contextual influence is critical as well, requiring the nurse's keen awareness and appreciation of the influence of clinical context on decision making. Both in the field of decision science and clinical decision making in the professions, normative decision models also have been developed to be applied in clinical decision making in an effort to improve the quality of decisions and bypass the natural human shortcomings in thinking processes.

There are three different sorts of clinical decisions in nursing:

1. Decisions regarding what and how to gain information from clients, families, and the environment, which may be termed *assessment decisions*
2. Decisions regarding the nature of conditions and problems in order to formulate clear ideas about the situations into diagnoses or problem identification, which may be termed *concept decisions*
3. Decisions regarding what actions to take such as informing a physician about a patient's symptoms or deciding upon a specific teaching plan for a patient, which may be termed *action decisions*

These types are a specification of clinical judgment that Tanner identifies as "an interpretation or conclusion about a patient's needs, concerns, or health problems, and/or the decision to take action (or not), use or modify standard approaches, or improvise new ones as deemed appropriate by the patient's response" (2006, p. 204). Often clinical decision making involves a serial relationship among these three types of decisions, starting with assessment decisions that result in a set of information, moving to concept decisions that formulate an idea about the nature of a clinical situation usually in linguistic forms (e.g., diagnoses) based on the information obtained, and then involving action decisions in relation to concept decisions that lead to specific nursing actions.

Assessment decisions have been neglected often, with a tacit understanding that clinical assessment would be carried out well. However, assessment decisions involving "what to assess" (content) and "how to assess" (method) result in specific information that is put forward for interpretation of its meanings and judgments regarding its implications. Assessment decisions in relation to content involve deciding upon what aspects of the reality are to be "noticed" (e.g., vital signs, facial expressions, body movements, verbal expressions, skin tone, etc.) through the discrimination of information in terms of criticality. It is selective attention and has to be based on the nurse's knowledge of what is critical and essential, thus the criteria for discrimination. For example, the assessment decisions for a patient one day after hip replacement would be quite different from the assessment decisions for a patient being admitted with a medical diagnosis of congestive heart failure.

Assessment decisions regarding method are oriented to selecting appropriate methods of assessment for the kind of data required for decision making. The nurse's knowledge and skills in applying specific assessment methods in relation to the type of information necessary in a given clinical situation influence the assessment decisions regarding methods. Accurate, reliable, and appropriate information is the objective in such decisions. Often nurses rely on known, familiar methods for data collection without resorting to active decision making in this regard.

A concept decision is arriving at an idea about a clinical situation, which culminates through the interpretation of the meanings of the information regarding that specific clinical situation. A concept decision as an idea can be illustrative as in "this patient does not understand the impact of being a diabetic on his lifestyle," "a diagnosis of disturbed sleep pattern" (NANDA Category #00198), or "this patient needs an immediate intubation." Concept decisions are formulations of ideas regarding given situations or phenomena, and are specified as "diagnoses" or "problem statements" in clinical professions.

Action decisions in practice, which usually follows concept decisions, refer to decisions regarding what behavioral actions including discourse actions to perform in given clinical situations. Actions in nursing practice range from carrying out various assessment activities to instituting therapeutic interventions, and from those performed in direct contact with clients such as teaching and respiratory care or activities carried out without direct involvement of clients such as in consulting with a physician or talking with the representative of a discharge destination. Action decisions of selecting and performing specific actions in situations are preconfigured by goals. While there are several different approaches to describe and explain actions from the philosophical perspectives of action, in general, the notion of action from the practice perspective accounts for intentions, goals, or reasoning as the preconditions of actions. In nursing, as a professional practice, actions are normatively oriented to "goals" specifically related to clients' well-being. Action decisions in nursing practice also presuppose action alternatives (choices) that include nonaction. As action decisions have to foresee the consequences of actions in terms of both goals and precarious consequences, practical reasoning and *phronesis* have been considered critical. The experiential basis of practical reasoning and *phronesis* has emphasized the role of experiences in action decision making. However, prior clinical experiences with certain actions especially with specific therapeutic actions that have produced expected outcomes may lead nurses not to consider alternatives in making action decisions. This can entrench nurses into habitual behaviors in practice.

As clinical decisions or judgments are outcomes of the primary step in the process of nursing practice, it is critical for nurses to acquire skills in clinical decision making in order to provide responsible practice to clients. In addition, because assessment decisions, concept decisions, and action decisions in nursing practice are connected together in a series, there are cascading consequences in these decisions viewed together in practice.

## Nursing Assessment

Nursing assessment as a general tool of nursing practice has its beginning in the concept of nursing process that became the model for nursing practice since the early 1960s. Assessment is the first step in the nursing process, and is defined as "a systematic, dynamic way to collect and analyze data about a client, the first step in delivering nursing care," including "not only physiological data, but also psychological, sociocultural, spiritual, economic, and life-style factors as well" (ANA, 2010b).

The term "nursing assessment" refers to assessment of clients not only in terms of health-related status, but also in relation to needs for nursing care, whereas the term "health assessment," although sometimes used interchangeably with "nursing assessment," refers to gathering health data in a general sense. Nursing assessment includes gathering, interpreting, and organizing information related to clients in terms of their current status, history, backgrounds, and resources from the nursing perspective. In nursing, assessment is often carried out in relation to an assessment form, a guideline, or a tool designed according to a specific framework such the Orem self-care nursing assessment tool, or the assessment tool designed for older adult care that incorporates five stages of assessment starting with three essential care components (Royal College of Nursing [RCN], 2004). Nursing assessment also has been tied to the concept of nursing diagnosis for pattern identification, especially applying the functional health pattern assessment framework (Gordon, 2007) or NANDA's 13 domains (Herdman, 2009). Nursing assessment has been structured within the development of classification systems for nursing diagnoses such as NANDA and the International Classification of Nursing Practice (ICNP).

Nursing assessment can be comprehensive (i.e., general) or focused as stated by Lunney (2009). General nursing assessment refers to assessment usually carried out at admission or at discharge involving comprehensive data gathering from various domains of the client's life including the current status and background. On the other hand, focused assessments are of different types, ranging from domain-specific (e.g., mobility or sleep), problem-focused (e.g., wound assessment or respiratory status assessment), event-specific (e.g., postoperative or postmedication), and progress orientation. While general/comprehensive assessment provides the baseline upon which general nursing care planning is developed, specific assessments are oriented to specific goals. Stanley and Joseph (2003) proposed a health assessment pyramid that includes holistic assessment, physical assessment, special/specific assessment, and health screening as a way to organize patient-care needs, suggesting that specific assessments are additional to a holistic assessment.

Nursing assessment whether it is general/comprehensive or focused involves gathering information, therefore requiring application of decision rules. Decision rules for nursing assessment can be specified in terms of domain, characteristics (quality), and meaning. The first set of decision rules for assessment pertains to domain as in "what" sorts of information are to be collected. Assessment tools are developed to specify domains of information, such as the functional pattern assessment framework (Gordon, 2007) for comprehensive assessment and a sleep assessment form for a focused assessment. Assessment tools usually consist of systems of categories identified or extracted based on certain frameworks, and delineate what domains of information are critical for assessment. Different concepts are introduced in assessment tools according to the framework chosen. For example, the RCN's assessment tool for older adults incorporates the framework of the essential care components that includes maximizing life potential, prevention and relief of stress, and promotion and maintenance of health as the major components (RCN, 2004). Often problem-focused assessment domains are determined through concept development and instrument development processes as in various pain assessment forms. Decision rules for assessment regarding domains are oriented to differentiating information in terms of critical from noncritical, essential from nonessential, meaningful from insignificant, and necessary from unnecessary. Even if a practitioner does not use an established assessment tool, she or he must apply an assessment guideline that has been established by applying a set of decision rules.

The second set of decision rules for assessment pertains to the dimension of characteristics of information. The dimension of information characteristics refers to not only quality (i.e., degree, strength, character, etc.), but also how it presents itself in relation to stability in terms of continuity/fluctuation, its presence (present/past), and its meanings specifically to clients. In assessment tools, this dimension is often incorporated into the domains to identify domain-specific characteristics.

The third set of decision rules for assessment has reference to nursing care needs. The orientation in this set of decision rules is in determining the types of nursing care needs the assessment data point to, for example, in terms of therapy, support, or surveillance, and in terms of problems versus resources or strengths versus weaknesses.

The fourth set of decision rules for assessment pertains to methods of information gathering, including from what source information should be gained and what detection methods (i.e., instrumental, discursive, physical, etc.) should be applied to gather information. Assessment procedures may be differentiated according to the domains of information and characteristics.

The fifth set of decision rules for assessment is related to interpretation of data. Because assessment usually has to be communicated in nursing practice situations, interpretation of data involves what data are retained and highlighted as opposed to discarded or deemphasized. In addition, meanings of the data both from the perspective of clients and practitioners are brought into interpretation, and this requires a decision rule that would put values into specific meanings.

Both general/comprehensive and focused assessments need to be guided by these five sets of decision rules, which often have to be established prior to assessing clients. There are three specific concepts that are closely related to nursing assessment and are critical tools of nursing practice: "knowing the patient," "outcomes assessment," and "surveillance."

### *Knowing the Patient*

The concept of knowing the patient defined as a process of understanding and treating the person as a unique individual (Radwin, 1996) has been considered a critical asset in nursing practice both in patient-care decision making and nurses' approaches in their relations with clients. Fairhurst and May (2001) in their study of general practitioners differentiate "knowing the patient" from "knowing about the patient" as the former is couched in understanding the patient in a personal way, whereas the latter refers mostly to biomedical or biographical knowledge of the patient. In this sense, knowing the patient goes beyond having the data about the patient and means having an understanding of the patient to be a unique individual. Morrison and Symes (2011) found "knowing the patient" as one of the characteristics of expert nursing practice as was earlier suggested by Tanner, Benner, Chesla, and Gordon (1993), which makes it possible for nurses to provide individualized and person-centered care to clients. Knowing the patient is a generative process in which the practitioner gains increasingly personal understanding of clients and becomes a frame that guides all sorts of clinical decision making, including decisions in nursing assessment (Ellefsen & Kim, 2005). However, knowing the patient and nursing assessment are intertwined as a process, because nursing assessment involves looking closely into various aspects of clients often through interaction and communication. Nursing assessment feeds into the emergence of knowing the patient, and knowing the patient, in turn, becomes a frame by which further nursing assessment may proceed and further clarification in the assessment may occur.

### *Outcomes Monitoring and Assessment*

One specific type of assessment is related to assessing patient outcomes. Nursing care outcomes as a total set or specific outcomes resulting from a therapeutic action are assessed in order to find out the effectiveness and efficacy of nursing care or of a specific therapeutic regimen. The concept of nursing-sensitive outcomes has become one of the central pieces in the structuring of the process of nursing practice in a systematic way in the effort to make systematic connections among clients' health or nursing care needs and problems (diagnoses), interventions applied to resolve problems (nursing interventions), and results of nursing care. This has culminated into the development of the NANDA, the NIC, and the NOC systems in the United States and the classification system for nursing practice (ICNP) at the international level by the International Council of Nursing. Outcomes assessment utilizing a comprehensive data tool that contains all appropriate outcomes in clients from nursing (NOC or ICNP) has been recommended as a way to monitor the results of nursing care, whether general or specific both for individual clients and for collectives (i.e., populations). The concept of evidence-based outcomes is the basic assumption undergirding the development of any outcomes guidelines.

Outcomes assessment in nursing is complex as nursing care of patients is configured by both general goals, such as improving health status and well-being, and specific ones associated with nursing problems (e.g., pain, fatigue, etc.). Therefore, it is possible to view outcomes assessment in terms of general and focused as in nursing assessment. While general outcomes assessment is oriented to general status of health and well-being, focused outcomes assessment is oriented to specific sets of nursing diagnoses and nursing intervention.

"Outcomes monitoring" is an associated term, which is usually used in relation to assessments at a collective level in the context of outcomes monitoring systems. Outcomes monitoring systems have been developed to evaluate the effectiveness of interventions through a systematic collection of outcomes data, for example, in an auditing system.

### *Surveillance*

The concept of surveillance, which is often used interchangeably with monitoring, has been respecified in nursing with its inclusion in the NIC as a nursing intervention, differentiating it from monitoring. Surveillance as a nursing intervention is defined in the NIC as "the purposeful and ongoing acquisition, interpretation, and synthesis of patient data for clinical decision-making" and additionally as "the purposeful and ongoing collection and analysis of information about patients and their environment for use in promoting and maintaining patient safety" (Bulechek et al., 2013). The focus in the second definition is in relation to patient safety and risk reduction. This focus of surveillance has made this concept differ from monitoring, which is oriented to assessment in a general sense. Although its application as an intervention has been suggested mostly in acute-care settings, it is applicable across various nursing care situations.

Kelly and Vincent (2010) in their concept analysis of surveillance adopted a theoretical definition of the concept as "a process to primarily identify threats to patient health and safety through purposeful and ongoing acquisition, interpretation and synthesis of patient data for clinical decision-making" (p. 658). Henneman, Gawlinski, and Giuliano (2012) also emphasize the focus on patient safety in nursing surveillance as an intervention applied in critical and emergency care settings. The concept of surveillance therefore encompasses the foreseeing of potential risks, harms, danger, and changes in patients' conditions and in the relevant environment as the starting point for monitoring and vigilance.

## Nursing Vigilance

Vigilance is a concept referring to careful attention to possible threats to safety with readiness to act. This concept is related to the concept of surveillance, but goes beyond surveillance in its orientation to "risks" in patient-care situations. Nursing vigilance is defined by Meyer and Lavin (2005) as a state of being scientifically, intellectually, and experientially grounded with (a) attention to and identification of clinically significant observations/signals/cues, (b) calculation of risks inherent in nursing practice situations, and (c) readiness to act appropriately and efficiently to minimize risks and to respond to threats. Vigilance is a safeguarding work in anticipation of problems, adverse events, disturbances, or emergencies in clients. It involves conscious and watchful attention to clients regarding changes, happenings, and reactions with a keen concern for safety and well-being.

## Tailoring

Tailoring is a concept central to the ideology of person-centered practice, and points to the process of matching various aspects of nursing practice with the individuality of clients. The term *tailoring* has been often used interchangeably with individualization, and is differentiated from customizing, targeting, and personalizing (Park, McDaniel, & Jung, 2009). Tailoring is tied to interventions, messages, approaches, and instructions in nursing, and is based on modifying nursing strategies to align with individual-specific characteristics. Redman and Lynn (2005) also suggest tailoring nursing care according to patients' expectations and needs.

Tailoring as a concept was coined by Cox (1982) in her Interaction Model of Client Health Behavior to mean adjusting nurses' communication style and contents in alignment with the individuality of the client. Brown (1992) found tailoring by expert nurses to fit nursing actions of assessment and management for clients with client individuality. In recent years, there have been many approaches for tailoring interventions, messages, and instructions in nursing practice and health care. Tailoring requires knowing the client's individual characteristics and putting that knowledge into making adjustments in interventions, messages, instructions, and programs so that there would be a match between client singularity and nursing approaches, which is thought to produce better outcomes in clients. In addition, tailoring requires the knowledge of effective variations in delivering nursing strategies in relation to client characteristics. Various methods of tailoring applying computer technology have been developed, most significantly for "tailoring interventions" (Ryan & Lauver, 2002) and tailoring health information (Park et al., 2009). Tailoring as a nursing tool is especially critical in the current health care scene where professional practitioners often have to work with practice guidelines and clinical pathways that offer standardized approaches to patient care.

## Critical Path Development

Critical path development is defined in the NIC system as "constructing and using a timed sequence of patient-care activities to enhance desired patient outcomes in a cost-efficient manner" (Bulechek et al., 2013). It is a tool to be used to project and plan for patient care in a systematic, sequential process with a view toward goals in patient outcomes. It is based on scientific evidence and practice guidelines developed for clinical problems tailored to specific patients' needs.

## Program Development

Program development is a generic strategy aimed at producing changes or introducing new forms of life applied in various disciplines including nursing, education, social service, and public health. In nursing, program development is oriented to developing a program for a client or a group of clients, designed to produce changes in behaviors to enhance health and healthful living. Often programs in nursing involve multiple actors including professionals, clients, family, and others in order to address a problem or an issue that requires an organized approach for resolution. It is defined in the NIC system as "planning, implementing, and evaluating a coordinated set of activities designed to enhance wellness, or to prevent, reduce, or eliminate one or more health problems for a group or community" (Bulechek et al., 2013).

Program development as a nursing tool encompasses a process involving several steps, which are generally specified to include: (a) preparation, (b) design, and (c) evaluation plan. The stage of preparation involves identifying and fully describing the problem, determining the goals of a program to be developed, and searching for available approaches to meet the goals. While identifying the problem and setting the goals involve intimate understanding of clients or situations for which a program is to be developed and emerge from this understanding, searching for strategies involves a systematic investigation of the evidence base (research/theory base) and past experiences. In addition, at this stage, information gathering regarding available resources and possible constraints has to be done. The second stage of design involves a decision regarding specific approaches (strategies) to be applied in the program, a determination of change theory to be applied in the program, determination of contents (activities and materials), specification of procedures for the program, and specification of resources for the program implementation. Often pilot testing is critical in program development. The third stage of evaluation plan involves specification of the plan for both formative and summative evaluations both during its implementation and at its conclusion. Saettler (1990) suggests that while formative evaluation is used to refine goals and evolve strategies for achieving goals, summative evaluation tests the validity of a theory or determines the impact of a program in order to change or modify future applications.

In nursing, program development may target individual clients, groups, or communities varying from lifestyle-change programs, such as an exercise program for older adults, to educational programs, such as a self-care program for diabetics. Program planning as a tool involves communication not only as embedded within programs, but also in relation to communicating its design and contents for implementation by others besides the program developer.

In line with the perspective of person-centered practice in nursing integrated into the current health care arena, there has been a growing emphasis on program development that is collaborative/participatory, especially involving clients. Fraenkel (2006) suggests a collaborative relationship between professionals and users in his Collaborative Family Program Development Model, in which users (family members) are involved in every phase of program development from initiating the project to implementation. Involving clients' collaboration in program development ensures the input and integration of clients' goals, preferences, needs, and insights into program development, and limits the possibility of program's failure due to misalignments in goals and approaches.

## Referral

Referral as a tool involves an organized system of communication in interprofessional and interorganizational relationships to obtain expert opinions or special services on behalf of the client. Referral is defined in the NIC system as "arrangement of services by another care provider or agency" (Bulechek et al., 2013). Nursing referrals are either made to specialists in order to obtain recommendations regarding nursing care programs, especially for clients with complex health issues, or to service organizations in order to obtain specialized services for clients, such as cardiac rehabilitation or hospice care. Coordinating referral and ongoing access to primary and other health care services for patients has been upheld as one of the key functions of nursing, especially in mental health nursing (National Panel for Psychiatric Mental Health NP Competencies, 2003).

There are specific aspects to be included in referrals: (a) a clear idea regarding the purpose of a referral, (b) a statement of relevant information about a client for whom a referral is sought, (c) a clear statement of expectations sought from a referred party, and (d) a follow-through. Because referrals are made to specific individuals (i.e., professionals) and service organizations, the first requirement for referral is the knowledge of available expertise and specialized services to which referrals can be made. However, the patterns of referral are influenced by many factors including the aspects of the professional and the contexts of health care. Foster and Tilse (2003) propose a model of referral for post–acute care following traumatic brain injury that puts "the processes of interpreting the characteristics of the individual, the interaction with the contexts of care" at the center, which is framed and influenced by the characteristics of the individual requiring a referral and the contexts of care that include the organization and health care environment. These authors conceptualize the interpretative processes of health professionals as "the processes of selecting information (grounds), interpreting information (warrants) and determining referral (conclusions)" (Foster & Tilse, 2003, p. 2206).

Such processes of interpretation in referrals therefore involve interpreting the client's needs reflected upon and negotiated with the available resources in the contexts of care. In addition, the professional's orientation regarding problems and the type of solutions considered by the professional influence the processes of interpretation, and the interpretations communicated to referred persons or agencies are thus affected. The nature of decision making in the interpretive processes of referral determines responses by the recipients (professional or agency) of the referral as it is the interpretations that are communicated to the recipients.

## CARING AND PERSON-ORIENTED ESSENTIAL TOOLS

Nursing practice guided by the philosophy of care has to incorporate caring and person-oriented approaches and strategies to promote health and well-being of clients. There are several essential tools of nursing with this orientation. These tools are intrinsically tied to client–nurse relationships, and are strategies of person-to-person contact and communication. The goals of these tools are not orientated to specific clinical problems, but are for enhancing clients' well-being and protecting clients in their vulnerability. These caring and person-oriented tools are to be applied in all nursing care situations in order to uphold clients' humanity, individuality, and personhood and to protect clients in their vulnerability.

### Caring

Caring as an essential nursing tool can be differentiated from the philosophy of caring by strictly focusing on professional strategies of care. Caring as a strategy is behavioral (bodily and communicative), based on a commitment to other's uniqueness, humanity, individuality, and autonomy. It is the ways nurses approach and connect with a client (i.e., the other) in their relationships. Finfgeld-Connett (2008b) in her meta-synthesis study of caring identified it as a process involving expert nursing by which the nurse has "the ability to identify the nuances and meanings accurately of another's situation" (p. 199), interpersonal sensitivity reflected by the trenchant, intuitive, and empathic insight into another's suffering, and intimate relationship of trust and protection. There have been many attempts to identify activities within the concept of caring. For example, McCance (2003) specified the following activities: providing for patient's physical and psychological needs, being attentive, getting to know the patient, taking time, showing respect, being firm, and doing the extra touch. Wu, Larrabee, and Putnam (2006) in their instrument development study identified four activities: being readily available to a patient's need and security, demonstrating conscience and competence, attending to the dignity of the person, and providing constant assistance to patients with readiness.

Several theoretical or conceptual models of caring in nursing practice have been proposed. Watson (2012), from the framework of the human caring science, offers the concept of transpersonal caring relationships experienced through "caritas consciousness" and the concept of "clinical caritas process" as a way of caring engagement with clients. The transpersonal caring relationship involves the nurse entering into and staying "within the other's frame of reference for connecting with the inner life world of meaning and spirit of the other" in which the nurse and the client "together join in a mutual search for meaning and wholeness of being and becoming to potentiate comfort measures, pain control, a sense of well-being, wholeness, or even spiritual transcendence of suffering" (Watson, 1996, p. 153). Swanson's theory of caring (1991) specifies caring with five subprocesses of knowing, being with, doing for, enabling, and maintaining belief. Edwards (2001) considers these types of caring approaches as "intentional care" as opposed to "ontological care," which has been advocated in the hermeneutic phenomenological perspective such as by Benner and Wrubel (1989) on the primacy of care. From the perspective of considering caring as an essential tool of nursing practice, the manifest orientation of caring would be an intentional one. However, the argument can be made for the notion that intentional caring is only possible because of ontological caring, especially in the context of professional caring as in nursing practice.

## Empowerment

Empowerment is a concept that is oriented to helping persons to flourish in difficult situations by exercising control over choices. It is a concept that emerged with the postmodern awakening in health care in regard to the power inequality between the professionals and clients and dependency-fostering modes of health care practice in modern times. It is a process that also aligns well with the ideology of person-centered practice in which the clients' voices, needs, preferences, and approaches are central in health care practice. Empowerment in nursing practice is defined variously, but is in general agreement with Gibson's definition (1991) as a process of helping people to assert control over the factors that affect their lives, and is aligned with informed choice, promotion of independence, and active partnership in care. However, there are different theoretical underpinnings for empowerment pointing to different ways of delineating strategies of empowerment, ranging from the emancipatory processes, fully disclosing information to clients, and helping with decision-making processes. Empowerment as a nursing tool is applied in nursing practice both for a general sense of independence as well as for control over specific decision-making situations.

## Presence

Presence is defined in the NIC system as "being with another, both physically and psychologically, during times of need" (Bulechek et al., 2013). Although the concept of presence is often either included within the process of caring or coined in conjunction with caring, this concept is viewed to have a unique conceptual property (Finfgeld-Connett, 2006). Finfgeld-Connett (2006) through a meta-synthesis of work on presence suggests that the concept of presence is an interpersonal process involving a nurse being with another (client) in an intimate way characterized by interpersonal sensitivity regarding the person's unique needs and situation, holistically concerned with the individual's physical, psychological, and spiritual well-being, and projecting trust and sensitivity for vulnerability. Presence as a nursing tool involves nurses "being with" clients consciously, which can transmit their acceptance of clients' humanity in their uniqueness and circumstances and their willingness to go through physical, psychological, and spiritual difficulties together. Presence as a process involves the nurse as a whole to "exist" for a client in the time and the situation with full attention and involvement as a person (Osterman & Schwartz-Barcott, 1996).

## Support (Emotional and Spiritual)

Throughout its modern history, the concept of support in nursing has been a mode of helping clients. Support connotes both materialistic (i.e., physical) and nonphysical, that is, psychological and spiritual helping to enhance the strengths clients have and to supplement what are lacking in clients. In the NIC system, support is differentiated into emotional support as "provision of reassurance, acceptance, and encouragement during times of stress" and spiritual support as "assisting the patient to feel balance and connection with a greater power" (Bulechek et al., 2013). Usually physical, materialistic support is considered to be a part in the provision of what is lacking in clients, such as providing mobility aids or finding sources of financial funding for specialized services such as respite care for clients and their families. For this sort of support, the process is straightforward, moving from an identification of needs and types of support necessary to meet needs, finding sources of support, and securing needed support for clients. On the other hand, emotional and spiritual support requires processes that are complex, involving personal and interpersonal aspects.

Based on the concept that health and illness experiences involve an integration of physical, psychological, social, emotional, and spiritual facets of one's living, support from the emotional and spiritual perspectives is viewed to enhance human well-being, especially when clients are in vulnerable and needful states. Emotional and spiritual support as a nursing tool provides assistance to enhance clients' emotional and spiritual processes of well-being through interactive processes.

## Active Listening

Active listening is defined in the NIC system as "attending closely to and attaching significance to a patient's verbal and nonverbal messages" (Bulechek et al., 2013). It is a critical communication skill necessary to gain in-depth understanding of patients as individuals and of patients' meanings of their experiences. The ideology of person-centered practice mandates application of strategies that will assist nurses to gain patients' perspectives and subjective meanings of their experiences.

## Client Advocacy

Advocacy by nurses on behalf of clients is expressed in several different ways such as nursing advocacy, nurse advocacy, client advocacy, and patient advocacy, referring to the same concept. ANA's definition of nursing identifies "advocacy in the care of individuals, families, communities, and populations" (ANA, 2010c) as one of its responsibilities, and client advocacy is specified in the *ANA's Code of Ethics for Nurses* in its statement that "the nurse promotes, advocates for, and strives to protect the health, safety, and rights of the patient" (ANA, 2015).

Bu and Jezewski defined the concept of patient advocacy as "a process or strategy consisting of a series of specific actions for preserving, representing and/or safeguarding patients' rights, best interests and values in the health-care system" (2007, p. 104), and identified the core attributes of patient advocacy as (a) safeguarding patients' autonomy, (b) acting on behalf of patients, and (c) championing social justice in the provision of health care. It is a professional responsibility of nurses, further specified as "voicing responsiveness" with active commitment to engage in a continued expression and support of patients' needs and wishes (Vaartio, Leino-Kilpi, Salantera, & Suominen, 2006). Client advocacy as a nursing tool involves speaking for, interceding, and representing clients in order to promote and protect clients' well-being, rights, and interests. The aim for client advocacy is to empower clients in their decision making, to ensure that clients are able to exercise their rights, and to seek out and provide the best services to meet their needs.

## Client–Nurse Alliance

Client–nurse alliance is described as forming a partnership to move toward mutually agreed goals of care (Wills, 1996). Client–nurse alliance is a concept that is broader than therapeutic alliance that has its background in psychotherapy viewed as a form of positive transference (Zetzel, 2004). It is defined as the conjoining of two partners (a client and a nurse) in a bond of understanding, knowledge, power, and goals, being united in mutual goals through empathy, mutuality, and coalition (Kim, 2010). Client–nurse alliance as an interactive process oriented to the attainment of goals for the client is characterized by (a) a feeling of mutual understanding, (b) a mutual appreciation of possibilities and limitations that exist in the situation of nursing care, (c) a culmination into mutual acknowledgment of the client's health and health care goals, (d) a sharing of power and knowledge for the client's health and health care goals, and (e) an achievement of a joint "voice" for the client's health and health care goals (Kim, 2010, p. 164). As a nursing tool, client–nurse alliance is developed and utilized in the client–nurse processes for defining goals for the clients, gaining a mutual understanding of goals, and being partners in nursing care.

## Nursing Aesthetics

Nursing aesthetics (used here to refer to the concept art of nursing) as a nursing tool refers to application of various modes of incorporating creativity and artistry into nursing practice in order to enhance the effects of nursing actions by raising an awareness for individual's unique existential experiences in nurses' practice. Nursing aesthetics is present in self-presentations of the nurse through expressions in client–nurse relationships. Expressions take up the characteristics in relation to sublimity, beauty, empathy, and sensibility, and are in verbal, bodily, and whole-person modes. Chinn (2001) specifies the art of nursing as narratives creating living stories in practice and embodied synchronous movements. Finfgeld-Connett offers a synthesized view of art of nursing by specifying that it is "relationship-centered," involving "interpersonal sensitively and intimacy" and creativity in the care to meet the needs of individual patients, and adapting "empirical and metaphysical knowledge of self and others" as well as the values of holism and individuality (2008a, pp. 383–385). Nursing aesthetics are to be infused into the practice of nursing in order to enhance positive outcomes in clients.

## ESSENTIAL TOOLS OF GENERAL NURSING THERAPEUTICS

Various strategies in nursing are therapeutically oriented, but are applicable nonspecifically to clients' problems. These are "therapeutic" as the goals of these strategies are to remedy, treat, or address clients' problems in a general way. These general nursing therapeutics may be adapted to fit more specifically to circumscribed problems; however, as general tools, they are applicable in nearly all nursing care situations. Nursing tools in this category include those to address clients' learning needs (i.e., anticipatory guidance, counseling, and teaching), dealing with multicultural issues (i.e., cultural brokerage), for maintaining comfort and safety (i.e., comforting, safety management, and environment management), and for managing symptoms of distress (i.e., symptom management). These are tools that are applied often to clients regardless of their health status, and therefore are designated as the general repertoire of nurses' therapeutic tools.

### Anticipatory Guidance

Anticipatory guidance is a clinical strategy often ascribed to the process of preparation for what to expect, most notably used in pediatric care during the past several decades to prepare parents to parenting issues. It is defined in the NIC system as "preparation of patient for an anticipated developmental and/or situational crisis" (Bulechek et al., 2013). Pridham (1993) notes that anticipatory guidance in pediatric care refers to providing information about what to expect and how to deal with unwanted or challenging events or conditions related to developmental or life change. As a nursing tool, its application can be extended to clients who are faced with developmental phases (e.g., menopause), life changes (e.g., retirement or widowhood), new events (e.g., hospitalization or surgery), and new experiences (e.g., new diagnosis of a chronic disease or first-time parenting). This tool is applicable at various points of health-related transitions in a person's life. It involves guiding clients for anticipated experiences by providing reality-oriented information about an anticipated state often using illustrations, discussing possible variations in expectations, and guiding through various ways of addressing both expected and unexpected occurrences. The essence of anticipatory guidance is in being informative, enabling and empowering, and supportive of clients' concerns.

## Supportive Counseling

In the NIC system, counseling is defined as the "use of an interactive helping process focusing on the needs, problems, or feelings of the patient and significant others to enhance or support coping, problem solving, and interpersonal relationships" (Bulechek et al., 2013). Supportive counseling as a nursing tool is applicable for clients in difficult or unstable situations, with nonspecific problems of living (such as the loss of independence or contracting social network), and sometimes with problems that require clarification, understanding, deliberation, and decision making. Supportive counseling as a helping process requires not only an expertise in interactive and relationship building processes, but also in the knowledge of the client. The goal of supportive counseling is to help clients to understand difficulties in their lives so that the clients themselves may be able to arrive at solutions regarding their difficulties.

## Teaching

Teaching as a general process is a tool used by many professionals to meet the learning needs of clients, most notably in education, but also in nursing, medicine, and other health professions. Clients' learning needs related to health, well-being, and health care vary widely from general ones, such as learning to having a fulfilling life, to very specific ones, such as learning how to carry out testing for blood glucose levels. In the NIC system, teaching as a strategy is listed for various specific teaching needs in addition to a general strategy of "individual teaching" defined as "planning, implementation, and evaluation of a teaching program designed to address a patient's particular needs" (Bulechek et al., 2013). Teaching as a nursing tool involves a goal-oriented process of transmitting information and knowledge to clients and applies theories of learning and teaching to fit into client individuality and clients' learning needs.

## Culture Brokerage

In the NIC system, culture brokerage is defined as "the deliberate use of culturally competent strategies to bridge or mediate between the patient's culture and the biomedical health care system" (Bulechek et al., 2013). It is a nursing strategy developed to address problems of health care access and in clients' communication and interaction within the health care system in the current culturally diverse population. Cultural brokering is defined as the act of bridging, linking, or mediating between groups or persons of differing cultural backgrounds for the purpose of reducing conflict or producing change (Jezewski, 1990), and a cultural broker acts as a go-between, one who advocates on behalf of another individual or group (Jezewski & Sotnik, 2001). Culture viewed broadly as a system of language, beliefs, attitudes, norms, customs, and traditions is not only specific to race, ethnicity, and religion, but also to groups sharing such a system as medicine and health care. Clients with varying cultural backgrounds often experience difficulties in their negotiations and interactions with professional providers and systems of care because of cultural differences especially in terms of language, norms, and values. Clients not only experience misunderstanding, frustration and conflicts, but also withdrawal, resistance to change, and rejection. Culture brokerage therefore is a strategy to prevent such problems and promote understanding between clients and health care professionals and the system of health care through mediation and advocacy.

## Comforting and Comfort Measures

The feeling of comfort is often jeopardized in illness and during health care experiences with distress and suffering. Comfort refers to both bodily and emotional feelings of well-being. Comforting and comfort measures are essential in promoting the feeling of well-being and in relieving discomfort, distress, and suffering. Morse (1992) suggests that comforting involves direct actions such as touching, talking, and listening and indirect actions such as manipulating the environment. Although the sources of discomfort, distress, and suffering are varied, it is the use of general comforting and institution of comforting measures that can produce the feelings of well-being in clients.

## Security Enhancement

In the NIC system, security enhancement refers to "intensifying a patient's sense of physical and psychological safety" (Bulechek et al., 2013). Security enhancement as a nursing tool is carried out through interactive processes of reassurance and support. It is carried out through an understanding of a patient's sense of and concerns regarding physical and psychological safety, and providing information and support to enhance the sense of safety.

## Client Safety Management

Client safety refers to being in a state of protection from potential harm in being clients of health care. Clients in health care are exposed to potential harm and injury, having safety risks related to being away from home and receiving health care. The Joint Commission adopted the National Patient Safety goals in 2002, which has been reviewed annually for various health care settings. The National Patient Safety goals for 2015 include those related to: (a) improving the accuracy of patient identification, the effectiveness of communication among caregivers, and the safety of using medication, (b) reducing the harm associated with clinical alarm systems, the risk of health care–associated infections, and the risk of patient harm resulting from falls, (c) preventing health care–associated pressure ulcers, and (d) ensuring organizations identify safety risks inherent in its patient population (The Joint Commission, 2015). Client safety management as a nursing tool encompasses assessing risks for harm in individual clients, ensuring nurses' own practice of adhering to safety criteria for the accuracy of patient identification, effective interprofessional communication, and medication procedures, and to make provisions to prevent patient harms such as self-injury, infection, falls and injury, and pressure ulcers.

## Environmental Management

Environmental management is defined in the NIC system as "manipulation of the patient's surroundings for therapeutic benefit, sensory appeal, and psychological well-being" (Bulechek et al., 2013). Environmental management is a part of the holistic patient care in which clients' experiences in institutions of health care are viewed to be influenced by environmental facets. It involves making provisions for therapeutically enhancing, emotionally satisfying, and appealing environments for clients in institutional care.

### Symptom Management

Although different clinical symptoms require therapeutic strategies that align specifically with the characteristics of given symptoms, symptom management as a general nursing tool refers to the patterned processes in addressing symptoms individually or in clusters. Clinical symptoms are experiences of distress usually associated with diseases or pathologic changes that are experienced subjectively. In various diseases, symptoms occur in clusters as in cancer, stroke, diabetes, and so on. Managing symptoms refers to dealing with symptoms in order to be relieved of the experiences. Often symptom management refers to self-management of symptoms. Fu, LeMone, and McDaniel state that symptom management emerges as "individuals perceive the occurrence of the symptom, set goals, and direct certain activities to relieve or decrease symptom distress or prevent symptom occurrence" (2004, p. 67). Symptom management can be carried out by the individual experiencing symptoms or by others including health care professionals and family members. In health care situations, usually nurses are responsible for therapeutically attending to patients' symptoms. Symptom management as a nursing tool is a dynamic process involving (a) assessment of presenting symptom(s) in terms of its occurrence, distress, and experience, especially in relation to coexisting symptoms or existence of a cluster of symptoms; (b) determining its impacts on clients' well-being, activities, and feeling states; (c) seeking therapeutic strategies available for symptom management; (d) determining the best strategy to be applied through a collaborative decision making with clients; (e) instituting selected strategies; and (f) evaluating outcomes.

## PROFESSIONAL ROLE–RELATED ESSENTIAL TOOLS

In the repertoire of nursing tools, there are those related to nurses' professional responsibilities as an individual professional and as a member of a health care organization. The professional role of nursing requires nurses to communicate about their activities and results of their work, and to take on responsibilities as a member of nursing and health care teams. Nursing tools to fulfill such professional role responsibilities range from documentation, information management, handover communication (shift reporting), inter- and intraprofessional consultation and collaboration, delegation, and patient-care management. The major goals of these nursing tools are to provide an integrated, coordinated nursing care to clients, to mobilize the best health care possible for clients, and to ensure a high level of quality of care.

## Documentation

Documentation as a nursing tool refers to "recording of pertinent patient data in a clinical record" (Bulechek et al., 2013) in order to maintain comprehensive data regarding patients' experiences, status, progress, changes, and outcomes as well as in relation to nursing care that has been instituted for clients. Nursing documentation is for an evidential record of patients' experiences during an incidence of health care providing sequential data regarding patients' status and care received along with statements of progress and outcomes. It serves as the basis for maintaining a continuity of patient care, effective communication among members of a health care team, assessing patients' progress and outcomes of care, and providing legal evidence of care. In the *Principles of Documentation*, the ANA states that "clear, accurate, and accessible documentation is an essential element of safe, quality, evidence-based nursing practice" and that "it is how nurses create a record of their services for use by payors, the legal system, government agencies, accrediting bodies, researchers, and other groups and individuals directly or indirectly involved with health care. It also provides a basis for demonstrating and understanding nursing's contributions both to patient-care outcomes and to the viability and effectiveness of the organizations that provide and support quality patient care" (ANA, 2010a).

Jefferies, Johnson, and Griffiths (2010) in their meta-analysis of the literature on nursing documentation identified seven essentials of quality nursing documentation: (a) to be patient-centered, (b) to contain the actual work of nurses including education and psychosocial support, (c) to reflect the objective clinical judgment of the nurse, (d) to be presented in a logical and sequential manner, (e) to be written contemporaneously, or as events occur, (f) to record variances in care within and beyond the health care record, and (g) to fulfill legal requirements. According to the ANA's *Principles of Documentation*, documentation characteristics are to be (a) accessible; (b) accurate, relevant, and consistent; (c) auditable; (d) clear, concise, and complete; (e) legible/readable; (f) thoughtful; (g) timely, contemporaneous, and sequential; (h) reflective of the nursing process; and (i) retrievable on a permanent basis in a nursing-specific manner (ANA, 2010a). In the contemporary health care scene, both electronic recording systems and narrative writing have become parts of health care data within which nurses have to carry out documentation.

## Information Management

Information management in nursing practice includes the management of information at two levels: (a) at the client level in terms of clinical information systems including nursing information systems for collecting, recording, storing, and communicating data regarding clients and clinical work for clients, and (b) at the decision-support level in terms of knowledge systems designed to support clinical decision making in nursing practice (Phillips, 2005). The first-level information management is oriented to maintaining precise, accurate, relevant, timeless, necessary, economic, and readable data in patient information systems pertinent to nursing and to selectively communicating information in such systems for quality patient care. Information systems currently tend to be electronic data systems; however, they include data in nonelectronic forms. Information management at this level requires nurses to have competency in information technology as well as communication skills. Information management at the second level is oriented to accessing, organizing, and utilizing decision support systems and knowledge (e.g., scientific evidence) in the public domain relating them to patient data for nursing care decision making in order to provide safe and effective patient care. The American Association of Colleges of Nursing (AACN, 2008) views knowledge and skills in information management critical to deliver quality patient care by nurses.

## Handover Communication

As nursing is continuously practiced in a team environment rather than as a solo practice in most situations, handover communication is critical for the continuity of care. In the NIC system, shift handover is defined as "exchanging essential patient care information with other nursing staff at change of shift" (Bulechek et al., 2013). However, handover communication in nursing includes shift handover between nurses, departmental handover that is usually termed "transfer" such as from an emergency department to a ward, interprofessional handover, and discharge handover.

Handover involves transferring information by a professional to another regarding patient data to ensure the continuity of care and patient safety. It can be carried out verbally or in written forms. There has been a great deal of development for electronic handover tools in recent years in order to ensure the transmission of essential information. Handover as a nursing tool requires nurses' selection and communication of essential and relevant data regarding patient care so that recipients of handover information obtain it clearly, without any possible distortions in meaning, and receive information critical for continuing care and safety. Information loss and information distortion have been the major issues in the application of this strategy in practice.

## Consultation

The role of consultation has often been attributed to advanced practice nursing. However, it is a tool for general nursing that is applicable in various nursing practice situations as a method to make available one's expertise, whether it is a general expertise or a situation-specific expertise, to those who can benefit. In the NIC system, consultation is defined as "using expert knowledge to work with those who seek help in problem solving to enable individuals, families, groups, or agencies to achieve identified goals" (Bulechek et al., 2013). Although nursing consultation is utilized between nurses and other health care professionals, it can be applied in nurses' relationships with clients, families, and client groups. Consultation as a nursing tool requires nurses to have a clear assessment of his or her own expertise regarding the issues at hand, an understanding regarding the goals of consultation, and the ability to use communication skills appropriately to work collaboratively with those seeking consultation.

## Delegation

Nurses, in delivering nursing care to clients, often have to delegate tasks to other nursing personnel in order to fulfill patient-care responsibilities. Delegation in nursing involves making decisions regarding what types of nursing-related tasks and activities are to be delegated to nonprofessional personnel, to which type of specific personnel delegations are to be made, and the extent to which nurses' supervision with the performance of tasks or activities is to be in place. Because delegation has a legal ramification for nursing, it is circumscribed by the profession of nursing and the licensing organizations. Delegation is defined in the NIC system as "transfer of responsibility for the performance of patient care while retaining accountability for the outcome" (Bulechek et al., 2013), and the ANA's *Principles for Delegation* states delegation as involving "assignment of the performance of activities or tasks related to patient care to unlicensed assistive personnel while retaining accountability for the outcome" (ANA, 2012a). The National Council of State Boards of Nursing (NCSBN) defines delegation as "transferring to a competent individual authority to perform a selected nursing task in a selected situation" (NCSBN, 1995, p. 1).

These principles of delegation (ANA, 2012a; NCSBN, 1995) are the base for making delegation in practice. Delegation involves (a) a decision regarding which task is to be delegated, (b) a decision regarding to whom the task is to be delegated, (c) delegating the task with a discussion of additional directions/information, (d) checking on the completion of the task, and (e) assessing the outcomes (Curtis & Nicholl, 2004; Eason, 2000). Timm in her analysis of the literature identified the key attributes of delegation as "selected tasks ... transferred from one person in authority to another person, involving trust, empowerment, and the responsibility and authority to perform the task, where communication is succinct, guidelines are clearly delineated in advance, progress is monitored constantly, and where the person in authority remains accountable for the end results" (2003, p. 263). Delegation as a nursing tool requires the nurse's understanding of the dynamics of nursing care demands, the roles and capabilities of assistive personnel, a view of total patient care, and nursing accountability.

## Care Management

Health care has become complex, multifaceted, and diversified in terms of settings of health care, modes of health care delivery, engagement of various health care professionals, and the dynamics among various sectors and modes of care. The major concern in this context has been ensuring continuity of care, prevention of fragmentation of services, and ensuring the best possible client outcomes in terms of effectiveness, safety, and well-being. The concerns regarding the gaps in patient care, patient safety concerns, poor continuity and quality of care, and poor financial outcomes were addressed in the Patient Protection and Affordable Care Act passed by the Congress in 2010 in the United States. Nursing has taken up the responsibility of care management for clients in order to fulfill the gap created by fragmentation and to ensure high-quality care for clients throughout health care experiences (ANA, 2012b). The concept of care management, often in conjunction with the concept of case management, refers to coordinating health care for individuals throughout the care process. The National Committee for Quality Assurance (NCQA) defines care management as "a collaborative process of assessment, planning, facilitation, care coordination, evaluation and advocacy for options and services to meet the comprehensive medical, behavioral health and psychosocial needs of an individual and the individual's family, while promoting quality and cost-effective outcomes" (NCQA, 2014). In the NIC system, case management is defined as "coordinating care and advocating for specified individuals and patient populations across settings to reduce cost, reduce resource use, improve quality of health care, and achieve desired outcomes" (Bulechek et al., 2013).

Care management involves developing an individualized coordinated plan of care and implementing a process for: (a) attaining continuity of care, high quality of care, and patient safety and satisfaction; (b) limiting duplication of services through coordination of care; and (c) facilitation of communication among involved professional caregivers and clients/family. Care management as a nursing tool is applicable both at a micro level (i.e., for individual clients in specific health care settings) and at a macro level as a part of organizational programs for safe, effective, and cost-effective health care to groups of clients.

## SUMMARY AND QUESTIONS FOR REFLECTION AND FURTHER DELIBERATION

Essential tools of nursing practice are those that are applicable across client types and health care settings. Nurses need to develop competency in these essential tools in order to provide quality nursing care. While these essential nursing tools are required for providing quality nursing care to clients, these have to be supplemented by other specific strategies that focus on clients' specific clinical problems and needs in order to provide comprehensive nursing care. Furthermore, the application of these essential nursing tools in nursing practice has to be configured by the ideology of holism and person-centeredness. There still is a great need to develop these tools further conceptually, theoretically, empirically, and methodologically in order to identify their essential structures, modes of institution, and factors that influence variations in their applications.

- What do you consider the essential tools necessary for your practice? Do you apply the essential tools presented in this chapter routinely in your practice? Would you consider them essential for your practice?

- Are there additional essential tools that are critical for your practice? In which category among the four categories identified in this chapter do these belong?
- What additional knowledge and research are necessary to further develop these essential tools?
- Are these essential tools taught to meet the demands of general nursing practice in undergraduate education? In what ways is the teaching of these essential tools extended at the graduate level of education in nursing?

# CHAPTER 9

# Collaborative Practice

COLLABORATIVE PRACTICE IS THE KEYSTONE IN the current health care system in which health care is provided by various professionals and in diversified settings, each with somewhat distinct goals and orientations. Interprofessional collaboration in health care provision became the major form of collaborative practice, especially in the 1980s and 1990s during which a surge of advanced practitioners in nursing, specialization in health care professional disciplines, and professionalization of various health care providers occurred (Campbell, 1997). The emphasis on collaborative practice has also been a response to fragmentation of services and a lack of continuity in health care. Furthermore, this development has expanded in recent decades to include clients, families, and consumer groups along with multiple health care professionals in the collaborative provision of health care, with the increasing concern for self-determination, consumerism, and participatory governance. In the spirit of person-centered practice, the World Health Organization (WHO) embraced the inclusion of clients by adopting a stance that "collaborative practice in health care occurs when multiple health workers provide comprehensive services by working together synergistically along with patients, their families, caregivers and communities to deliver the highest quality of care across settings" (WHO, 2010). The Interprofessional Education for Collaborative Patient-Centred Practice (IECPCP) developed for Health Canada adopted the position that service users are active partners in the interprofessional collaborative practice framework, being located at the center of the process and acting as active partners in service provision (D'Amour & Oandasan, 2005). Health Canada (2004) states that interprofessional collaborative practice "is designed to promote the active participation of each profession in patient care.

It enhances patient and family centred goals and values, provides mechanisms for continuous communication among caregivers, optimizes staff participation in clinical decision making within and across professions, and fosters respect for disciplinary contributions of all professionals" (p. ii). Collaborative practice in the current health care scene therefore embraces collaboration among various health care professionals with clients and their families as the focal point of collaboration.

The WHO Study Group on Interprofessional Education and Collaborative Practice states that collaborative practice strengthens health systems and health outcomes, and envisions interprofessional health care teams to optimize the skills of their members, share case management, and provide better health services to patients and the community (WHO, 2010). From the WHO perspective, collaborative practice is to be integrated into every aspect of practice that includes "both clinical and nonclinical health-related work, such as diagnosis, treatment, surveillance, health communications, management and sanitation engineering" (WHO, 2010). In both acute and primary care settings, Mickan (2005) found higher levels of patient satisfaction, better acceptance of care, and improved health outcomes following treatment by a collaborative team.

The term "collaboration" is often used in conjunction with coordination and partnership, and refers to a complex process in relationships in which competence, confidence, and commitment on the part of all participants are required with a shared vision (Henneman, Lee, & Cohen, 1995). Although collaboration can occur naturally, it is often an intentional process to produce better outcomes. Collaborative practice is present in engagements of various individuals and/or agencies in the delivery of care either in established, formal teams or in situation-specific involvement of different people and agencies. Collaborative practice has been hailed as the mode of practice appropriate in the current health care scene, both as a philosophy and an approach.

Collaborative practice from the perspective of nursing practice encompasses four levels of collaboration, beginning with collaboration between the client/family and the nurse, intranursing collaboration, interprofessional collaboration, and interagency collaboration linked to the context of both formal health care system and teams and independent service arrangements (Figure 9.1). Collaborative practice in this framework puts the client/family at the core, involving them in collaborative processes as active players providing voices and participating in decision making.

The goal of collaborative practice is to achieve better goal attainment for clients through coordinated service relationships in terms of planning, provision, and evaluation of health care. Collaboration has to occur at the immediate interaction level between the client/family and the nurse, which becomes the

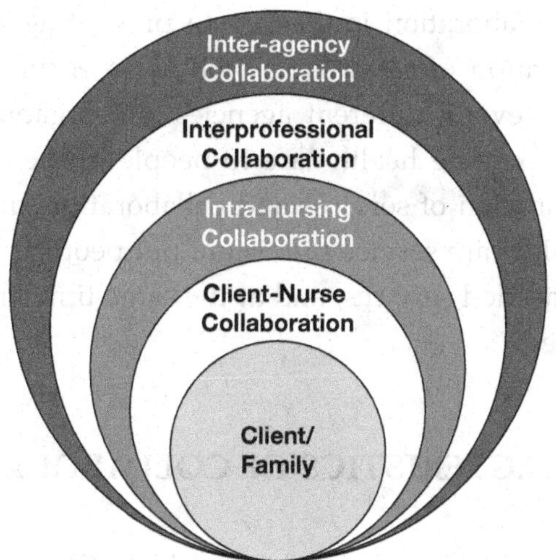


**FIGURE 9.1** Levels of collaboration in nursing practice.

baseline for collaboration at other levels and makes such collaboration more readily possible. It is the permeation of collaborative spirit and attitude that leads to collaboration at various levels, especially viewed from the nursing context in which nurses play the role of advocate for their clients. Client–nurse collaboration sets the tone for the actualization of person-centered care.

Institutional nursing practice involves an organizational arrangement of nurses in groups for the care of clients in various nursing care delivery models. The formal team-nursing as a nursing care delivery model organizes nurses in teams to provide care coordinated through a team approach. While this approach has waned and has been replaced by the professional model, nursing care delivery in institutional settings, in which the delivery of nursing care has to be coordinated among several nurses, involves an "informal" team approach with collaboration as the key process. Collaboration among nurses in the intraprofessional context involves shared decision making regarding nursing care and participating in the delivery of nursing care within the dynamics of a team approach.

On the other hand, interprofessional collaboration for nursing goes beyond the focal concerns for nursing care, extending to the delivery of total health care. Thus, as interprofessional collaboration involves various health care professionals, it is complicated by different sets of contributions toward client outcomes by various health care professionals. Interprofessional collaboration has been problematic from the lack of understanding regarding respective expertise and role responsibilities of various professional practitioners involved in such teams and delivering care, and power differences among health care professionals.

Interagency collaboration is the key to preventing fragmentation and unnecessary duplication of services as well as to ensuring a continuity of care to people. As several different agencies and organizations are invariably involved in providing health care to people in the current health care system, it is coordination of services and collaboration among agencies that can streamline health care service provision, put people in the right place at the right time for needed services, and at the same time know each agency's contribution to care.

## CHARACTERISTICS OF COLLABORATION

Characterization of collaboration has been identified as components and elements of collaboration by various authors. Henneman et al. (1995), in their concept analysis of collaboration, extracted nine attributes of collaboration as joint venture, cooperative endeavor, willing participation, shared planning and decision making, team approach, contribution of expertise, shared responsibility, nonhierarchical relationships, and shared power based on knowledge and expertise. In a review of the literature, D'Amour, Ferrada-Videla, San Martin-Rodriguez, and Beaulieu (2005) found the concepts of sharing, partnership, interdependency, and shared power as the core concepts of collaboration. Warburton, Everingham, Cuthill, Bartlett, and Underwood (2011) characterized collaborative relationships as those founded on trust, respect, and mutual understanding, and having clear and stable roles and arrangements among participants. Bronstein (2003) proposes five components of interdisciplinary collaboration as collective ownership of goals, interdependence, flexibility, newly created professional activities, and reflection on process. Five essential components of collaboration identified by Reilly (2008) characterize collaboration as having an established central purpose with a shared vision and a structure that has clearly established roles, agreed upon ground rules, open and frequent communication, and access to credible information that supports problem solving. Shared identity, information congruence, and spontaneous communication as well as distance are also seen as the elements of collaboration (Hinds & Kiesler, 2002; Kiesler & Cummings, 2002). The characteristics of collaboration are also depicted as: cooperative endeavor; team approach; partnership and willing participation; interdependency; sharing in planning, decision making, intervention, and responsibility; mutual respect and trust; symmetric empowerment and power sharing; understanding and respecting others' perspectives, values, and philosophies; and colocation (Banfield & Lackie, 2009; Bronstein, 2003; Craven & Bland, 2006; Henneman et al., 1995;

Reese & Sontag, 2001; Way, Jones, & Baskerville, 2001). These findings and others from the literature suggest the essential characteristics of collaboration to be interdependence and mutuality, sharing of information and expertise, sharing of goals and decisions, and a sense of partnership through power equalization.

## CRITICAL PREMISES OF COLLABORATION

Collaboration is embedded in interaction among people, and has to be guided by premises inherent in interactive work. There are many records of failed or abandoned collaborative projects in scientific fields resulting apparently from differences in perspectives, knowledge, and culture, misunderstandings or difficulties associated with procedures or structure of projects, or the failure in the process of collaboration. Premises of collaboration are the foundation upon which the collaborative process can occur successfully. Premises of collaboration have been identified by many authors as principles, assumptions, and foundations, which include equal partnership, interdependence, and shared decision making; accountability for consistency in the service of outcomes; commitment to developing effective and sustainable interventions; commitment to agreed upon outcomes rather than approaches; open, clear, and respectful communication; and shared values, mutuality, and nurturing (Clarke & Mass, 1998; Metzler et al., 2003; Owen & Grealish, 2006).

Four critical premises of collaboration are identified from the literature as self-understanding, mutual understanding, shared values and goals, and open communication. Self-understanding as the first premise directs people to have a firm grasp of their own perspectives, knowledge, motivations, and biases. As collaboration requires getting into a project or a program involving two or more individuals with different backgrounds and orientations, variations in knowledge and expertise, and sometimes with differences in vested interests, the first step has to be self-understanding. The concept of personhood is critical in social interaction in which the questions of how one regards oneself and others and how one wishes and expects to be regarded by others are addressed (Mokros, Mullins, & Saracevic, 1995). Pullon (2008) found in a study of interprofessional relationships between physicians and nurses in primary health care settings the development of professional identity among members of the interprofessional team to be one of the bases for improved collaborative practice. The basis of self-understanding in this context is "professional personhood" acquired through the integration of practice experiences and professional role expectations into one's personal identity and experiences (Dombeck, 2003). Self-understanding is the basis for a sense of personal and professional security, and of self-confidence that is critical for collaboration (Henneman et al., 1995). Self-understanding especially associated with one's professional identity is critical to form the basis for an understanding regarding the extent to which one's own contribution is possible in working toward goals either alone or as a member of a team. Before launching on a collaborative project, one must assess oneself to lay bare the specific perspectives and knowledge relevant to the project, one's strengths and weaknesses, one's motivations related to the project, and one's specific biases (e.g., regarding what should be done, what is desirable, or what are expected outcomes). Self-understanding is necessary because people usually think and act according to what they are. It is often useful to write out such assessments for a clear self-understanding. Self-understanding is the basis for making oneself available for collaboration with one's knowledge and expertise.

The second premise, mutual understanding, is based on Habermas's critical philosophy. Habermas in his theory of communicative action espouses mutual understanding as the primary basis for avoiding or correcting distortions, domination/oppression, and coercion in the conduct of social life. In order to achieve mutual understanding, people must be engaged in communicative actions to tease out differing validity claims of truth, rightness, and truthfulness (Habermas, 1990). Mutual understanding allows people to gain and appreciate differing perspectives, values, motivations, and expertise. Mutual understanding especially in interprofessional context requires an understanding of and respect for different professional roles, the complex interplay between them, and the factors that affect each one's role (Salvage & Smith, 2000). Mutual understanding is the base for developing mutual respect and interpersonal trust, which are critical to collaborative process. Mutual respect refers to the recognition of complementary contributions and the knowledge of different expertise of various professionals, and stems from the acceptance of interdependency among professionals (Baggs & Schmitt, 1997; D'Amour et al., 2005; Gage, 1998; Way & Jones, 1994). The lack of understanding, respect, or appreciation of the contribution of other professionals is a critical barrier to collaboration among health care professionals (Bradford, 1989; Stichler, 1995). Mutual respect also leads to mutual trust that is another essential element for successful collaboration (Evans, 1994; Henneman et al., 1995; San Martin-Rodriguez, Beaulieu, D'Amour, & Ferrada-Videla, 2005; Stichler, 1995; Warren, Houston, & Luquire, 1998; Way & Jones, 1994). This is why people often spend a great deal of time together to thrash out differences in preparation for collaborative projects, and why people who know each other well can collaborate more successfully.

The third premise of shared values and goals is a necessary condition for any collaborative work because when people in a collaborative project work with differing values or goals, interpersonal processes for collaboration may not occur and may be frozen at the initial stage. A shared goal or vision is a basic precondition for a successful collaboration (Johnson, Zorn, Tam, LaMontagne, & Johnson, 2003; Thompson, Socolar, Brown, & Haggerty, 2002). For health care professionals, the common goals relate to the promotion of health and well-being of clients. Sharing such common goals can lead to a commitment to collaboration as the professionals can acknowledge both the needs for and the advantages of collaboration (Liedtka & Whitten, 1998; Sicotte, D'Amour, & Moreault, 2002). An essential shared value for collaboration is a commitment to collaboration, that is, a willingness to work in collaboration (Baggs & Schmitt, 1997; Henneman et al., 1995; Liedtka &Whitten, 1998; Sicotte et al., 2002; Stichler, 1995). It is a value of openness for teamwork, which is closely related to holding common goals inherent in relationships and projects. McLeish and Oxoby (2011) found that people with a shared identity tend to be more cooperative in negotiations. Health care professionals assembled to provide services to clients with common goals share identity, which propels them to be collaborative than antagonistic.

The fourth premise is open communication, which is fundamental to the processes of collaboration. Open communication requires a precondition of what Habermas calls "ideal speech situation" in which participants have speech competence, and are free to express their opinions and ask questions without constraints. Under ideal speech conditions, communicative action occurs by which "participants coordinate their plans of action consensually with the agreement reached at any point being evaluated in terms of the intersubjective recognition of validity claims" (Habermas, 1990, p. 58). Harbermas's concept of communicative interaction thus presupposes open communicativeness in participants' willingness to speak freely and hear others without prejudice and constraints leading to binding/bonding among participants toward some goals. Open communication refers to a state free of constraints that have the potential to bring about domination, conflicts, devaluing, embarrassment, depersonalization, or punishment. Open communication as a premise lays the groundwork for interactive processes in collaboration to occur. Baggs and Schmitt (1997) identified two critical conditions for collaboration—being available and being receptive. "Being receptive" requires an interest in collaboration that can be conveyed through the adoption of active listening, openness, and questioning.

These four premises form the foundation for collaboration to occur in various social situations involving two or more individuals. Collaborative culture that has integrated these premises will exhibit a commitment to common shared goals, respective of each other's knowledge, expertise, and contributions, and a willingness to work together to attain the goals by dealing with differences in opinions and approaches. This means that any project or work relationship that requires collaboration has to ensure the presence of these premises as the initial step. Thus, often it is necessary to launch a collaborative work with a preparatory stage to establish the collaborative culture. Education of and enculturation into these four premises for various health care professionals are the first steps, as has been endorsed by the WHO via the Interprofessional Education for Collaborative Practice project.

## PROCESSES OF COLLABORATION

Processes of collaboration have been identified in the literature in terms of stages, procedures, and strategies. Although there are various ways of conceptualizing processes of collaboration, there are two essential types of processes involved in collaboration: processes of progression and processes of interaction for achieving collaboration. While the processes of progression refer to the stages starting with an initial state of recognizing the need for collaboration and ending either with continuation of a collaborative relationship or a resolution of problems, the interactional processes for achieving collaboration refer to ways of operating in collaborative work involving participants. Warburton et al. (2008) refers to this second type of processes as the processes, procedures, and ways of operating that involve agreed and effective ways of working such as division of labor, communication, problem solving and decision making, and knowledge sharing.

The processes of collaboration from the staging perspective are oriented to establishing collaboration among people initially working through to establish a collaborative culture and moving to achieve joint actions. Kahn and Prager (1994) identified four stages in establishing relationships for interdisciplinary collaboration: (a) listening across the gulf in search of a common theme, (b) a conceptual translation in order to establish a shared conceptual vocabulary, (c) the onset of collaboration involving activities of consultation, with a high degree of mutual tolerance and mutual helpfulness, and (d) a joint project in which a goal is being met. This means that an interdisciplinary team moves through these stages in identifying critical concerns, defining an interdisciplinary approach to solve problems, and developing and instituting a program of action in a collaborative manner. Gardner (1999) on the other hand identified (a) information exchange, (b) joint projects, (c) changing the rules, and (d) changing the system as the stages of collaboration in interagency collaboration. De Stampa et al. (2012) identified initiating collaboration, developing real two-way collaborations, and developing interdisciplinary teamwork as the stages of collaboration for geriatric care teams with different dynamics at play in different stages. Somewhat differently, Abma and Broese (2010) consider exploration, consultation, prioritization, integration, programming, and implementation as the six phases in the establishment of collaborative relationships. In a phenomenological study of collaboration in rehabilitation teams, Croker, Trede, and Higgs (2012) found "engaging" as the central aspect of the experience of collaboration that melds together the stages of "establishing," "envisioning," "effecting," and "entering" into reciprocity. From the literature, the stages of collaboration can be specified in general as:

- The initial stage at which participants are engaged in sharing information about themselves and their perspectives, efforts for understanding each other, and forming working relationships
- The problem-oriented stage at which participants identify the nature of problems to be solved or addressed, decide upon shared goals regarding identified problems, and address various questions related to problems such as availability of and needs for resources or to contextual issues surrounding problems
- The solution-oriented stage at which participants discuss various approaches to problem solving and arrive at mutually agreed approaches or programs for problem solution including the identification of forms of collaborative/participatory engagement necessary for implementation
- The implementation stage at which selected joint approaches or programs are implemented and evaluated

This stage view of the processes of collaboration specifies how collaborative relationships progress in order to address problems or projects. However, it does not give insights into how this progression occurs, that is, it does not specify the interactive processes that have to be in place in order for the stages to progress, which are referred to in the second conceptualization of the processes of collaboration.

Processes of collaboration as the processes of "workings" include open dialogue (Abma & Broese, 2010; Baggs & Schmitt, 1997; Ness et al., 2014; Probandari, Utarin, Lindholm, & Hurtig, 2011; Schwartz, 2007), partnership, or team building (Baggs & Schmitt, 1997; de Stampa et al., 2012), participatory engagement (Ness et al., 2014), and sharing (Alt-White, Charns, & Strayer, 1983; Baggs & Schmitt, 1997; Bronstein, 2003). The dialogue model proposed by Abma and Broese (2010) is based on the assumption that participants in collaborative projects have unique and relevant perspectives and that mutual understanding and shared action programs supported by all participants will result only from dialogic exchanges that incorporate openness, respect, trust, and commitment of participants. Open and genuine dialogue makes it possible for participants to listen to each other, learn from each other, and jointly create new ideas, approaches, and experiences. Probandari et al. (2011) also suggest that open dialogue is useful for articulating each partner's expectations and for defining shared partnership objectives. Open and active communication with active listening is critical for collaboration, as it makes mutual knowledge possible among team professionals and is a vehicle through which professionals share critical information (Alt-White et al., 1983; Baggs & Schmitt, 1997). Open communication allows participants to engage in developing a common ground for shared information and to deal with differences and problems immediately in order to continue in group work with as little conflict as possible.

Ness et al. (2014) specifically propose two essential processes as open dialogue and participatory engagement. Seikkula and colleagues (2003, 2006) proposed the process of open dialogue for mental health care constituting unconstrained back-and-forth exchanges of meanings, voices, and interpretations, through which common understandings regarding situations, problems, goals, and approaches are developed and shared. Ness et al. (2014) suggest valuing uncertainty and tolerance for uncertainty as two key elements within open dialogue, which generate the freedom in participants to address different options and choices in meanings, interpretations, and courses of action. Open dialogue that allows valuing uncertainty and tolerance for uncertainty leads to symmetric empowerment and a sense of affinity with the generative nature of a group's work. The second process for collaboration advanced by Ness et al. (2014) is participatory engagement, which is defined as the process of sharing in all aspects of a group's work by its participants willingly, without feeling constraints or prejudices, and bringing in "expertise" of each participant. Participatory engagement is an active sharing involvement and refers to being directly and personally engaged in sharing every aspect of a group's work whether it is dialogue or action and whether it is for understanding, goal-setting, planning, or intervention. While open dialogue is a process of medium through which collaboration occurs, participatory engagement is an active involvement of participants in every aspect of joint work as partners in action requiring open dialogue as its key medium.

## DETERMINANTS OF COLLABORATION

There are many factors found to influence the success of collaboration. Such factors as determinants of collaboration have been conceptually classified into (a) interactional factors, (b) organizational factors, and (c) systemic factors by the IECPCP (WHO, 2010) and in a review paper by San Martin-Rodriguez et al. (2005). In a similar approach, Kim (1983) identifies three structures—participants, context, and interaction—in which variations can influence the quality of collaboration. San Martin-Rodriguez et al. extracted from the review of the literature the following factors as determinants of collaboration (2005, pp. 136–140):

- Systemic factors
  - The social system—collegiality (+); power differences (−); a nondemanding approach by the nurse and a nonabusive approach by the physician (+)
  - The cultural system—different perspectives on collaboration (−)
  - The professional system—understanding the practice of other professionals (+); awareness and valorization of other professionals' contribution (+); fragmentation of care along professional jurisdictions (−); different values, work styles, and personality traits among the professions (−); awareness of other professionals contribution (+); adhesion to professional logics (−); adhesion to collaboration logics (+)
  - The educational system—socialization into a strong professional identity (−); limitation in the exposure for understanding and acknowledging the nature of various professionals' expertise and contribution (−)
- Organizational factors—organizational philosophy in terms of climate of openness and positive conflict management (+) and of an approving atmosphere (+); administrative support with leadership (+) and realistic objectives (+); resources in terms of physical proximity (+), space and time (+), and small patient units with primary care nursing (+); and coordination mechanisms in terms of standardization of work and skills (+), group discussion (+), formalization of rules and protocols (+), and division of work and common rules (+)
- Interactional factors—willingness to collaborate (+); trust (+); active and open communication (+); and mutual respect (+)

Warburton et al. (2008) identified six domains for successful collaboration: (a) procollaborative sociopolitical climate and history of the environment and favorable locale; (b) partner characteristics such as diverse cross-section of stakeholders possessing a range of relevant skills and knowledge; (c) processes, procedures, and ways of operating that are agreed on and effective; (d) structures with clear definitions of roles that are stable and relationships founded on trust, respect, and mutual understanding; (e) a shared vision and establishment of concrete attainable goals; and (f) sufficient material and other resources. Reilly (2008) similarly considers aspects for successful collaboration in terms of: (a) a central purpose incorporating a shared vision and a critical need for action; (b) a broad-based participant group representing needed expertise and interests; (c) a structure with well-established role relationships, rules, accessibility to critical information, and open communication; (d) a process of open communication, monitoring, and feedback; and (e) material and social resources to support collaboration. As pointed out by San Martin-Rodriguez et al. (2005), the results of many studies suggest that a successful collaboration is related to the attributes of participants in terms of appropriateness of expertise, a sense of personal and professional security, commitment to collaborative work, and an appreciation for and willingness to work with the complexities of carrying out collaborative projects. For collaborative practice to be successful, it is necessary to have not only the support from participants in their beliefs, attitudes, expertise, skills, and efforts, but also the support in the immediate and broader contexts in terms of cultural elements, systems' institutionalized forms of social practice, and system support and resources.

## COLLABORATIVE PRACTICE IN NURSING

### Client–Nurse Collaboration

Collaboration between the client and the nurse is the hallmark of person-centered care, and has been considered an ideal approach that can result in positive client outcomes. The prevailing view in the current health care arena is that shared decision making (SDM), a process by which a health care choice is made jointly by the practitioner and the patient, is central to patient-centered care, and "policy makers perceive SDM as desirable because of its potential to (a) reduce the overuse of options not clearly associated with benefits for all (e.g., prostate cancer screening); (b) enhance the use of options clearly associated with benefits for the vast majority (e.g., cardiovascular risk factor management); (c) reduce unwarranted health care practice variations; (d) foster the sustainability of the health care system; and (e) promote the right of patients to be involved in decisions concerning their health" (Légaré et al., 2010). SDM through collaboration thus has consequences both at the client level in terms of positive outcomes in individual clients and at the system level in terms of system effectiveness. High level of collaboration between the client and the nurse has shown to result in such client outcomes as high levels of satisfaction with care, feelings of control over health, feelings of well-being, and compliance with prescribed treatments (Barsevick & Johnson, 1990; Krouse & Roberts, 1989; Mahler & Kulik, 1990; Paavilainen & Åstedt-Kurki, 1997).

The phrase "client–nurse collaboration" has been used in the literature interchangeably with patient participation in care and client–nurse cooperation, and refers to collaboration in decision making and care planning, and client participation in care activities. In general, the definition of client–nurse collaboration is in line with the definition adopted by Clarke and Mass, which states that it is "a joint communicating and decision making process with the expected goal of satisfying the patient's/client's wellness and illness needs while respecting unique qualities and abilities of the client and nurse" (1998, p. 218). The focus is on joint decision making in interaction, which not only results in specific decisions for the client, but also leads to client participation in ensuing care processes. However, Cahill (1996) suggests a hierarchy of the client–nurse relationship in terms of collaboration as: (a) the highest level as partnership, (b) the intermediate level as patient participation, and (c) the lowest level as patient involvement/collaboration. Millard, Hallett, and Luker (2006) found in their study of community health nurses that nurses as the controlling agents for client relationships were engaged in five different levels of involving clients in decision making ranging from completely involving, partially involving, forced involving, covert noninvolving, and to overt noninvolving. These studies suggest that the concept of collaboration has to be viewed in a continuum of varying levels of client involvement in decision making and care processes.

Kim (1983) proposed a theory of collaborative decision making in nursing practice that delineates (a) the context of participants including factors related to the client and the nurse, and (b) the context of situation in terms of the organization of decision-making situation and decision types, which influence how collaboration occurs resulting in varying levels of collaboration to take place as the primary outcome, and influence client outcomes in relation to goal attainment, autonomy, and satisfaction as the ultimate outcomes. The client's and the nurse's attitudes and willingness for collaboration, role expectations, subjective definition of situations, and personal traits are the key factors that are proposed to influence their participation in the collaborative process. A critical requirement for a successful collaboration is related to the attributes of participants in terms of appropriateness of expertise, a sense of personal and professional security, and commitment to, appreciation for, and willingness for collaboration. Clarke and Mass (1998) found several factors related to the clients and the nurses as the antecedents of collaboration: (a) readiness to work collaboratively including willingness to give up control, share information, share power, and interpersonal trust; (b) respect for each other's knowledge, abilities and experiences, and communication skills;

(c) attitudes for independence and autonomy; and (d) understanding own and other's roles, obligations, and power in relationships. In addition, the factors in the organization of decision making influencing collaboration include the established organizational structure and processes in place, the characteristics of the care delivery system, and the established forms of decision making in the situation. Clarke and Mass (1998) found the organizational philosophy of fostering cooperative environment, nonhierarchical relationships, and shared planning, decision making, and responsibilities as the organizational antecedent for collaboration (Clarke & Mass, 1998). Decision types that are the focus for collaboration are also considered to influence collaboration, as different decision types (e.g., program decisions, agenda decisions, and operational-control decisions) have different meanings and are oriented to different outcomes (Kim, 1983).

Because there is an evidence that client–nurse collaboration does not occur naturally (Clarke & Mass, 1998; Kim, 1987; Millard et al., 2006; Paavilainen & Åstedt-Kurki, 1997), it is critical that interventions are developed to increase the level of client–nurse collaboration. However, the Cochrane review of SDM as a process of making health care choices jointly by the practitioner and the patient indicates a paucity of research testing interventions that are aimed at promoting or increasing SDM (Légaré et al., 2010). As the first-level interventions, developing mutuality among participants (Probandari et al., 2011) and integrating procollaborative attitudes (Kim, 1983) have been suggested, and an intervention to transform nurses' attitudes and interactive behaviors in practice has also been proposed based on critical philosophy and action science (Kim et al., 1993).

## Intranursing Collaboration

Nursing's intraprofessional collaboration involves nurses working together to plan and provide care to clients either within a same clinical setting or across different settings. Intranursing collaboration within a given clinical setting often involves jointly working together to provide care to patients in order to coordinate and address patients' needs that are diverse. Examples of such collaboration are for critically ill patients in critical care units involving critical care nurses and clinical specialists such as oncology nurses, for elderly patients involving general staff nurses and gerontological nurse specialists, or for general patients with special psychological needs involving staff nurses and mental health nursing specialists. Although sometimes such relationships are specified as "consulting," the process is collaborative as such relationships are for joint decision making in relation to plans of care or approaches to solving clients' problems. Ruesch et al. (2012) suggest that collaboration between bedside nurses and remote nurses with the use of tele-ICU program technology improves critical care patient outcomes, while Hull and O'Rourke (2007) indicate that collaboration between critical care nurses and oncology nurse liaisons promotes the continuity of care for patients and better plans of care resulting from joint decision making. Intranursing collaboration at a given clinical setting is enhanced by reciprocal support and mutual respect for respective expertise and knowledge. Moore and Prentice (2013) further suggest that an organization's supportive culture for collaboration is a critical requirement for such collaboration to occur in clinical settings.

Intranursing collaboration across clinical settings usually occurs during handover or transfer of clients from one setting to another, and requires an understanding and appreciation of others' expertise, knowledge, and service capabilities. Because such collaboration often occurs not as direct face-to-face contacts, communication skills used in interactions play a critical role. Involvement of clients and/or families in intranursing collaboration has become a mandate in upholding the ideal of person-centered practice in nursing, and it means any joint decision making among nurses should be guided by client preferences and needs from the client's perspective through team collaboration that includes clients/family members as active participants.

## Interprofessional Collaboration

Interprofessional collaboration from the nursing practice perspective was historically introduced formally as collaboration between physicians and nurses with the advent of nurse practitioners and clinical specialists in the 1970s. However, interprofessional collaboration means a variety of collaborative relationships among health care professionals both as one-to-one collaboration and as team collaboration, with a growing emphasis on team collaboration in health care provision. Interprofessional collaboration within health care systems has been emphasized as a critical process in health care for improving people's health outcomes through coordinated, high quality, and safe care to clients, because increasingly health care is provided to people with a team approach involving many different health care professionals, each of whom has different sets of expertise, knowledge, and skills necessary for a comprehensive, safe care (AACN, 2008; Health Canada, 2004; IOM, 2003a; WHO, 2010). In order to make interprofessional collaboration among health care professionals become effective, there has been a growing emphasis on the Interprofessional Education for Collaborative Practice (CAIPE, 2002; Canadian Interprofessional Health Collaborative, 2007; IOM, 2014; WHO, 2010). Creating a culture for collaborative practice in both at micro and macro health care levels along with socialization and education of health care professionals for interprofessional collaboration is thought to be the first-level grounding for improving collaborative practice among professionals.

D'Amour and Oandasan (2005) defined "interprofessionality" as "the process by which professionals reflect on and develop ways of practicing that provides an integrated and cohesive answer to the needs of the client/family/population ... [I]t involves continuous interaction and knowledge sharing between professionals, organized to solve or explore a variety of education and care issues all while seeking to optimize the patient's participation ..." (p. 9). Interprofessional collaboration encompasses an establishment of shared goals, understanding, and appreciation of competencies and expectations regarding various health care professional roles within health care teams, a decision-making process that is flexible, and an establishment of open communication patterns and leadership (AACN, 2008). Open communication among members of health care teams is critical for making mutual knowledge possible among team members, sharing clinical information, and contributing to building team approaches for best patient care (Baggs & Schmitt, 1997; D'Amour & Oandasan, 2005; Melville-Smith & Kendal, 2011; Schwartz, 2007). Open communication to develop a common ground for shared information and frequent contacts among members to resolve differences and problems immediately seem to be the mechanisms through which collaboration can continue without as little conflict as possible. In addition, trust and respect among team members are critical to sustain partnerships (Buse & Harmer, 2007; Hardy, Phillips, & Lawrence, 2003; Harris, 2008; Pullon, 2008; Shortell et al., 2002).

There is a variety of theoretical approaches to describe and explain interprofessional collaboration ranging from organizational theories to social and psychological theories in the literature with many models developed for specific types of interprofessional collaboration (D'Amour et al., 2005; Dow, DiazGranados, Mazmanian, & Retchin, 2013). Factors in participating professionals, organizational characteristics, and the nature of processes that get into place play critical roles in influencing the success of interprofessional collaboration. The major impact on interprofessional collaboration has been attributed to professional education with a strong emphasis on interprofessional education for development of the commitment to collaboration and critical processes in collaboration. In recent years, the mandate for an active involvement of clients in health care decision making has put clients at the center of interprofessional collaboration.

## Interagency Collaboration

Interagency collaboration refers to collaboration between or among agencies, organizations, or sectors in the community to provide better services to individual clients or a target population. Interagency collaboration involving a one-time relationship among two or more agencies for specific clients is often oriented to establishing comprehensive service plans or to solve specific service issues. For example, the case of an elderly client with multiple chronic diseases, financial and housing issues, and various health and social services needs requires an involvement, coordination, and collaboration among agency representatives from the health care, social services, housing, and welfare services in the community. Often such one-time interagency collaboration is initiated by a nurse or a social worker who works as a case manager, and is usually carried out especially when a formal protocol for relationships among agencies does not exist. For this type of interagency collaboration, nurses function as active advocates and coordinators for interagency collaboration in order to establish an integrated, comprehensive service provision for clients. Apparent compartmentalization of various agencies remains intact in such interagency collaboration, with a one-shot deal to create a collaborative program of services tailored to meet the specifics needs of the given situation.

Interagency collaboration in a formal sense goes beyond this one-time collaboration, and is oriented to establishing formal linkages, establishing protocols for integration of services, and developing collaborative programs. Collaboration is at the organizational level with a possibility that participants in collaboration are not fixed as members of teams. A prototypical example of an interagency collaboration is given in a study by Vogel, Ransom, Wai, and Luisi (2007) that examined the processes of collaboration regarding the health and social services for the elderly in New York City to implement the "Senior Wellness Project." The process for implementing this project, which involved the city's health department and housing authority, was examined by applying Gardner's model of the stages of collaboration. It involved four progressive stages, from information exchange, joint project, changing the rules, and changing the system, as the participating organizations moved toward an increasing program integration and commitment to the success of the collaboration. Their retrospective analysis indicates that although the development, implementation, and scale-up of the new integrated project was successfully carried out through the collaborative process, the conflicting organizational culture in the agencies, scarce resources available for the project, and managing expansion of the program influenced the process at different stages. As shown by this example, interagency collaboration when successfully carried out results in an integration of new coordinated approaches to clients' needs, often overcoming compartmentalized modes of services that were in place. Interagency collaboration thus changes the landscape in which service provisions are made to target populations. Especially because interagency collaboration involves changes at the system level, it has long-lasting influence on the relationships among involved agencies. Nurses can play an important role in interagency collaboration both by introducing the idea for integrated services to clients into organizations and also playing key roles in the collaborative process as active participants.

## SUMMARY AND QUESTIONS FOR REFLECTION AND FURTHER DELIBERATION

Collaborative practice in the context of nursing practice occurs at various levels, and nurses have to be able to play active roles at all levels in order to increase the effectiveness of health care and nursing services and to ensure the best client outcomes that are possible. Shared goals, trust, and respect among collaborating individuals are key attributes for successful collaboration, and the process of communication that is open, sharing, and mutually oriented is essential for collaborative practice at all levels. The ideal of person-centered practice has to be translated into the concept of collaborative practice as that involving clients and their families actively in the collaborative process. Nurses as proactive collaborators in health care need to develop and integrate values and attitudes for client involvement and participation and for collaboration in general. It is also necessary to help to create and sustain the health care environment to promote collaboration.

- What are the demands for collaborative practice present in your own practice? What forms of collaboration do you engage in your current practice?
- What are the key processes you have used in your experiences of collaboration at various levels such as client–nurse, intranursing, interprofessional, and interagency collaboration?
- What are the values you hold that are important for collaborative practice?
- How should nurses be taught to engage effectively in collaborative practice?

# CHAPTER 10

# Knowledge Application in Nursing Practice

## KNOWLEDGE-BASED PRACTICE

THE CONCEPT OF KNOWLEDGE-BASED PRACTICE REFERS to the requirement that nursing practice as a professional practice be guided by various types of knowledge. It is a much broader and more generic perspective regarding how nursing should be practiced than the currently espoused idea of "evidence-based" nursing practice (Kim, 2006). This semantic emphasis moving away from the term "evidence-based" to "knowledge-based" nursing practice is necessary for nursing in order to shift away from the focus on a specific type of knowledge, that is, "evidence-based" knowledge, as the primary type of knowledge for nursing practice. Nursing practice cannot be based solely on the evidence-based knowledge type, which refers generally to empirical, generalized knowledge, but has to rely on various types of knowledge encompassed within a more general, comprehensive view of knowledge to meet its mandate.

The idea of *knowledge-based nursing* adopted in this chapter is based on five key assumptions:

1. Knowledge for nursing practice refers to a body of specialized knowledge that is multidimensional, complex in its configuration, and derived from multiple sources
2. Knowledge use in nursing practice involves "being a nurse" and "doing in nursing"
3. Knowledge use in nursing practice situationally involves two interlinked but different foci—the first on the client's status as an

experiential one, involving the practice of assessment, and the second on the client's status as requiring nursing approaches and interventions, involving the practice of care, therapy, and professional work

4. The processes by which individual practitioners apply knowledge in practice are context specific, situated, and individualistic, in the sense that each practice instance is unique in the presentation of a client's conditions, problems, trajectory, history, and context
5. The practitioner is the user of knowledge who must adopt certain cognitive, strategic, and action processes

The five cognitive needs identified for the nursing epistemology fulfill how knowledge-based nursing practice can be produced in a comprehensive manner, and refer to the five different types of knowledge necessary for informed, responsible practice. The five types of knowledge for nursing practice are to be coalesced and synthesized in situation-specific instances of nursing practice, drawing from knowledge developed for phenomena in four different domains as discussed in Chapter 4.

However, the knowledge used in practice is the knowledge in the private domain, and that the knowledge in the public domain to be "actually" used in practice must first be integrated, transferred, transmitted, or incorporated into the private knowledge domain of individual nurses by what I term "knowledge synthesis." Public knowledge is the knowledge that belongs to a discipline (or a field of study) as a shared, validated and/or accepted, or emergent knowledge as opposed to private knowledge that belongs to individuals. When we talk about public knowledge of a practice discipline, there is an assumption that such knowledge is to be used/applied in practice by practitioners of the discipline. Thus, knowledge-based practice involves a process of linking the public knowledge of the discipline and the private knowledge of a practitioner. Knowledge application in a general sense consists of two interrelated but distinct processes—knowledge synthesis and knowledge use—knowledge synthesis dealing with how knowledge in the public domain comes to be incorporated, assimilated, or transferred to the private domain, and knowledge use addressing how knowledge in the private domain, that is, the knowledge acquired, stored, and cumulated by an individual, comes to be used in actual practice. This is depicted in Figure 10.1.

## Knowledge in the Knowledge-Based Nursing Practice

Knowledge-based nursing practice refers to what knowledge is necessary on which to base practice (*the content*) and how such knowledge is to be used in practice (*the process*). Knowledge-based nursing practice in the context of the

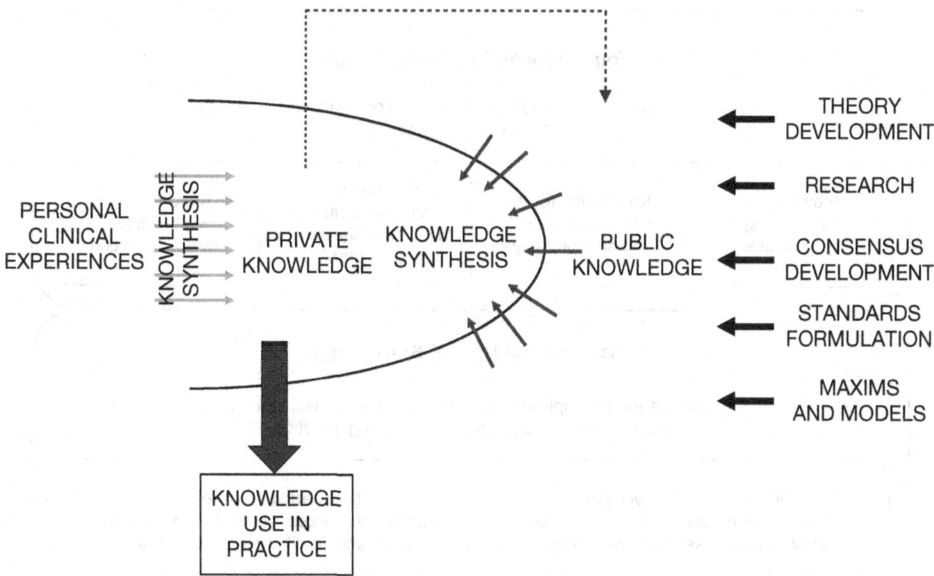


**FIGURE 10.1** Knowledge synthesis and use in practice: Relationship between knowledge in the public and private domains.

comprehensive characterization of nursing practice points to two distinct roles that knowledge plays in nursing practice: (a) a foundational role to shape and undergird how nursing has to be practiced in general regardless of the clinical situation, and (b) an instrumental role to respond to requirements of specific clinical situations for nursing practice. These two roles can be understood as two levels of knowledge use in practice—the general, unspecified one as the base level, with the attainment of the basic orientations, attitudes, commitments, as well as the general knowledge; and the particularistic, instrumental role as the second level to address unique knowledge requirements of specific clinical situations (Figure 10.2). Clinical nursing practice in specific clinical situations, therefore, assumes that the general, unspecified knowledge use establishes the foundation upon which nurses are "ready" to embrace the knowledge necessary to develop nursing-specific competencies to be applied in particular clinical situations at the second level. There is an ongoing process of integrating these two levels of knowledge use in practice. In this chapter, the two roles of knowledge in nursing practice are delineated to systematize the way knowledge is used in clinical practice by integrating into the model of nursing practice.

## The Foundational Role of Knowledge

Nurses need to embrace and integrate knowledge that provides the basis for understanding humans and nursing practice from the nursing perspective as well as builds up the philosophical commitment necessary for nursing

**Foundational Role of Knowledge**

Knowledge for building the philosophical and orientational foundation for nursing practice

| Knowledge for the nursing perspective | Knowledge for the philosophies of nursing practice | Knowledge for commitments to the five rationalities of nursing practice | Knowledge for the processes of nursing practice |
|---|---|---|---|

**Instrumental Role of Knowledge**

Knowledge for developing nursing specific approaches, strategies, Interventions, and programs for nursing practice

| Knowledge for developing the general modes of nursing practice applicable across clinical situations | Knowledge for developing various specialized modes of nursing practice applicable to different clinical situations |
|---|---|

**FIGURE 10.2** The roles of knowledge in knowledge-based nursing practice.

practice. This refers to the role of knowledge as a general one, as it provides the foundation for nurses in practice squarely and directly to be practitioners of nursing. This means that the foundational role encompasses the knowledge for building the philosophical and orientational foundation for nursing practice. It means that at the baseline nursing practice is guided by the knowledge that establishes nurses' commitments, orientations, attitudes, and values in the nursing perspective, the philosophies of nursing practice, and the values inherent in the performance of nursing practice.

This role of knowledge in nursing practice refers to the role of:

- General philosophical and theoretical knowledge that undergirds the nursing perspective encompassing holism, health orientation, person-centeredness, and caring
- The knowledge that supports the philosophies of practice delineated as the philosophies of care, therapy, and professional work
- The knowledge necessary to understand the philosophical underpinnings regarding the practice dimensions of nursing in terms of scientific, technical, ethical, aesthetic, and existential aspects
- The knowledge necessary to engage in the processes of deliberation and enactment in nursing practice as generic processes

The knowledge for the nursing perspective thus includes philosophical, theoretical, and conceptual frameworks regarding humans and human practice critical for nursing practice, which are oriented to delineate the foundational characteristics of humans, human health, and nursing practice in general ways. It also includes specifically the knowledge regarding the ideologies of holism, health-orientation imperative, person-centeredness, and caring to establish nurses' commitments to the specific practice perspective of nursing. Articulation of general knowledge regarding these ideologies drawing from the disciplines of philosophy, humanities, and general sciences as well as nursing is critical in order to build up the knowledge for nursing practice. The knowledge for the philosophy of practice including care, therapy, and professional work specifies the normative elements that configure these three philosophies in detail for nursing practice. Philosophical and theoretical knowledge that undergird these three philosophies of nursing practice forms the basis with which nurses establish commitments to and attitudes regarding these philosophies so that their practice reveals an integration of these philosophies.

The knowledge of the philosophical underpinnings regarding the scientific, technical, ethical, aesthetic, and existential dimensions of nursing practice builds up the value commitments and the evaluative criteria necessary to actualize a high-quality practice in these dimensions. The knowledge undergirding the scientific, technical, moral, aesthetic, and existential rationalities critical for nursing practice would establish nurses to be committed to the values inherent in these rationalities. In addition, the descriptive and normative knowledge regarding the processes of deliberation and enactment as general human processes is the foundational base upon which nurses can build specific methods of applying these processes in practice. The role of knowledge at this level is general, in the sense that the knowledge for this level is fundamentally required for nurses to practice nursing in the discipline-oriented ways. Knowledge at this level is necessary to establish nurses into the role of nursing and to build up commitments to the perspective and the philosophy for nursing practice as the foundation. Such knowledge is "used" in practice basically as "the undercurrents" (i.e., as the foundation) to affirm the role of nursing and to reflect the frames applied in everyday nursing practice. In general, when we discuss knowledge-based practice, this foundational role is usually overlooked probably with the assumption that it is a given. However, this role is critical as it is the base upon which nursing practice is built, and which infiltrates into every aspect of nursing practice.

## The Instrumental Role of Knowledge

At the second level, knowledge is necessary to address demands of a given clinical nursing situation. It is possible to conceptualize clinical nursing situations at varying degrees of specificity, such as a broadly defined nursing care situation of a patient who is hospitalized with a stroke to a narrowly defined nursing care situation of a patient on the day of being diagnosed for diabetes. However, at this level, a particular set of knowledge is necessary for nursing to respond to and address the specific nature of a given clinical situation of nursing practice. An assumption is that the characteristics of nursing practice in clinical situations are determined primarily by the application of knowledge at the first level for the generalized ways of practice, and secondarily by the application of knowledge in order to provide nursing practice addressing particular, situation-specific demands for practice. The role of knowledge at the second level addresses the five cognitive needs for nursing practice, as nurses engage in the processes of deliberation and enactment in practice in any given clinical situation. Therefore, the knowledge configured to address this role encompasses (a) the generalized knowledge for the inferential cognitive need, (b) the situated hermeneutic knowledge for the referential cognitive need, (c) the critical hermeneutic knowledge for the transformative cognitive need, (d) the ethical knowledge for the normative cognitive need, and (e) the aesthetic knowledge for the desiderative cognitive need.

The instrumental role of knowledge for nursing practice can be further differentiated into two types: one regarding the knowledge necessary for attaining general modes of practice applicable across all clinical nursing situations, and the other for the knowledge necessary to address specialized needs of particular clinical situations. Nursing practice involves applying general nursing approaches (such as those identified as the essential tools of nursing practice) that are applicable across various clinical nursing situations and at the same time applying specific strategies and methods to address specific and specialized needs apparent in each clinical nursing situation. Therefore, for this instrumental role of knowledge, there is a need for knowledge to be applied in carrying out general nursing approaches, and at the same time for knowledge to be applied with an orientation to address the specific nature of different clinical situations. Therefore, knowledge is applied instrumentally in general approaches, such as nursing process, clinical decision making, general assessment, clinical evaluation, caring approaches, comforting and protecting, nursing communication, teaching, advocating, and collaboration. In addition, knowledge is applied instrumentally to address particular situation-specific clinical issues, for example, pain assessment, respiratory care, and diabetic teaching.

The knowledge for this instrumental role encompasses both general and specialized knowledge in five types in order to address the five cognitive needs. For example, the knowledge necessary for application in nursing practice in the care of Mr. Baxter (see Chapter 7), with a focus on the instrumental role, is given in Table 10.1. While it is not exhaustive, it reveals many different

**TABLE 10.1 A List of Knowledge Applicable in the Care of Mr. Baxter in Relation to the Instrumental Role of Knowledge**

| COGNITIVE NEED TYPE | KNOWLEDGE FOR THE INSTRUMENTAL ROLE | |
|---|---|---|
| | **GENERAL** | **SPECIFIC** |
| **Inferential Cognitive Need** | Theories of human nature<br>Theories of health and illness<br>Theories of recovery<br>Theories of self-care<br>Theories of practice<br>Theories of nursing intervention<br>Theories of comfort and safety<br>Theories of caring<br>Theories of decision making<br>Theories of teaching and learning<br>Theories of communication | Theories of stroke, fatigue, and depression<br>Theories of stroke trajectory and recovery<br>Theories of stroke therapy<br>Theories of speech and speech therapy<br>Theories of pain and pain therapy<br>Psychosocial theories of disability and chronicity<br>Theories of stroke rehabilitation<br>Theories of prevention in relation to regurgitation, immobility, skin integrity, and musculoskeletal integrity |
| **Referential Cognitive Need** | Meanings of health and illness in life<br>Narratives of recovery<br>Narratives of support and caring<br>Narratives of personalization in practice | Stroke narratives<br>Chronic illness narratives<br>Stroke rehabilitation narratives<br>Narratives of pain, fatigue, depression, and communication difficulties<br>Narratives of sudden health changes |
| **Transformative Cognitive Need** | Critical theories of human communication<br>Critical theories of social roles<br>Critical theories of independence/dependence<br>Critical theories of professional domination<br>Theories of human comporting | Critical theories of role change in illness<br>Critical theories of stroke perception<br>Critical theories of dependence in stroke |
| **Normative Cognitive Need** | Ethical theories of therapy and care<br>Ethical standards for autonomy, beneficence, justice, dignity, fidelity, and care<br>Ethics of professional conduct<br>Standards for ethical decision making | Ethics of truth telling<br>Ethics of sharing information |
| **Desiderative Cognitive Need** | Theories of creativity<br>Theories of aesthetic expression and communication<br>Theories of empathy<br>Theories of sensibility | Theories of understanding stroke experience<br>Theories of tailoring communication with patients who have had a stroke |

types of knowledge that needs to be drawn in order to meet the demands of this clinical situation. The actual application occurs in the processes of deliberation and enactment in nursing practice for Mr. Baxter, and the knowledge becomes interwoven in the processes of deliberation and enactment in practice to reveal the dimensional characteristics. Application of knowledge in practice is therefore expressed with qualitative variations in nursing practice in terms of scientific, technical, ethical, aesthetic, and existential dimensions.

In singular clinical situations nurses need to draw knowledge that is characteristically identified in the five spheres (i.e., the generalized, situated hermeneutic, critical hermeneutic, ethical, and aesthetic knowledge spheres) in order to satisfy the cognitive needs for practice. The knowledge applied at the foundational level to develop commitments to the perspectives, the philosophies of practice, and the practice dimensions is also related to these five cognitive needs but with a broader, general orientation. Nurses must not only draw from such diverse bases of knowledge, but also must synthesize them to address demands of the clinical situation at hand. It means then that the ultimate synthesizer and knowledge user is the nurse in practice. Practicing nurses must be able to come to understand and analyze the critical aspects of her or his client, the situation, and her or his own practice by dissecting different aspects of them drawing on various sorts of knowledge. And this is followed by actions in *their practice* that are based on decisions for the goals established for nursing care by layering and knitting together this understanding/analysis and a complex set of knowledge for various nursing approaches. Professional practice needs to be intentional in this sense.

Synthesis of knowledge in practice involves bringing forth knowledge that exists in many different sectors (i.e., the knowledge in the public domain and the knowledge in their private domains) to bear relevance in specific situations, and knowledge use in practice involves incorporating various types of knowledge (i.e., content) into nursing work carried out in specific situations. The process of knowledge synthesis and knowledge use is not necessarily carried out consciously, systematically, programmatically, or overtly. This is carried out generally "without seams," sometimes systematically, and other times innovatively or haphazardly. Of course, this process is not too different from the knowledge synthesis and knowledge use done in our ordinary life situations—such as in parenting, working with our tools, or solving everyday problems. We do not necessarily talk about theory–practice linkage in ordinary life situations, although that could be the focus of study in cognitive science or human action studies. The reason why we need to address this issue in nursing is because our actions must be goal directed and based on specialized knowledge.

# PROCESSES OF KNOWLEDGE APPLICATION IN NURSING PRACTICE

## Knowledge Synthesis

As shown in Figure 10.1, knowledge application in nursing practice involves the processes of knowledge synthesis and of knowledge use. Knowledge synthesis that must occur in individual practitioners involves a three-step process. First, new knowledge is selected for possible incorporation into the private knowledge domain; second, it is evaluated to be valuable, essential, meaningful, and important for practice; and third, it is incorporated and integrated into the existing personal knowledge. This three-step process is analytically separated into three steps; however, the process may not occur serially or systematically in actual practice. There are two sources of knowledge for knowledge synthesis—knowledge in the public domain and knowledge in the private domain gained through personal experiences. In addition, the meaning of knowledge plays an important role regardless of whether it is in relation to the knowledge of the public or the private domain in this process of knowledge synthesis. Knowledge synthesis with three sequential steps of selection, evaluation, and integration is depicted in Figure 10.3.

Knowledge synthesis is a process involving the source and characteristics/meaning of new knowledge in individual's encounters and engagements with new knowledge. This framework can be used to examine knowledge synthesis from an individual perspective, with a possibility for addressing factors that may influence the process. A three-step process involving selection, evaluation, and integration is posed in relation to the three aspects of knowledge, that is, public knowledge, private knowledge, and the meaning of knowledge. In addition, these three processes (i.e., selection, evaluation, and integration) are guided by specific attitudinal variables as the governing principles. The process of selection is guided by the attitude of *openness*, which allows individuals to be either ready or closed for incorporation of new knowledge, whether it is new theory, new piece of research, or new experience. The openness of individuals is influenced not only by persons' individuality such as past experiences, commitment to certain philosophies and perspectives, or personality traits, but also by social structural forces that exist in the usual practice settings that foster either openness or closeness. The process of evaluation is guided by the attitude of *critique*, which is a discriminatory attitude toward new knowledge and guides determination of the value, relevance, utility, and fittingness of knowledge in general and to a nurse for his or her practice. The attitude of critique is influenced by analytical abilities as well as the

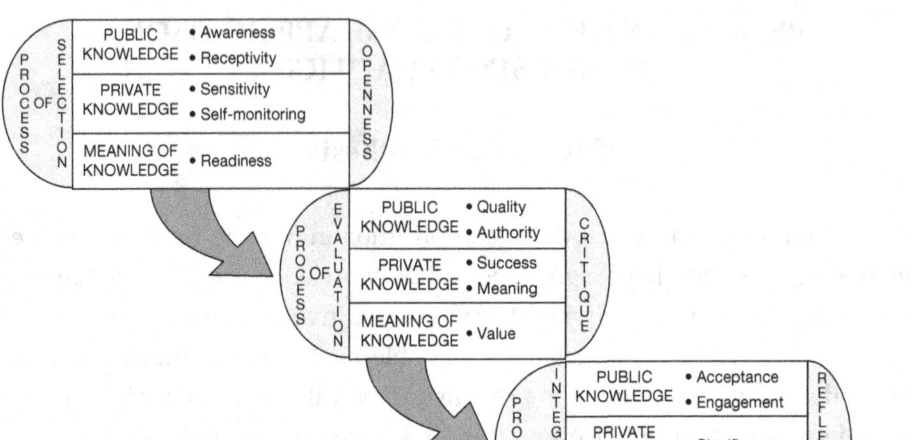


**FIGURE 10.3** The processes of knowledge synthesis.

nature of one's current personal knowledge, and supportive mechanisms that exist for evaluation (such as computer programs, journals, and peer-review groups). The process of integration is guided by the attitude of *reflection*, which allows a conscious posing of new knowledge in relation to what already exists. Reflection or reflexibility is influenced by a person's attitude toward himself or herself, reflexive habit, learning, and external support.

Knowledge synthesis involving knowledge in the public domain is viewed by many as critical for professional practice, since knowledge is continuously revised and expanded, and there is a need for professionals to be up-to-date in their knowledge base. Although knowledge synthesis of the knowledge in the public domain is an individualistic process, it is primarily influenced by the contents of the public knowledge. Contents of the public knowledge are continuously updated by the process of *evidence-based* codifying of knowledge. Here the term "evidence" is used to denote "facts" (or knowledge) out in the public domain, differentiated from those belonging to individual practitioners and local situations. Evidential knowledge in this sense refers to those that have been scrutinized for public displays (in print, presentations, or other forms) by various evaluative means such as peer review processes, consensus conferences, and expert panels. This use of the term "evidence" is different from various other ways of conceptualizing evidence in which individual expertise is also viewed as evidence.

Knowledge generation within a discipline is selectively done for various reasons, such as the maturity of a given subject matter or epistemic urgency for gaining answers to problems (e.g., the current emphasis on the problems of older age), funding resources, social mandates, researchers' orientations, fads, and public policy agendas or priorities. Knowledge accumulation is also influenced by selectivity, most often by language (e.g., non-English publications are often ignored), biases introduced by a prevailing scientific orientation (such as positivism) used to determine the quality of "evidence," and acceptance of certain review methods (e.g., a specific method of meta-analysis or the Cochrane formula). In addition, massive and continuing output of knowledge in the public domain needs to be reviewed and evaluated in order to update and systematize the knowledge base for practice collectively. Knowledge of all five types (generalized, situated hermeneutic, critical hermeneutic, ethical, and aesthetic knowledge) specified in Chapter 4, which are relevant to nursing practice and are developed and "evidenced" in the literature, must be evaluated continuously in order to revise, expand, and update them. Since the modes and methods with which different types of knowledge are developed differ considerably, there are different sets of criteria to judge the maturity of "evidence" in the literature rather than accepting the supremacy of one method of evidence generation (e.g., randomized controlled study) and evaluation for all types of knowledge.

Knowledge synthesis for individual practitioners involving the first step of selection in relation to the public knowledge, therefore, involves selectivity carried out at the disciplinary level as described previously, and selectivity at the individual practitioner level regarding selection of knowledge for integration into the practitioner's private knowledge domain. Selection of knowledge at the individual level is greatly influenced by the awareness of new knowledge through exposures and the receptivity toward new knowledge, which may encourage or discourage seeking of new knowledge by practitioners. The second step in knowledge synthesis involving the public knowledge is individual nurses' evaluation of knowledge in terms of quality and authority. When a nurse encounters new knowledge in books or journals, at conferences or in conversations with colleagues, or through the Internet, it is evaluated for its quality and authority. As this process in general is unsystematic in practice, most of the knowledge utilization models have advocated for the importance of this step by introducing various methods of knowledge (research) evaluation. Various criteria for evaluating the quality and authority regarding newly encountered knowledge have been suggested, and the continuing expansion of the Cochrane system is one approach to offer an "authoritative" evaluation that can be used to bypass individual practitioners' evaluations.

The third step in knowledge synthesis, which is the step of integration, is the focal process that brings knowledge into the private knowledge domain from the public arena. A great deal of this integration is accomplished through formal and informal learning. Learning occasions expose nurses to preselected knowledge that is transmitted for integration into private knowledge systems. Integrating specific knowledge to become a part of a person's private knowledge domain depends on the degree of individuals' acceptance of and familiarity with the knowledge. To individual practitioners, evidential knowledge that goes through the selection process at the first step in relation to substantive contents and the evaluation step for making judgments about values is again subject to selectivity at the integration step.

The Internet availability of up-to-date review information and practice guidelines/recommendations through the use of handheld computer tablets at bedside especially in health care practice has been one attempt to control such selectivity in synthesis, and make information readily available to be used in practice. Of course, reviews and guidelines that exist in such databases have also been collected through selective processes. Hence, knowledge synthesis involving knowledge in the public domain is influenced by both social and public forces and individual-specific factors. Because of such selectivity, it is imperative that each professional practitioner be aware of the nature of selectivity and become an astute and responsible knowledge synthesizer.

Knowledge synthesis of personal experiences has often been depicted as the process of expertise building or developing practical knowledge. Professional, clinical experiences are thought to be the most meaningful cognitive elements individuals retain as scripts, patterns, and information in various studies (see, for example, Benner, 1984; Dreyfus, 1979). Synthesis of personal experiences also goes through the steps of selection, evaluation, and integration. Personal experiences that become synthesized solidly in a person's private knowledge domain are those "registered" as significant experiences through one's own sensitivity and self-monitoring (the selection step), and inherently encompass the success achieved in fulfilling the goals associated with the experiences and a significance in the meanings of the experiences to the practitioner (the evaluation step). Such experiences become integrated into the individual's private knowledge domain (the integration step). The significance of the experiences to the practitioner is the major criterion of what experiences become integrated into the private knowledge domain. This process of synthesizing one's own personal experiences into one's knowledge domain is rather informal and unsystematic. Conscious registration of the meaning of personal experiences, whether they are ordinary life experiences or are those in professional practice, occurs neither in a systematic nor in an automatic fashion. Impressions of experiences are registered into our cognitive system with varying levels of our own awareness. There are disputes as to how this process occurs naturally in persons and whether or not "strong" evaluation regarding meaning and success is at the base for which experiences become integrated in personal domains. The notion of vicarious learning also complicates our understanding of this process. However, it is generally accepted that knowledge synthesis of personal experiences does not occur with all experiences. For example, action science proponents point out that practitioners may be stuck in Model I learning mode, repeating practice behaviors that are routinized (Argyris & Schön, 1974; Argyris, Putnam, & Smith, 1985). This means that there is a need for a specific process that encourages knowledge synthesis of clinical experiences. Kim (1999) suggests the method of critical reflective inquiry (CRI) as a conscious, intentional way of examining a professional's practice so that day-to-day experiences of practice are reflected and evaluated in order to determine good practice from bad and to be able to synthesize new learning that adds to the existing knowledge. This is presented in the last section of this chapter.

Knowledge synthesis as a way for professionals' knowledge base to be updated is critical in making the professional practitioner an effective and efficient knowledge-based practitioner. This depends upon the *content* of knowledge and evidence that is synthesized, which is critically influenced by the *process* of synthesizing. Knowledge synthesis involving the public and the private knowledge depends most critically upon the meaning of knowledge to individuals. Such factors as (a) receptivity and readiness to revise one's knowledge; (b) value, relevance, meaning, and fittingness of new knowledge with what already exists; and (c) one's philosophies and attitudes may impact the process of synthesis. Knowledge synthesis as the first step in the knowledge use in practice greatly determines what knowledge is used in actual practice.

This exposition gives us awareness that knowledge synthesis is complex as it involves individuals, context, experience, and knowledge, and is a continuing, individualistic process. Current controversies in cognitive science and philosophy of knowledge, especially regarding the workings of the mind and the relationship between thoughts and actions, complicate our understanding of knowledge synthesis as a process in professional practitioners. Although the representation-computational approaches of the mind in which thinking is conceptualized to be the workings of representational structures of the mind and computation based on the mind's syntactic, compositional, and combinatorial abilities has been the dominant approach for our understanding of thinking (Fordor, 1981, 2000; Pinker, 1997), there are various issues that are not accounted for in this purely cognitivistic approach to thinking. Some controversies, such as the role of free will, intentionality, and consciousness; the notion that human thinking is embedded within the environment in which it occurs; that human thoughts are not purely the workings of the mind but involving embodiment; the role of emotion on thinking; the social nature of human thoughts; and the mind viewed to work within a dynamic system process rather than on computations, complicate our understanding about how mind works and how learning and experience get into knowledge (Horst, 2011).

## Theory–Practice Gap

With the understanding from the depiction of the process that knowledge use depends greatly on the content of knowledge in the private domain, we can now turn to the major issue in the theory–practice gap discourse; that is, there is a great deal of disparity and distance between what is produced by scientists, researchers, and theorists enriching knowledge base in the public domain and what is integrated and incorporated into the private domains of practitioners. Frameworks for "innovation diffusion" used by Rogers (1983) or information dissemination try to mend the gap in practitioners' knowledge vis-à-vis the public knowledge. In nursing, many writers have focused on this aspect of theory–practice linkage in discussing the theory–practice gap. The fault (if we can call it "fault") has been attributed to practitioners' inability to understand research or their lack of exposure to new knowledge, as well as to the remoteness of new knowledge or research from practice problems, obtrusiveness of research, or abstract nature of theories (see, e.g., Hunt, 1996). In addition, social or structural forces that exist in the context of nursing practice, and the educational process of nursing, have also been thought to increase this gap (McCloskey, 2008; Rafferty, Allcock, & Lathlean, 1996; Stetler, 2003).

Nursing has attempted to remedy this gap with many different programs and models during the past several decades. Most of these programs and models are aimed at increasing assimilation of knowledge, which in turn would result in changes in practice. These models can be grouped into three types: (a) innovation diffusion models, (b) facilitation models, and (c) individual assimilation models. Most of the models proposed in nursing incorporate both the knowledge-synthesis and knowledge-use aspects, but consider the knowledge-synthesis aspect as an important dimension in the use of new knowledge in practice.

Innovation diffusion models are oriented to disseminating new innovations and research through organized processes, such as through continuing education or staff development programs that were institutionalized within the nursing service structure during the 1970s, as the source through which nurses are expected to gain new knowledge and assimilate them for use in their practice. Staff development programs at local institutions were considered a more appropriate source for knowledge, as the programs they offered were thought to be more relevant to local needs. In addition, several research utilization models developed in nursing in the 1970s and 1980s were oriented to selection, dissemination, and use of research findings. The models developed during this period, such as the Western Interstate Commission for Higher Education (WICHE) model, Nursing Child Assessment Satellite Training (NCAST)-related projects, Conduct and Utilization of Research in Nursing (CURN) project, and other hybrid models are basically oriented to selection and dissemination of research findings through organized processes, often involving nurses in practice directly in selection, translation, and dissemination of new findings and innovations. The major assumption for these models is that research findings and new knowledge must be made relevant to practice and brought closer to actual users by translating them to be understandable, incorporable, and readily usable. While the continuing education programs tended to be expert-oriented programs, these dissemination models used "bridges" to connect research to individual practitioners—bridges of people involvement such as selected staff as members of research review committees, and bridges of translation for easy understanding and local relevance.

Facilitation models are much more globally oriented to knowledge synthesis and knowledge use. Kitson (1998) has proposed one of the most comprehensive facilitation models. Kitson (in the Royal College of Nursing Institute project, Kitson, Ahmed, Harvey, Seers, & Thompson, 1996; Kitson, 1998) identifies three components within a conceptual framework for enabling successful implementation of research into practice: evidence, context, and facilitation. In the dimension of *evidence*, three components are viewed to be variables—research evidence must be systematic, clinicians must have consensus and a consistent view about the innovation, and clients must accept the innovation that is viewed to result from partnerships in its development. *Context* as the environment is considered within this model as the setting in which change through the use of new knowledge must come about. Context is identified in terms of culture, leadership, and measurement (routine monitoring of systems and services). *Facilitation* is a process through which key individuals work to bring about changes in staff, and involves characteristics, role, and style of facilitator.

This is a model that sees research implementation from an organizational and external perspective.

Unlike the innovation diffusion and facilitation models, individual synthesis models focus on individual practitioners as the primary target for knowledge gain and assimilation. Stetler (1994) and Brown (2013) have proposed prescriptive models to specify processes that can be used by practitioners to gain new knowledge, assimilate it, and use it in practice in a systematic way. Stetler (1994) specifies six phases in her individual-oriented model—preparation, validation, comparative evaluation, decision making for possible use, translation/application, and evaluation. Brown's model for research-based practice (2013) also specifies steps necessary for applying new evidence or research into practice. From a different perspective, Rolfe (1996, 1998) suggests that nursing must develop "informal" theories developed from practice within the reflexive praxis. His contention is that the primary type and source of knowledge for practice should come from reflexive practice, and would be personally "referential" in nature.

## Knowledge Use

While knowledge synthesis into one's personal knowledge base is diffuse and general, knowledge use in practice is specific and situation oriented. Knowledge is "used" in human practice, whether it is an ordinary, everyday practice such as cooking and communicating, or a highly specialized professional practice such as nursing and other health care practices. Knowledge use in professional practice is critical because it refers to the use of specialized, professional knowledge, and it has implications in practice outcomes.

The main question of how knowledge that one possesses is used in actual practice has been answered in various ways by theories and research. Recent development in cognitive science suggests, first of all, that the human brain as a store house and as a processing machine engages in various shortcut techniques to bypass elaborate processing of information within the constraints of short-term and long-term memory and the brain's computational capabilities (Pinker, 1997). For example, cognitive heuristics have been identified as shortcuts humans use in making decisions, selecting alternatives, and conceptualizing situations (Kahneman, Tversky, & Slovic, 1982). At the same time, retrieving and selecting knowledge for use in specific instances are influenced by various situational contingencies, personal characteristics such as likes/dislikes, emotional stability, fatigue, or competency level, and contextual factors as well as the content and structure of private knowledge and specific working knowledge incited in given situations.

Benner's work (1984, 2009) furthermore suggested that nurses' modes of engagement in clinical situations were quite varied in relation to different constellations of personal knowledge, in that expert nurses' interpretation of situations were based on exemplars and maxims obtained through their experiences while novice nurses were engaged with their clinical situations in an analytic mode of knowledge use. While Benner distinguishes these two forms of engagement in practice in terms of novice and expert, giving a sense of approval that the expert's way of engagement is "better" or more desirable, it is not yet clear whether or not these different forms of engagement have any influences on patient-care outcomes. In addition, novices' usual mode of engagement is limited by the content and nature of formal knowledge and degree of rigor applied to situational analytics, while experts' usual mode of engagement may also be limited by the nature of exemplars in terms of their relevance to situations. This also suggests that there is a close linkage between knowledge synthesis and knowledge use in practice.

Furthermore, Argyris and Schön (1974) found that practitioner's actions are governed by theories-in-use that tend to be in place without conscious awareness by practitioners, and often theories-in-use are quite different from the practitioners' espoused theories. Theories-in-use in general also tend to be what they call Model I type, oriented to self-interest and closed toward new learning. Routinization in practice is common, suggesting the repeated use of the same set of knowledge.

These findings and related theories suggest that humans' use of knowledge in practice is varied and constrained by both internal factors belonging to practitioners such as the quality of personal knowledge base and habits, and external forces that exist in the immediate and remote environments such as specific clinical settings, unit culture, professional value systems, or practice cultures. Furthermore, because knowledge in the private domain that includes both formal and experiential knowledge is not systematically structured, and is blended together into a global, unstructured integration, accessing and using knowledge may not be very systematic. In view of these issues, it is only possible to depict knowledge use in practice in an *analytic* model described by Kim (1993), which may be quite different from how it actually occurs. This analytic model specifies how practitioners may systematically access knowledge for different purposes in the process of nursing practice, and is offered in the absence of a credible descriptive model. An analytic model can be used as a frame to describe varying characteristics of the process, because the process is not at all linear and knowledge accessing is often not an overtly intentional act. This analysis will show how complex the process of knowledge use is in practice, and also that a practitioner's knowledge in its content and structure is an intricate part of that process (Figure 10.4).

As a nurse encounters a clinical situation, she or he postures herself or himself toward the situation based on her or his perspectives and orientations by registering and selecting relevant aspects of the situation in order to narrow its scope to fit into nursing, her or his role, and clinical practice. This first step (Step 1) results in the practitioner's view (perception or definition) of the clinical situation at hand, and is viewed to be guided by the nurse's commitment to and the characterization of the philosophies of practice, that is, the philosophies of care, therapy, and professional role as well as the nursing perspective. In Step 1, knowledge is used to select relevant aspects of the situation for attention, circumscribing the direction and scope of attention to the clinical situation. This selective attention can be narrow or broad, one-sided or

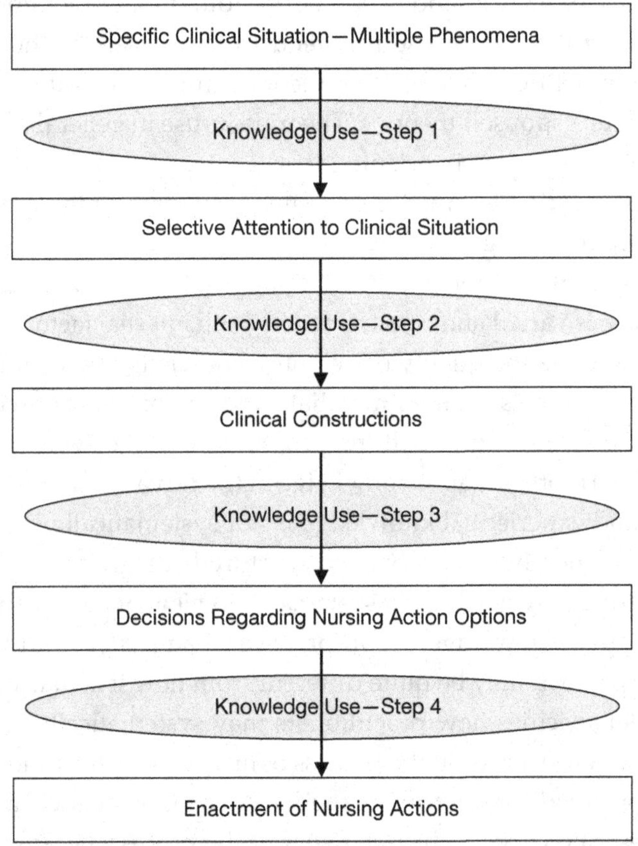


**FIGURE 10.4** Analytical steps in knowledge use in clinical practice.

comprehensive, depending on one's given perspective (including priorities) of viewing the clinical situation. To a degree, it is always a selective attention. In this step, the overriding sector of knowledge used may be foundational constituting one's philosophies and priority orientations.

In Step 2, the practitioner uses knowledge to deal with the perceptions of the clinical situation in order to understand the meaning and nature of the situation and arrive at framing of the situation resulting in clinical construction. This framing involves how the practitioner must understand the meaning of the situation within the perspective. Practitioners have to make inferences about the situation in order to understand and/or explain it, and incite references that can illuminate the situation further, and has been viewed as clinical construction by Ellefsen and Kim (2004) guided by the nursing gaze (Ellefsen, 2004; Ellefsen & Kim, 2005). The outcomes of Step 2, hence, are identification of problems, needs, and meanings of the situation gained through inferences and references made with the knowledge that is available to the person. The process at this step is conceptualized as clinical reasoning, clinical inferencing, or diagnosing in the literature, resulting often in problem formulations or diagnoses.

In Step 3, the practitioner is involved in selecting or making commitment to actions (i.e., strategies, approaches, or interventions) within the frame of identified problems, needs, and meanings of the situation. This step involves decision making in relation to selecting intervention strategies to solve specific problems, or selecting approaches for patient care. This step is most often identified as the core in evidence-based practice. Similarly, in Step 4, the practitioner, given the action choices, must bring about nursing actions by coordinating actions with what exist in the situation of practice. This again involves the use of knowledge, especially practical knowledge that guides behaviors, and for mediating enactments within given clinical contexts.

This depiction certainly is an extremely linear, rational, and rigid way of viewing the process. *No one would apply knowledge into practice in this way.* But, this analysis suggests two important points: Knowledge use depends on "what exists in the private domain of knowledge as an available source" and "how it is incited to have meanings to a given situation of practice." The first has to do with the content, while the second has to do with the modes of application. The content points to the richness or lack thereof, while the modes point to cognitive needs with which certain knowledge must be used—that is, to make inferences about, to gain insights through references, to arrive at meaningful human-to-human engagement in practice, and to attain the right and desirable forms of practice. This means that professional practitioners including nurses have to be concerned not only with the amount and variety of knowledge they must possess or develop, but also for what purpose that knowledge must be gained.

Examination of knowledge–practice linkage from this global perspective points to the need for us not only to examine how we synthesize and use knowledge in practice, but also to pay attention to what kinds of knowledge and for what purposes we must develop our knowledge. We must be cautioned, however, that not all knowledge is valuable or relevant, and this applies both to the knowledge in the public domain and that in the private domain. In general, there are in place various evaluative methods and processes to scrutinize knowledge in the public domain, while the knowledge from personal experiences is not naturally exposed to any specific evaluative methods, except by individuals. Experience-based knowledge must also be examined and considered with an equal skepticism for its value.

## CRITICAL REFLECTIVE INQUIRY IN NURSING PRACTICE[1]

The critical component in the knowledge synthesis for practice is the nurse's personal knowledge and the public knowledge of all types. The work of Benner (1984, 2009) has suggested that nurses at various levels of expertise are engaged in this synthesis with different processing. Gadow from a different perspective suggests a "clinical epistemology" to describe practitioners' synthesis in nursing assessment in which both general and particular knowledge are brought together to another level at which "knowledge is co-authored by client and nurse together in their relational narrative" (1995, p. 26). It means that nursing practice as it occurs in clinical situations is a rich source for developing clinical personal knowledge. However, it is also clear from our commonsense understandings that clinical personal knowledge is not necessarily all good and exemplary. It is only through a specific process of inquiry that we can gain access to the nature of clinical personal knowledge and be able to engage in improving our practice. The hallmark of knowledge-based practice is in the conscious assessment of the knowledge applied in practice, and such assessment can be accessed only through an intentional process of self-examination of one's practice. From this premise the approach of CRI (Kim, 1999) was proposed to be used for an in-depth, post hoc analysis and critique of one's own practice.

Kim (1999) proposed the method of CRI as an analytic approach based on narrativity of human activity, reflection, critique, and emancipation. This method of inquiry is founded upon the ideas in action science (Argyris & Schön, 1974; Argyris et al., 1985), Schön's reflective practice (1983), critical philosophy (Habermas, 1986), and critical reflection (Freire, 1970/1992). This method is focused on not only discovering new, synthesized knowledge of good practice, but also understanding the nature and meaning of practice to

| PHASE | I Descriptive Phase | II Reflective Phase | III Critical/ Emancipatory Phase |
|---|---|---|---|
| PROCESSES | • Description of practice events (actions, thoughts, and feelings)<br>• Examination of descriptions for genuineness, completeness, and comprehensiveness | • Reflective analysis against espoused theories (inferential, referential, transformative, ethical, and aesthetic theories)<br>• Reflective analysis of situation<br>• Reflective analysis of intentions, attitudes, values, and emotions | • Critique of practice regarding inadequacies, conflicts, distortions, and inconsistencies<br>• Engagement in emancipatory, transformative, and change processes<br>• Description of practice models |
| PRODUCTS | • Descriptive narratives (scripts) | • Knowledge about practice processes and applications<br>• Self-awareness and self-understanding | • Learning and change in practice<br>• Self-critique and emancipation<br>• Synthesized models of practice |

**FIGURE 10.5** Phases in critical reflective inquiry.

practitioners, and correcting and improving the practice through self-reflection and critique.

The method includes: (a) the *descriptive phase* for narratives or scripting, (b) the *reflective phase* for reflection and analysis, and (c) the *critical/emancipatory phase* for critique and emancipation as three distinct but interrelated phases (Figure 10.5). Through these phases a clinician gains critical knowledge of synthesis in practice, attains insights into inadequacies and shortcomings in practice, and engages himself or herself in self-corrective learning.

The descriptive phase (Phase I) involves a thorough narrative description by the practitioner of a specific instance, situation, or case of practice. The reflective phase (Phase II) involves a careful analysis of the narrative in a reflective mode with three different foci: (a) reflecting against standards or the "espoused theories" in the action science perspective, (b) reflecting on situation, and (c) reflecting on intentions. From the knowledge development perspective, this phase is involved in identifying how the synthesis of knowledge occurs in practice. From this phase, models of "good" practice, theories of application, and knowledge regarding the process of practice can be identified and constructed. It is also possible to discover omissions, deviations from the optimum, systematic inconsistencies, "poor" practice, or ineffectual routinization that exist in practice. The third phase is the critical/emancipatory phase (Phase III), which is oriented to correcting and changing less-than-good or ineffective practice, or moving forward to future assimilation of new innovations emerging in practice. This phase involves critical discourses that are aimed at discovering the nature and sources of distortions, inconsistencies, and incongruence between the actual practice and the expected, desired, or optimal practice. The process using self-dialogue, critique, and argumentation can lead to self-emancipation regarding practice and change in practice.

Three phases of CRI are carried out by practitioners, addressing specific questions relative to each phase. The questions are guidelines for description in the descriptive phase, for assessment and reflection in the reflective phase, and for evaluation and critique in the critical/emancipatory phase. The following are guiding questions to be addressed in each of the three phases of CRI in clinical application (taken from Kim, Lauzon Clabo, Burbank, Leveillee, & Martins, 2010).

### Descriptive Phase—Construction of Narratives of Practice (Scripting)

1. Is this an accurate description of what existed in the situation (features, circumstances, and other environmental aspects) at the time?
2. Is my preunderstanding of the situation accurately depicted?
3. Does this depict a truthful and accurate description of actions of myself and others (behaviors, happenings, speech, and interactions)?
4. Is this a truthful and accurate description of my thoughts of the time? Did I invent any of the thoughts included in this description? Did I omit any of the thoughts that existed at the time?
5. Is this a truthful and accurate description of my feelings at the time? Did I invent any of the feelings included in this description? Did I exaggerate or minimize my feelings at that time in any way? Did I omit any of my feelings that were felt at the time?

### Reflective Phase—Reflection on Action in Relation to Espoused Theories, Situations, and Intentions

1. What did I believe guided my actions (or inactions)?
2. What do I think guided my actions as I think back now?
3. What knowledge informed my actions?
4. What was the knowledge that was important in this situation? Why was this knowledge important?
5. Did I possess the knowledge required in this situation?
6. What sorts of values or ethical standards guided my actions?

7. How did these values or ethical standards determine my actions?
8. How was my "self" revealed in this situation?
9. Were my actions harmonious with the situation? How so?
10. What did I think were the salient features of the situation I faced?
11. Why did I think those were the salient features?
12. What aspects of the situation influenced my actions? In what ways and why?
13. What were my intentions in that situation? What did I want from my actions?
14. Were my intentions in agreement with the client's goals?
15. Why did I carry out the actions in the way I did in that situation?
16. What were the outcomes of the situation I wanted?
17. Did I get the outcomes I wanted in this situation?
18. To what extent did I not get the outcomes I wanted? Why not?

## Critical Phase—Critique for Change and Improvement, and Identification of Good Practice

1. Were my actions in this situation the best, most appropriate, and successful? If so, what caused them? If not, what were the reasons?
2. To the extent that I got the outcomes I wanted in this situation, were the outcomes the most appropriate and desirable ones? From whose perspectives? Were there other outcomes that I should have considered?
3. Did I use the knowledge appropriately? Do I know what I did not know in the situation?
4. Were the types of knowledge applied in the situation the most appropriate ones?
5. Do I need to revise my knowledge base? If so, in what ways and why?
6. Did I apply the most appropriate set of ethical values and standards in the situation? Are there other ethical values and standards with which I should have acted in the situation? If so, what are these and why are they important? Why did I miss them?
7. Do I need to rethink my values and attitudes? If so, about what, how, and why?
8. What have I learned from this situation?
9. How could I change my practice in the future?
10. Do I need to seek to become authentic in myself? If so, how can I accomplish it?
11. What were the critical factors that got in the way of my doing a better job? Why?

Application of CRI in clinical practice is an important approach for both clinicians and students to remain in a learning mode, to facilitate what Argyris and colleagues (1985) refer to as Model II learning, in which one is open to self-monitoring, self-correction, and generativity in practice. CRI not only provides opportunities for clinicians (or students) to examine their use of knowledge in practice, their attitudes and values that enter into practice, and their competence, but it also leads them to rethink their relationships with clients, awakening them to clients' perspectives and bringing clients' knowledge and meanings into the design and action in practice. Through the application of CRI in clinical practice, a clinician becomes what Schön (1983) calls a "researcher-in-practice." The goal is in line with the notion that "when a practitioner becomes a researcher into his own practice, he engages in a continuing process of self-education" and "when he functions as a researcher-in-practice, the practice itself is a source of renewal" (Schön, 1983, p. 299). This process of integrating the method into practice is important as both reflection and self-critique are not necessarily the intrinsic modes of our usual actions. An assimilation of this mode of inquiry as a part of a clinician's practice is a way to promote learning mode as a natural stance in practice. By assimilating this mode of inquiry into one's practice, the clinician practices in an open learning mode, continuously scripting, reflecting, and critiquing his or her practice. The clinician becomes a critically reflective practitioner who is engaged in discovering self in practice in terms of actions, thoughts, feelings, and attitudes, and is able to look upon his or her own actions in a detached, open stance so that his or her own practice is evaluated for quality, satisfaction, and completeness. As the clinician becomes well assimilated into this inquiry method, it also is possible for him or her to identify clinical personal knowledge that is exemplary. As the clinician practices in the mode of CRI, he or she is less likely to become entrenched with closed-end routinization and unilaterally oriented to self in relationships, and more likely to stay open to learning and self-correction in practice.

## SUMMARY AND QUESTIONS FOR REFLECTION AND FURTHER DELIBERATION

Orienting nursing practice as *knowledge-based practice* can awaken the discipline to accept the pluralistic nature of nursing knowledge needed for practice, and to develop understandings about knowledge synthesis and use, which are critical for responsible professional practice. The processes depicted in the preceding sections regarding both knowledge synthesis and knowledge use are complex and require individual practitioners' intentional engagements.

This means that ultimately it is individual nurses who are responsible for shaping and updating their personal knowledge necessary for responsible practice, and who are using knowledge in practice with varying degree or intention. As analytic models the models only provide the logic of the processes and cannot give full accounts of variations in professionals' knowledge synthesis and use in nursing practice. Although there is a need to develop descriptive theories regarding knowledge synthesis and use, what is necessary more urgently is the commitment of practitioners (nurses) to being responsible agents of knowledge synthesis and use. This will lead to continuous seeking of better methods of review and evaluation and open-mindedness regarding all sorts of knowledge as well as engaging in a critically reflective mode of practice for more effective and efficient use of knowledge embedded in continuously changing clinical situations.

- Can you point out differences between knowledge-based practice and evidence-based practice? Are these two concepts only semantically different? If not, what is your position regarding these two concepts?
- In thinking about a recent incident of nursing practice involving a client, can you list the types of the knowledge that were applied? Can you think about the ways in which you accessed the knowledge? In what ways were the knowledge used; for example, for enlightenment, understanding, explanation, design of nursing actions, implementations, and evaluative decisions?
- How do you involve yourself in the process of knowledge synthesis to advance your practice? What processes of review and critique do you use to assess the value of newly encountered knowledge such as new research?
- How do your experiences in nursing practice become your knowledge base for practice?
- What is your understanding of phronesis and your views on the role of phronesis in nursing practice?
- What is the stock of knowledge you hold that is ready for application to your practice?

## NOTE

1. This section is adapted from Kim (1999).

# CHAPTER 11

# Competence and Expertise in Nursing Practice, and Quality of Nursing Practice

THE CONCEPT OF PROFESSIONAL COMPETENCE IS fundamentally based on the concept of personal competence for individuals for effective functioning in their personal and social lives. The Organisation for Economic Co-operation and Development (OECD) member countries in 1997 launched the Programme for International Student Assessment (PISA), which generated the OECD's Definition and Selection of Competencies as the outcomes of mandatory education at the international level, which include competencies that "must contribute to valued outcomes for societies and individuals, to help individuals meet important demands in a wide variety of context, and to be important not just for specialists, but for all individuals" (OECD, 2005). This report specifies three generic competencies: (a) ability to use a wide range of tools for interacting effectively with the environment, (b) ability to engage with others in an increasingly interdependent world, and (c) ability to take responsibility for managing individuals' own lives, situate their lives in the broader social context, and act autonomously (OECD, 2005). Although these are competencies at the general and preprofessional level, it is possible to apply them to conceptualize professional competence. Professional competence viewed from this framework can be considered in terms of the use of specialized tools of the profession, the demands for interaction and relationships in the context of professional practice, and the specialized responsibilities associated with professional roles.

The concepts of competence, expertise, and quality in relation to nursing practice refer to how well nurses practice in meeting the demands of their roles

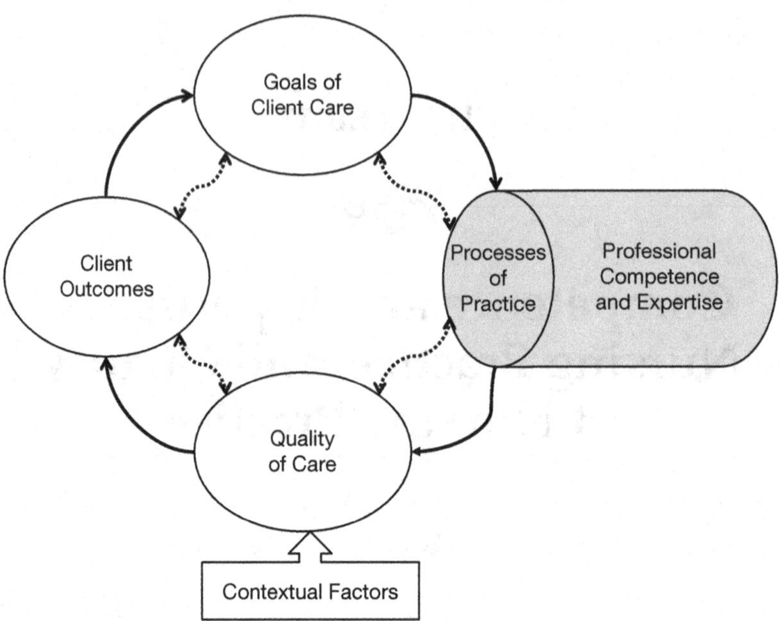


**FIGURE 11.1** Relationships among goals, practice processes, quality, and outcomes.

in nursing practice and in producing expected outcomes in clients. While nursing competence refers to the achievement of qualities in knowledge, skills, and attitudes to produce effective, safe, and meaningful nursing practice, nursing expertise is usually viewed in terms of a higher level of such qualities that goes beyond the level of standard achievement. The interrelationships among these concepts are shown in Figure 11.1.

Competence in professional practice is action oriented, which is a melding of knowledge, attitudes, and skills, and is expressed in terms of "competencies" in various action domains such as decision making, interactions and relationships, knowledge use, clinical approaches, and so forth. In a professional practice such as nursing, competence at the beginning level of practice is gained through education, and is legally governed by either licensure or professional standards or both. Competence and expertise are in the same domain of professional performance, which are the property (or capability) in professional practitioners. How the processes of professional practice occur in clinical situations depend upon the competence and expertise of professionals in addressing situation-specific goals, demands, and needs of which the goals of client care play the pivotal role. The processes of practice assume variations in the quality of care in nursing practice, which is intrinsically related to client outcomes. Competence and expertise are generic in the sense that these remain as the properties of the nurse, and only through how these are actualized in the processes of practice in specific clinical situations are they translated into the quality of practice. Hence, competence and expertise are generic qualities, whereas the quality of practice is in the actualization of such qualities in clinical situations and is connected to outcomes, most critically client outcomes.

## COMPETENCE IN NURSING PRACTICE

Most of the health professions have been struggling with the concept of professional competence during the past several decades, and have addressed this issue with fervor during the past two decades especially in relation to professional education, regulation, and quality and safety in patient care. Epstein and Hundert (2002) define professional competence in the context of medicine as "the habitual and judicious use of communication, knowledge, technical skills, clinical reasoning, emotions, values, and reflection in daily practice for the benefit of the individual and community being served," and further note that competence "depends on habits of mind, including attentiveness, critical curiosity, self-awareness, and presence" (pp. 226–227). In 2003, the Institute of Medicine (IOM) published *Health Professions Education: A Bridge to Quality* (Greiner & Knebel, 2003), which advanced the notion of core competencies for health professions. Core competencies are thought of as a common set of competencies for various health professions representing a set of knowledge, skills, and attitudes necessary for the comprehensive practice of clinical care. The core competencies identified by the IOM are (a) delivering patient-centered care, (b) working as part of interdisciplinary teams, (c) practicing evidence-based medicine, (d) focusing on quality improvement, and (e) using information technology (Greiner & Knebel, 2003). This has charted a way for nursing as well as other professions, including medicine, to identify profession-specific competencies and ways to achieve such competencies through educational programs. The American Council on Graduate Medical Education (ACGME) through its Outcome Project has established six areas of general competency for the graduates of medical training that include patient care, medical knowledge, practice-based learning and improvement, interpersonal and communication skills, professionalism, and systems-based practice. Similarly, for Canadian medical education, the CanMEDS framework has been developed that identifies seven thematic groups of competencies (i.e., "roles") for physicians including the roles of medical expert, communicator, collaborator, manager, health advocate, scholar, and professional, which are then specified in terms of essential competencies for each role (Frank, 2005). The American Psychological Association (APA) Task Force on the Assessment of Competence in Professional Psychology adopts the definition of professional competence as "complex and dynamically interactive clusters of integrated knowledge of concepts and procedures, skills and abilities, behaviors and strategies, attitudes, beliefs, and values, dispositions and personal characteristics, self-perceptions, and motivations ... that enable an individual to fully perform a task with a wide range of possible outcomes..." (APA, 2006, p. 11).

In nursing, the concept of competence has been articulated with some confusion with Benner's work on skill acquisition (1984, 2009) that identified "competent" as the third level following the levels of "novice" and "advanced beginner" and preceding the levels of "proficient" and "expert" within the Dreyfus model of skill acquisition (Dreyfus, 1979; Dreyfus & Dreyfus, 1986). In this context, "competent" is viewed as a nurse who, with 2 to 3 years of experience, sees and acts in terms of conscious, deliberate plans and adapting to varied clinical situations with a feeling of mastery and the ability to cope with and manage the many contingencies of clinical nursing incorporating previous experiences in decision making (Benner, 1984, 2009). This position has placed "competence" not as the required level of capability as beginning professional nursing practitioners, but the quality acquired through clinical experiences. Although this conceptualization continues to be applied especially in the assessment of nurses' progress toward expertise, the concept of competence in the past two decades has been identified in relation to educational achievement. Furthermore, the definition of nursing competence usually is referred back to the professional standards of nursing practice formulated by the American Nurses Association (ANA), and is considered in terms of how well nurses are able to meet these standards at the basic level (Schroeter, 2009).

Competence in nursing is generally viewed as having qualities in terms of knowledge, skills, and attitudes in nurses to practice within complex health care systems assuming the roles of professional nursing. Raines states, "competency is more than just clinical skill or theoretical knowing; it is the crossroads of knowing, doing, and being that is nursing care" (2010, p. 163). In recent years, nursing has adopted the idea of core competencies in health professions advanced by the IOM (Greiner & Knebel, 2003) as the reference point to identify competencies in nursing (AACN, 2006; Cronenwett et al., 2007). The Quality and Safety Education for Nurses (QSEN) project funded by the Robert Wood Johnson Foundation has delineated nursing-specific definitions of the five core competencies for health professions identified by the IOM to be applied in nursing education programs for curriculum development and student evaluation for competence assessment (Cronenwett et al., 2007). The American Association of Colleges of Nursing (AACN) as the major educational accrediting body in nursing has adopted competence in nursing in terms of the requirements for the attainment of profession-specific knowledge, skills, and attitudes, linking it to the design of nursing educational programs and in relation to educational outcomes, articulating also the core competencies for health professions suggested by the IOM. The AACN identified the following eight areas of competency in nursing at the generalist level (from baccalaureate education), the master's level for the clinical nurse leader role, and the doctoral level for advanced nursing practice in its publication on the essentials of nursing education (AACN, 2006, 2008, 2013):

1. General and specialized knowledge base relevant for practice
2. Organizational and systems leadership for quality care and improvement, and patient safety
3. Scholarship and evidence-based practice
4. Information and health care technologies
5. Health policy and advocacy
6. Interprofessional collaboration for improving patient and population health outcomes
7. Clinical prevention and population health
8. Knowledge, skills, and attitudes for the delivery of level-specific nursing practice (generalist, clinical nurse leader, or advanced practitioner)

The AACN identifies specific qualities in each area (i.e., knowledge, skills, and attitudes) that would indicate the level-specific competencies. The AACN clarified further the incorporation of competencies addressing the proposal by the IOM (2004a) to incorporate competencies in relation to "high quality and safe patient care" in the areas of critical thinking, health care systems and policy, communications, illness and disease management, ethics, and information and health care technologies (AACN, 2006).

The most controversial issue in relation to professional competence is how to assess competence. Competence assessment, also considered as the outcomes assessment in the educational perspective, has led specifically to the conceptualization of competence in terms of "competencies" and operationalization of them. The QSEN project delineates knowledge, skills, and attitudes for six competency areas for nursing associated with the core competencies for health professions identified by the IOM for the prelicensure nursing education (Cronenwett et al., 2007; Sullivan, Hirst, & Cronenwett, 2009) and for advanced practice nursing (Cronenwett, Sherwood, & Gelmon, 2009). From a different perspective, the Quad Council of community and public health nursing organizations established a compilation of competencies for public health nurses adopting the core competencies for public health professionals developed by the Council on Linkages (COL) between Academia and Public Health Practice (Council on Linkages between Academia and Public Health Practice, 2014). This set is specified in eight domains: (a) analytic and assessment skills, (b) policy development/program planning skills, (c) communication skills, (d) cultural competency skills, (e) community dimensions of practice skills, (f) public health science skills, (g) financial management and planning skills, and (h) leadership and systems thinking skills, identifying competency statements for each of these domains for three tiers of functioning in public health nursing.

Two approaches to competence assessment in nursing practice adopt the general categories or dimensions of nursing practice to anchor quality assessments. Meretoja, Isoaho, and Leino-Kilpi (2004) developed the Nursing Competence Scale (NCS) consisting of 73 items based on the Benner's seven domains of nursing practice for quantitative competence assessment. On the other hand, Enburg, Klein, Abdur-Rahman, Spencer, and Boyer (2009) identified eight core areas of competency as assessment and intervention skills, communication, critical thinking skills, human caring/relationship skills, teaching skills, management skills, leadership skills, and knowledge integration for their Competency Outcomes Performance Assessment (COPA) model. In addition, most educational programs are developing and applying competence assessment methods based on the operationalization of the AACN's Essentials for nursing education programs.

One major component of professional competence, which is often left out of various conceptualizations, is the competence in self-monitoring of one's own practice. Self-monitoring or reflection is a metacognitive ability to anticipate and reflect on one's own behavior. Although it is more often identified as a quality in experts, metacognition of self-monitoring and reflection is a critical aspect of professional competence. Epstein and Hundert (2002) suggest that the habits of mind including "self-awareness" influence professional competence by making professionals to evaluate, modify, and improve their practice through reflection. Reflective practice in nursing, adopting it from Schön's work (1983), has been viewed as a key mode of developing clinical competence (Kim, 1999; Liimatainen, Poskiparta, Kahlia, & Sjögren, 2001; Rolfe, 2005; Smith, 1998; Wallace, 1996). Reflectiveness in practice therefore is both a way to develop clinical competence as well as an aspect of nursing competence. It means that through nurses' critical reflections of their own practice they are able to learn from experiences, and that it is an ability that has to be cultivated and applied in practice routinely. Kim's critical reflective inquiry (1999) is one approach for self-monitoring, and its routine application in practice is critical in developing clinical competence. Competence assessment of nursing practice therefore should integrate self-monitoring and reflection as a critical component.

## EXPERTISE IN NURSING PRACTICE

Benner's work on the development of expertise in nursing (1984, 2009) has created a great deal of controversy regarding the concept of nursing expertise (Cash, 1995; Jasper, 1994; Kim, 2010). Benner (1984, 2001), drawing from Dreyfus (1979) and Dreyfus and Dreyfus (1986), considers nursing expertise from the skill development perspective. In this conceptualization, expert practice is skillful comportment that is shaped through experiences and characterized by the use of a mode of pattern recognition based on paradigm cases and intuitive knowing. Intuitive knowing is viewed to develop from the holistic grasping of situations and understanding. Intuitive knowing that is only possible through experiences is the basis of skillful comportment (i.e., excellence in practice), different from formal knowledge. Because nursing expertise from this perspective is domain-specific and situational, one can only conjecture that nurses who practice with excellence repeatedly and in varied situations often would be called experts (Benner, Tanner, & Chesla, 2009). As the focus of this work was to depict how experts practiced rather than what expertise is, the characteristics of "excellence" in expertise are not identified and are not well articulated. Expertise in Benner's model thus is process oriented rather than quality oriented. The focus on evidence-based practice in the recent years may be counter to the concept of expertise based in intuition.

From the cognitive perspective, expertise refers to the acquisition of an advancing series of knowledge structures critical for professional practice (Schmidt, Norman, & Boshuizen, 1990). Different knowledge structures are developed sequentially, beginning with the elaborated causal networks, building up to a compilation of abridged causal networks, a network of event scripts, and a network of instance scripts. Development of a series of knowledge structures becomes the basis for drawing situational decisions and selecting approaches with an increasing level of competence, leading to expertise. On the other hand, the action science perspective by Argyris and Schön (1974) and Argyris, Putnam, and Smith (1985) suggests experts as those who are in the double-loop learning mode in their practice. The APA Task Force on the Assessment of Competence in Professional Psychology states that "... experts notice features and meaningful patterns of information, have considerable content knowledge that is organized in a fashion indicative of a deep understanding of the material, possess knowledge reflective of contexts of applicability rather than isolated facts, flexibly retrieve salient knowledge with minimal attention effort, know their discipline thoroughly, and demonstrate varying levels of flexibility in dealing with novel situations" (APA, 2006, p. 13). This position incorporates the roles of knowledge, knowledge application, and skillfulness in experts. Christensen and Hewitt-Taylor state that expertise "includes knowledge, experience, the assimilation of these, which contributes to intuition and the ability to use this to make appropriate and prompt clinical decisions" (2006, p. 1534). Hardy, Titchen, Manley, and McCormack (2006) also state that expertise is "an ability to use multiple forms of knowing, plus use of self, in a seamless way, to promote care that is tailor-made for the patient" (p. 264). The literature on nursing expertise indicates that the essential features of clinical expertise in nursing include skillfulness in technical execution of nursing activities, possession of advanced knowledge, ability to produce correct outcomes, use of intuition, and recognition by peers (Kim, 2010). Donnelly (2003) quotes the Canadian Nurses Association's position that the cornerstone of advanced nursing practice is expertise characterized by an ability to assess and understand complex patient responses; significant depth and knowledge and intervention skills and strong intuitive skills in the practice area; and specialized practice that concentrates on a particular aspect of nursing that may have as its focus age, medical diagnostic grouping, practice setting, or type of care. Advanced practice nursing is a culmination of clinical experiences and advanced knowledge. Similarly, the AACN's publication, *The Essentials of Doctoral Education for Advanced Nursing Practice* (AACN, 2006), also states that practice-focused doctoral programs are designed to prepare experts in specialized advanced nursing practice.

A new approach to delineate the essential features of expertise in nursing practice may be to use the structure of practice dimensions and the philosophies of practice in the model of nursing practice advanced in this book as the guideline. In the model of nursing practice, the scientific, technical, ethical, aesthetic, and existential dimensions of nursing practice characterize nursing practice as it occurs in clinical situations with orientations in three philosophies of practice (i.e., care, therapy, and professional work). The specific mode that characterizes each dimension in relation to the three philosophical orientations can be used as the starting point to determine competence and expertise that can be revealed in each dimension as shown in Table 11.1.

Characteristics of competence and expertise for each dimension can be identified, which will then be culminated into a holistic picture of competence and expertise in nursing practice. In this way, expertise can be conceptualized

**TABLE 11.1 Expertise in Nursing Practice Delineated in the Five Dimensions of Nursing Practice and Three Philosophical Orientations of Nursing Practice**

| DIMENSIONS OF NURSING PRACTICE AND KEY MODUS OPERANDI | KEY FUNCTIONING ATTRIBUTES | PHILOSOPHICAL ORIENTATIONS OF NURSING PRACTICE | | |
|---|---|---|---|---|
| | | CARE | THERAPY | PROFESSIONAL WORK |
| **Scientific**: Knowledge Translation and Application | Knowledge acquisition<br>General and situational knowledge assessment and evaluation<br>Clinical decision making applying the principles of logic, explanatory power, and experiential relevance | Holistic orientation | Problem orientation | Organizational orientation<br>Professional orientation |
| **Technical**: Performance of Techniques | Performance in terms of optimization, coordination, contextualization, and flexibility | Caring approaches<br>Communication and interaction | Clinical strategies and interventions | Intra- and interprofessional relations<br>Organizational actions and strategies |
| **Ethical**: Choice Selection | Assimilation of moral, cultural, and professional values, attitudes, and sensitivity<br>Ethical decision making applying the principles of holistic understanding, contextuality, truthfulness, and compassion | Holistic, person-oriented ethical decisions | Problem-specific ethical decisions | Work-oriented ethical decisions |
| **Aesthetic**: Expression in Self-Presentation | Creativity and aesthetic sensibility<br>Self-presentation (verbal, nonverbal, bodily, and managing) guided by the principles of unity, harmony, and finesse | Self-presentation in caring | Self-presentation in clinical approaches | Self-presentation in work relationships and organizations |
| **Existential**: Comportment | Establishment of self-identity in relation to commitment, freedom, and choice<br>Comportment in relation to authenticity, particularism, and understanding | Holistic | Problem focused | Work oriented |

to encompass both the processes applied in practice and the attributes of expertise. Benner's findings regarding pattern recognition and intuition in clinical decision making can be placed in the processes of practice in nursing expertise, while knowledge, skills, and attitudes can be placed in the attributes of expertise in order to identify their characteristics in expertise. The five key attributes of expertise extracted from the literature by Hardy et al. (2006) include holistic practice knowledge, skilled knowledge, knowing the patient/client, moral agency, and saliency. They also added through their investigation the attributes of "creative risk-taking" and "being catalyst for change" to this list (Hardy et al., 2006). This set identifies the specific characteristics of the attributes of expertise, not focusing on the nature of the processes of practice evident in expertise. Because various models of nursing expertise in the literature only deal with either the processes or attributes, it is critical to have a model of nursing expertise that identifies both the nature of the processes used in expertise and the attributes of expertness in practice. The model suggested here can identify the form and character of expertise in the processes of practice for each dimension and at the same time essential attributes that identify "expertness" in practice as well. Expertise in nursing practice conceptualized in this model may then be specified for various specialty areas or different practice roles as well as for the development of competence and expertise assessment.

## QUALITY OF CARE AND QUALITY OF NURSING PRACTICE

The concept of quality of nursing practice has to be viewed from the wider perspective of quality of health care of which nursing is one contributing component. The health care system designs are socially and politically determined, shape the processes of health care, and eventually affect patient outcomes. In the publication by the IOM regarding the quality of health care for the 21st century, it identifies six national quality aims in health care as *safety*, *effectiveness*, *patient-centeredness*, *timeliness*, *efficiency*, and *equity* (IOM, 2001a). The IOM (2001a) considers the quality of health care in these six areas to be influenced by "high performing patient-centered teams" that exist within "organizations that facilitate the work of patient-centered teams" in care systems. This means that the quality of health care is influenced not only by the practice of health care providers, but also by the organizations within which health care occurs. In addition to the six quality aims, the report gives 10 general principles that are to be used to improve quality in health care, addressing both the processes of practice and the organizational culture. These are:

*1.* Care is based on continuous healing relationships.
*2.* Care is customized according to patient needs and values.
*3.* The patient is the source of control.
*4.* Knowledge is shared and information flows freely.
*5.* Decision making is evidence based.
*6.* Safety is a system property.
*7.* Transparency is necessary.
*8.* Needs are anticipated.
*9.* Waste is continuously decreased.
*10.* Cooperation among clinicians is a priority (IOM, 2001a).

In addition, the adoption of the Patient Safety and Quality Improvement Act (Patient Safety Act) in 2005 has also stimulated the development of voluntary, provider-driven initiatives to improve the quality, safety, and outcomes of patient care, especially through the efforts of professional organizations and accrediting bodies such as the ANA, the AACN, and specialty organizations in nursing, and the AAMC and the ACGME in medicine. These quality aims of health care produce outcomes in clients, and point to how health care should be practiced in order to achieve the best possible outcomes from health care. Hence, this proposal has become the guidepost for identifying the quality of health care and outcomes especially at the national aggregate level. The Agency for Healthcare Research and Quality (AHRQ) has been publishing the National Healthcare Quality and Disparity Reports on these six quality areas and two additional areas of care coordination and health system infrastructure annually since 2003, which provide findings at the national level regarding both the processes (i.e., health care activities) and the outcomes related to the areas in order to gauge the quality of health care evident at the aggregate level. At the individual level, these areas of quality of care translate into the quality of care received by a client as to *how effective* the care was in meeting his or her needs, *how safe* it was in preventing untoward adverse events and errors, whether the care was *timely*, whether the care was *patient-centered*, and how *efficient* the care was. Because health care for individuals for any given service occasion (e.g., office visit, hospitalization, emergency visit, long-term care admission, or rehabilitation visit) is usually provided by several different health care professionals through various forms of health care processes, the quality of care in this regard has to be in relation to the aggregate (i.e., the totality) of care received for that occasion. From the individual client perspective, the quality of care has also to be considered in terms of how *salient* the care is in addressing the client's needs, and how the care *fits* into the total client care. This means that the quality aims for nursing practice may be conceptualized to align with the six quality aims identified by the IOM with additions of *saliency* and *fittingness*.

Quality of nursing practice is a component of the total quality of care resulting from interdependent, connected parts of a total system of patient-care processes. As nurses are the key contributors, quality of nursing practice affects the total quality of care, and eventually health care outcomes in clients. While the quality of care from the nursing perspective has to be viewed within this general orientation, there is a need to delineate the quality of nursing practice more specifically addressing the specific features of nursing care delivery. Nursing is practiced as both an organized service and an individual practice. Nursing service delivery is made within the health care system as an organized service. Organizational characteristics (i.e., structure and functioning) vary according to types and goals of health care settings such as hospitals, long-term care institutions, community health care agencies, and ambulatory care settings as well as according to institutional characters such as size, complexity, location, and so forth. In addition, nursing service is a sector within a system of total patient-care services that is currently based on differentiation and coordination, commonly established, yet partitioned goals, complementary relationships, and policy mandates. The work of "Magnet hospitals" in relation to the quality of nursing practice has focused specifically on organizational characteristics that foster best practices and high quality of nursing service (Aiken, Havens, & Sloane, 2000; ANCC, 2008; Lundmark, 2008). Quality of care from the nursing perspective therefore needs to be conceptualized in terms of both individual practice and organized service. Quality of care for individual practice can be termed "quality of practice" considered in terms not only of practice performances, but also of practice activities' saliency and coherence within the total structure of patient care. As stated earlier, quality of individual practice refers to the quality associated with what nurses "do" in practice, that is, in terms of *effectiveness, safety, timeliness, efficiency, saliency,* and *fittingness*. Two concepts in the IOM quality aims, *patient-centeredness* and *care coordination*, are viewed as practice processes rather than as quality indicators. These practice processes affect the quality of practice by the variations in their application in practice. The unit of analysis is the nurse in her or his practice for a group of clients or individual clients.

The organized service of nursing can be viewed as "coordinated practice" in this conceptualization of quality of practice. Quality of care for coordinated practice must be considered in relation to *cumulation, complementarity,* and *contiguity* for individual clients and groups of clients. Cumulation in care refers to the processes of nursing practice in a coordinated system, resulting in summative effects of nursing care provided by different caregivers. A coordinated system must be oriented to progressively adding the effects and influences. It means that each nurse's practice independently can be of quite high quality, but may be paralleling each other in its effects rather than building on to each other. Complementarity refers to the processes of nursing practice in a coordinated system resulting in complementary effects of nursing care provided by different caregivers. What different caregivers are doing for patients must not be contradictory or replacing of each other's effects. Although nurses who are involved in nursing care of a specific patient are often members of care teams manifestly in an organization of health care, they must also establish an "invisible team" to coordinate their work so that their practice influences patients in complementary fashion. Contiguity in practice in a coordinated system means that what different practitioners (caregivers) are doing are connected together as a network so that there is a movement toward progression in a systematic fashion rather than moving uncoordinated or in random arrangements. Contiguous practice is one in which there are rational, systematic connections among nursing care provided by different practitioners so that there is a continuity in progression as well as streamlined harmony among various activities. When practice is contiguous, it is possible to avoid omissions and unnecessary duplications. Emphasis on specific areas of patient-care needs can be followed through in a contiguous process through coordinated effort.

In addition, there are three different perspectives with which the quality of care can be considered: "quality of care delivered," "quality of care performed," and "quality of care received." "Quality of care delivered" is contextualized to the organization of care with an orientation to nursing practice as an organized service, whereas "quality of care performed" is contextualized to practitioners. On the other hand, "quality of care received" is a view in the context of patients. Quality of care from the organizational perspective is the orientation used in the assessment of quality of care in the system of nursing care delivery (e.g., wards or hospitals). From this organizational orientation, quality of care is usually considered in terms of meeting the standards of care as a collective delivery, not differentiating how each individual practitioner within a nursing service system practices nursing. When the perspective is practitioner "providing" care or "performing" nursing activities, the focus is on the character of nursing practice as it is carried out by individual nurses either for a given client or for a group of clients. Williams found in her qualitative study of nurses' perception of quality of nursing care that "quality is viewed in terms of therapeutic effectiveness as the degree to which patients' needs (i.e., physical, psychosocial, and extra care needs) were met by nurses specified by the types of care given to meet individual patient's needs" (1998, p. 811). Hence, according to Williams (1998), nurses' criterion of value for quality of practice assessment is therapeutic effectiveness in relation to patients' needs. On the other hand, from the patient's perspective, the quality of nursing care is found to be process oriented, and has been identified in eight process characteristics by Radwin (2000) in terms of using professional knowledge, establishing rapport, supporting a partnership with the patient, treating the patient as an individual, showing a caring approach, demonstrating an attentive manner, providing continuity of care, and promoting coordinated care. Usually from the patient's perspective, the quality of care refers to nursing care received not just from one nurse, but also from all nurses providing the care. These two studies indicated that nurses seem to be emphasizing the practice process associated with the philosophy of therapy while patients seem to be emphasizing it more in terms of the philosophy of care when they view quality of nursing practice. Furthermore, nurses seem to be more oriented to outcomes while patients seem to focus on processes. If we frame the results of these two studies on the quality aims identified by the IOM, then the quality of care "provided" seems to focus on effectiveness, while the quality of care "received" seems to focus on the patient-centeredness and care coordination. This is in line with the diversity in which quality of nursing practice has been conceptualized both in terms of outcomes and process measures in the literature, as well as the two bifurcating orientations of quality aims—one that is oriented to outcomes (effectiveness and safety) and the other oriented to processes (patient-centeredness, timeliness, efficiency, and care coordination). The assumption is that the process-oriented quality affects client outcomes as well.

There is a paucity of specifications in the literature regarding how to describe quality of nursing practice. Most of the empirical work use simple quality ratings, and some works refer to patient satisfaction or nurse satisfaction with care as the quality measures. There is a need in nursing to delineate specific aspects of quality aims of health care in relation to the conceptualization of quality of nursing practice for individual practice and organized service as well as for the three perspectives with which it is addressed. As pointed out in the preceding section, the quality aims offered by the IOM are in two different orientations—outcomes and processes. Therefore, it is necessary to clarify the meanings of the quality aims of "outcomes" and "processes" in relation to nursing practice. One approach is to apply a framework to align these general quality aims of health care with the philosophical orientations of nursing practice in identifying specific attributes for the quality of nursing practice as shown in

**TABLE 11.2 Specification of Quality of Nursing Practice: Linking the Quality Aims of the IOM and the Philosophical Orientations of Nursing Practice**

| QUALITY AIM AREAS | PHILOSOPHICAL ORIENTATIONS OF NURSING PRACTICE | | |
|---|---|---|---|
| | THERAPY | CARE | PROFESSIONAL WORK |
| **Effectiveness** | Prevention of nursing problems<br>Treatment of nursing problems<br>Management of nursing problems | Upholding human flourishing<br>Healing relationships | Completion of designated patient-care responsibilities |
| **Patient Safety** | Prevention of nursing-sensitive errors and accidents | Upholding human integrity | Organizational surveillance and evaluation of patient safety |
| **Timeliness** | Timely provision of nursing interventions | Timely attentiveness to clients as persons | Timely accomplishment of organizationally oriented nursing responsibilities (recording, communicating, etc.) |
| **Patient-Centeredness** | Person-centered intervention decision making<br>Application of person-centered interventions<br>Tailoring of interventions | Upholding individuality<br>Upholding autonomy<br>Mutuality and mutual decision making | Fostering of the person-centered culture |
| **Care Coordination** | Collaboration in therapeutic health care | Coordination of caring and healing | Intra- and interprofessional communication, coordination, and collaboration |
| **Efficiency** | Efficient application of nursing interventions | Efficient use of the self in practice | Efficient delivery of nursing service |
| **Equity** | Equitable application of nursing interventions | Cultural sensitivity | Application of the value of distributive justice |

Table 11.2. The framework offers a way to identify nursing-specific quality attributes in terms of the generally accepted quality aims that are in place.

## CLIENT OUTCOMES IN RELATION TO QUALITY OF CARE

Client outcomes refer to the results associated with the ultimate goal of health care in terms of making "a difference in the state of health of people" (Strickland, 1997). The notion of patient outcomes in relation to health care has become a buzzword since the 1980s as the nation is struggling to handle the rising cost of health care and deal with quality of care. Notions of *outcomes*, such as "the changes in a patient's health status that can be attributed to antecedent healthcare" by Donabedian (1988), "the end result of care or a measurable change in health status or behavior of patients" by Harris (1992), or "that representing the cumulative effect of one or more processes on a patient at a defined point in time" offered by the Joint Commission on Accreditation of Healthcare Organizations (JCAHO), suggest the basic agreement on the term outcomes. However, there are various interpretations and applications of this term in practice and research. Jennings and Staggers (1998) in their analysis of "the language of outcomes" suggest that the concept "outcomes" is used in various meaning contexts, such as "outcomes studies, outcomes research, outcomes management, performance measures, and outcomes indicators." The Nursing Outcomes Classification (NOC) work (Moorhead, Johnson, & Maas, 2004; Moorhead, Johnson, Maas, & Swanson, 2013) has proceeded to codify nursing outcomes in a classification system to unify the disarray of the conceptualizations regarding nursing outcomes. The National Quality Forum (2004) published a list of National Voluntary Consensus Standards for Nursing-Sensitive Care for patient-centered outcome measures, nursing-centered outcome measures, and system-centered measures, in which patient-centered outcome measures include:

- Death among surgical in-patients with treatable serious complications (failure to rescue)
- Pressure ulcer prevalence
- Falls prevalence
- Falls with injury
- Restraint prevalence (vest and limb only)
- Urinary catheter-associated urinary tract infection for intensive care unit (ICU) patients
- Central line catheter-associated blood stream infection rate for ICU and high-risk nursery (HRN) patients
- Ventilator-associated pneumonia for ICU and HRN patients

All of these "nursing-sensitive" outcomes are related to patient safety outcomes and are oriented to the organizational level. In health care, the concept of *outcomes* is used in two different but interrelated contexts: outcomes in individual patients and outcomes in patient aggregates or systems. There is confusion in addressing outcomes from these two separate but interrelated perspectives, especially in talking about measuring outcomes. From the outcomes management perspective, outcomes are measured from the systems or aggregate basis using such terms as "performance measures," "report cards," and "instrument panels" developed into such programs as JCAHO's IMSystem.

For individual patients, outcomes have been conceptualized from various perspectives in general and specifically in nursing. Strickland (1997) alludes that patient outcome measures in the nursing context must be concerned with identifying key physiological, psychological, and social variables as the nursing profession focuses on "the whole person and is concerned with addressing biologic, psychological, and social aspects of patient care needs." Similarly, Ditmyer, Coepsell, Branum, Davis, and Lush (1998) report the development of the "Health Status Outcomes Dimension Instrument" that is organized by self-care ability/functional status, engagement in health care management, and psychological distress/mental and social well-being components. The NOC system in its latest publication uses seven domains of outcomes (i.e., functional health, physiologic health, psychosocial health, health knowledge and behavior, perceived health, family health, and community health) to codify 490 patient outcomes into 32 classes (Moorhead et al., 2013). Such conceptualizations view health status as composed of multiple states that can assume certain values at a given time. Thus, when patient outcomes are considered as the "products" of nursing care, for example, at the point of discharge after a hospitalization, they are viewed in terms of how the values have changed over the course of nursing care from the input point on preexisting states or what are gained with certain values in new states. This is a mechanical view of patient outcomes.

A more dynamic approach to conceptualizing patient outcomes will have to be framed within a nursing perspective of clients. Various conceptual models in nursing regarding humans and health can be adopted as frames for patient outcomes. One approach is to consider a patient's position in a health care setting as a transition within the life-course trajectory. Patient outcomes therefore can be viewed as transitory states within the trajectory perspective by framing it within the framework of human living as the framework. Kim's model of human living (2000, 2010) is an example in which human living is considered to have four integrative dimensions: living with one's body, living of oneself, living with others, and living in situations. Living in these four dimensions is oriented not only to existential characters (status), but also to continuity, fulfillment, independence, cohabitation, interdependence, and feeling good. Living with one's body, both in physical and embodied senses, refers to such aspects as rhythms, intactness and appearance, capacities and limitations, body feelings, and sensations. Living of oneself, on the other hand, encompasses history, genealogy, desires and wants, dreams and hopes, ideas and opinions, choices, habits, and knowing. Living with others refers to connecting, interacting, relating, and communicating for instrumental, symbolic, and affective needs, while living in situations includes responding to, accommodating to, adapting, managing, engaging, choosing, and creating contexts of one's existence. Patient outcomes at any given point from the human living framework therefore are transitional and trajectorial. This view is close to the conceptualization of chronic illness in terms of "biographical disruption" (Bury, 1982; Reeves, Lloyd-Williams, Payne, & Dowrick, 2010). Continuity in one's life as a biographical streaming seems critical in considering an individual's health care outcomes. Nursing's concern with patient outcomes in the perspective of trajectory, therefore, has to focus on "how well the patient is able to 'live' through *this* episode of health-care" (i.e., the current states of living) and "what the prospect is for the trajectory of living" (i.e., the shape of trajectory of living). These may be termed as "readiness" outcomes referring to the client's position in his or her trajectory of living through the episode of care and "prospective" outcomes referring to how current status is likely to shape the trajectory of living for the client. Nursing, as the major care provider, affects patients' living in health care situations significantly and much more than any other health care providers. This view also redefines patient outcomes not as statuses to be measured at a point of discharge without regard for patients' positions in living, but as connected, continuous experiences of living that must be accounted for as nursing impacts. Hence, the processes of nursing care for patient outcomes in this perspective are concerned with the "present," that is, targeting patients' actual needs and requirements associated with health problems and with the prospect for the future in terms of patients' trajectory of living.

Figure 11.2 illustrates the interrelationships among the four components within nursing practice related to the conceptualization of quality of care, identifying specific aspects of the components. Quality of care and client outcomes are not independent of each other, but are interconnected in a system of goals, processes, quality, and outcomes in a dynamic way as was suggested in Figure 11.1.

From the nursing perspective, the goals of care can be viewed to have three components: (a) goals related to health problems oriented to treat, remedy, or reduce them or their effects; (b) goals related to healthful living oriented to ensuring, promoting, or improving living of one's body, of oneself, with others, and in situations; and (c) goals related to health care service such as success with health care, speedy recovery, satisfactory experiences, and expediency in the services. These general goals are the frames with which various practice processes are put into effect in nursing care, involving both individual practice processes and coordinated practice processes. The processes identified in this framework are general types that are critical in addressing these goals. The individual practice processes that take up the orientations of five dimensions

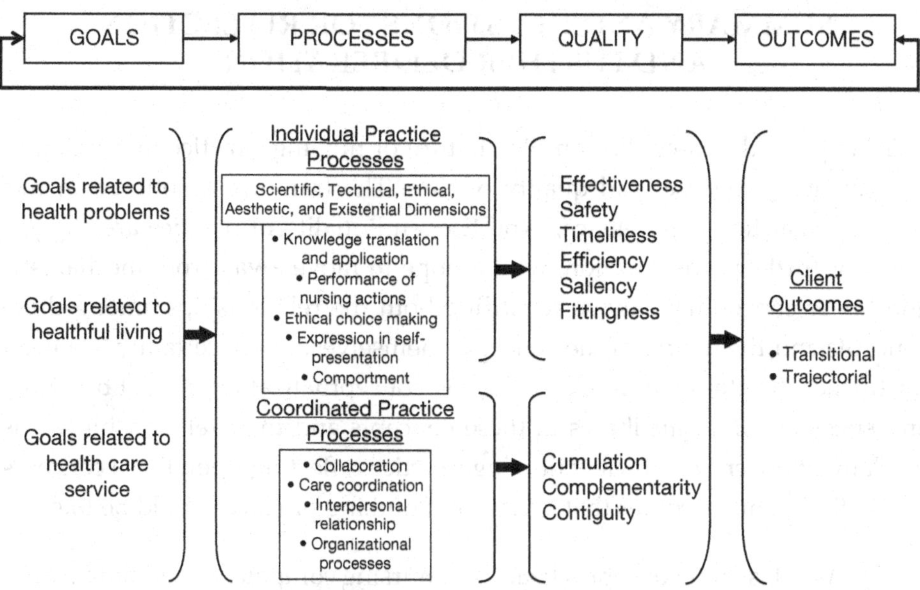


**FIGURE 11.2** A framework connecting practice processes with quality of care and client outcomes.

of practice (i.e., scientific, technical, ethical, aesthetic, and existential) to be applied in all nursing care situations are knowledge translation and application, performance of nursing actions, ethical choice selection, expression in self-presentation, and comportment. As these processes are interweaved into nursing practice, they result in applying knowledge in clinical decision making, being technically competent, ethically responsible, aesthetically compatible with clients and client situations, and existentially humanistic. The ways individual practice processes are applied in nursing practice then results in the qualitative differences in nursing practice in terms of effectiveness, safety, efficiency, timeliness, saliency, and fittingness. At the same time, nursing practice as coordinated practice (i.e., organized service) utilizes the processes of collaboration, care coordination, interpersonal relationships in intranursing and interprofessional contexts, and organizational processes for information sharing, work organization, and distribution of responsibilities. The nature of coordinated practice processes influences the quality of care related to cumulation, complementarity, and contiguity in care. Characteristics of the quality of care on these two dimensions (from the individual practice processes and the coordinated practice processes) therefore influence client outcomes in terms of the characteristics of transitional states and in trajectorial forms and positions. It is possible to specify further the elements in this framework to clarify the conceptualization of nursing practice in relation to goals, processes, quality, and outcomes in a dynamic system.

## SUMMARY AND QUESTIONS FOR REFLECTION AND FURTHER DELIBERATION

This chapter addresses the complex nature of nursing practice in relation to competence, expertise, and quality of care. The frameworks offered in this chapter regarding competence, expertise, and quality of practice are suggestions for further consideration, with a hope to move away from mechanistic and linear conceptualizations regarding both the relationships among these concepts and the nature of the concepts themselves. There certainly is a need for further development in clarifying the conceptualization, model building, and specification of attributes in these concepts and their relationships. It is fundamentally critical to view nursing practice reflecting upon these concepts as it is the client outcomes that drive what nursing practice should be like.

- What is your conceptualization of nursing competence and how would you characterize your nursing practice in terms of competence?
- How do you differentiate competence from expertise? Is general nursing expertise different from advanced practice nursing expertise? Does advanced nursing practice assume there is nursing expertise?
- What is your model of quality of practice? What are factors that influence quality of practice?
- What is your conceptualization of client outcomes? How can nursing control client outcomes through nursing service that involves collective provision of nursing care?
- What do you consider are the most critical issues in the current emphasis on quality and safety in health care from the nursing perspective?

# CHAPTER 12

# Concluding Remarks

## FUTURE OF NURSING PRACTICE

THE NATURE OF NURSING PRACTICE HAS gone through many changes in the past several decades not only because of the changes within the profession of nursing but also in response to the changes in health care systems and societal needs. Nursing practice in this age occurs in the midst of strong currents that are producing an unprecedented complexity in the health care system, especially in the United States. The aging of the population, the dominance of chronic illness for health care needs, and the societal consciousness for quality and safety concerns are pushing for reexaminations and innovations for health care system from social, political, economic, organizational, scientific/ technological, and professional perspectives. The prevailing ideological commitments to cost containment and cost efficiency, accountability, scientific base of health care, and quality have been in force to redesign the health care system and the provision of health care. With the passage of the Affordable Health Care Act (ACA) the political message is also for establishing ways to ensure quality health care in every sector of the health care system. In addition, the acceptance of the values of person-centered practice, evidence-based practice, and interprofessional collaboration in health care practice espoused at the national and world levels (Institute of Medicine [IOM] 2014; World Health Organization [WHO], 2010) has become the cornerstone in reshaping the characteristics and structures of health care practice in the recent years. The nursing profession is also experiencing forces that require it to reexamine its educational system and training, specialization, organization of services, and knowledge development.

In the IOM report on the future of nursing, the Committee on the Robert Wood Johnson Foundation Initiative on the Future of Nursing envisions a future health care system "that makes quality care accessible to the diverse populations of the United States, intentionally promotes wellness and disease prevention, reliably improves health outcomes, and provides compassionate care across the lifespan," which is driven centrally by primary care and prevention, and in which interprofessional collaboration/coordination and the delivery of patient-centered care responding to individuals' needs and desires are its critical characteristics (IOM Committee on the Robert Wood Johnson Foundation Initiative on the Future of Nursing, 2014, p. 22). The committee envisioning nurses as the central players in the transformation of the health care system made eight recommendations for the future of nursing among which the following four are viewed as the major messages: (a) practice of nursing reflecting nurses' education and training, especially for advanced practice; (b) educational reform in nursing, especially for "seamless" academic progression and advanced training; (c) nurses' participatory role in health care policy making; and (d) a comprehensive information infrastructure for health care policy and workforce planning (IOM Committee on the Robert Wood Johnson Foundation Initiative on the Future of Nursing, 2014).

These four key messages by IOM and the first three points, more specifically, have implications regarding how nursing practice should advance through:

1. Revising and formulating the standardization of the scope of nursing practice in order to transform nursing practice, especially the advanced level of nursing practice, to align well with the health care needs of the population
2. Remodeling of nursing's educational system to meet the health care demands of the future and a transformed health care system, which would require not only a rigorous advancement in the nursing knowledge system but also creative approaches to address the learning needs at all levels
3. Assigning a greater role to nursing as a partner in transforming the health care system, which would require nurses to be better prepared for leadership and policy making and become active partners in meeting the demands of a transformed health care system

The latent issue embedded in these three points is clinical specialization and advanced practice in nursing. Clinical specialization and advanced practice in nursing have to be examined carefully and redesigned in order to respond to the changing and complex needs of the population. The linkage among clinical specialization, advanced practice, the health care system, the educational system, and advancing nursing knowledge has to be reconfigured to meet the demands of the future.

These agendas for advancing nursing practice need to be taken up at the institutional level (i.e., by the nursing profession at large and other public organizations such as governmental, legal, and educational systems). However, individual nurses must also be engaged in advancing nursing practice at the everyday practice level. Advancing nursing practice at the practice level requires nurses to engage in a continuous self-monitoring of their practice in order to move toward an increasing level of competence and expertise and to engage in developing and codifying clinical knowledge that emerges from personal practice. Practicing nurses are the makers and the purveyors of clinical knowledge. Knowledge generation from clinical experiences has to become an institutionalized form of knowledge codification in nursing.

## KNOWLEDGE DEVELOPMENT TO ADVANCE NURSING PRACTICE

The essential aspect in advancing nursing practice is knowledge development in nursing. Nursing as a knowledge-based practice proposed in this model has to have a comprehensive, rich, and advancing knowledge base in order for the practice to meet its demands for responsible, goal-oriented practice. Nursing knowledge development has progressed greatly during the past several decades, and with an ever-increasing number of nurses prepared and engaged in knowledge development (theory development and research) as their primary focus, nursing knowledge is being developed in diverse areas addressing various epistemic questions at the macro and micro levels such as grand theory development as well as narrowly circumscribed questions such as management of postoperative pain. Although there is no formal, comprehensive codification of the status of nursing knowledge, it is possible to state that the advancement is remarkable but at the same time unsystematic. This means that there still are many epistemic questions that have not been addressed, for which there is a paucity of systematic knowledge development, or for which a confusing and conflicting disarray of knowledge continues to exist.

The issues regarding knowledge development to advance nursing practice are addressed in this exposition with the focus on epistemic questions. Two interconnected spheres of knowledge development are specified here: one in relation to the nursing perspective and the philosophy of practice identified in the model of nursing practice, for which knowledge development is foundational, and the other in relation to the five cognitive needs in practice specified in the nursing epistemology that addresses knowledge development regarding critical phenomena of the practice domain.

## Knowledge Development Regarding the Nursing Perspective and the Philosophy of Practice

As discussed in Chapter 3 (the nursing perspective) and Chapter 5 (the philosophy of practice), these two components of the model of nursing practice advanced in this book are foundational and provide for establishing general beliefs, commitments, attitudes, and postures that become immersed and integrated into nurses' engagement in nursing practice. Therefore, the epistemic questions in relation to these two foundational aspects of nursing practice (the perspective and the philosophy of practice) are of three types: (a) the contents (i.e., the features), (b) enculturation in practitioners, and (c) emergence in practice. The following epistemic questions as a set of key examples need to be addressed critically in order to gain a full understanding of how these foundational aspects are essential for and integrated into nursing practice. Both philosophical analyses and empirical approaches are appropriate to address these questions.

The questions related to the issues of the nursing perspective specified in the model as four ideologies (holism, health-orientation, person-centeredness, and caring) on two dimensions as the currently valid ones making up the nursing perspective for practice are:

- Are these the generally accepted ideologies undergirding the nursing perspective currently in the profession? (Content)
- What are the philosophical values embedded within the four ideologies of the nursing perspective? How relevant are they to nursing practice? (Content)
- What are the origins and the trajectories of change of these ideologies? (Content)
- What is articulated by nurses as the nursing perspective guiding their practice? What are the variations and the sources of the variations? (Enculturation)
- What are the processes of enculturation applied in relation to the nursing perspective? (Enculturation)
- What are the variations in the nursing perspectives held by practicing nurses in terms of nurses' characteristics, settings of practice, and other social–institutional variations? (Enculturation)

- What are the nursing perspectives embedded in clinical practice? And how different or similar are these with the generic ideologies identified in the model? Why are there variations? (Emergence)

The epistemic questions related to the philosophy of practice identified in the model as the philosophies of care, therapy, and professional work can also be extracted in relation to the content, enculturation, and emergence. These are:

- Do the three philosophies of nursing practice (caring, therapy, and professional work) represent the philosophy of practice in the nursing profession? (Content)
- What are the elements of the philosophy of nursing practice? (Content)
- How reflective is the philosophy of nursing practice of the current philosophical, political, and professional culture? (Content)
- What philosophy of practice is articulated by nurses as guiding their work? What are the variations and sources of the variations? (Enculturation)
- What are the processes of enculturation applied in relation to the philosophy of practice? (Enculturation)
- What philosophy of nursing practice is embedded in clinical practice? And how is the philosophy of practice articulated in clinical practice? How different or similar are these with the espoused philosophy of practice? (Emergence)

The knowledge regarding these foundational components is necessary not only to gain an understanding about the perspective and the philosophy of practice, but also to assess the nature of their articulation in clinical practice. It is especially critical to gain knowledge regarding the relevance, appropriateness, acceptance, and workability of these foundational components in relation to clinical practice, because these are viewed normatively as essential components for practice.

## Knowledge Development for the Practice Domain Phenomena

The practice domain as the one conceptual area of nursing knowledge (Kim, 2010, and discussed in Chapter 4) is the area of study regarding nursing practice. The domain of practice "embraces" what and how nurses carry out and perform those actions called "nursing" and the focus is on "understanding

**TABLE 12.1 Types of Theories for the Modes of Practice Specified for the Domains of Nursing Practice**

| COGNITIVE NEEDS | DIMENSIONS OF NURSING PRACTICE AND MODES OF PRACTICE | | | | |
|---|---|---|---|---|---|
| | SCIENTIFIC: KNOWLEDGE TRANSLATION AND APPLICATION | TECHNICAL: PERFORMANCE OF TECHNIQUES | ETHICAL: CHOICE SELECTION | AESTHETIC: EXPRESSION IN SELF-PRESENTATION | EXISTENTIAL: COMPORTMENT |
| Inferential | Descriptive, explanatory, normative, and prescriptive theories regarding the modes of practice in each domain | | | | |
| Referential | Heuristic theories, scripts/narratives, and constructions regarding the modes of practice in each domain | | | | |
| Transformative | Theories of interpretation, critique, and transformation/change regarding the modes of practice in each domain considered as the forms of social practice<br>Critiques of the values and principles undergirding the five rationalities identified for the domains of practice | | | | |
| Normative | Descriptive, analytic, and normative theories of ethical and moral standards of practice embedded in the modes of practice in each domain | | | | |
| Desiderative | Descriptive, analytic, and normative theories of aesthetics associated with the modes of practice in each domain | | | | |

and explaining nursing practice and on improving the way we practice nursing" (Kim, 2010, p. 170). Therefore, knowledge development for the practice domain phenomena is central to advancing nursing practice, and it can be addressed in terms of the five cognitive needs in nursing practice (i.e., the inferential, referential, transformative, normative, and desiderative cognitive needs). The first approach is to examine the need for knowledge development to meet these five cognitive needs in relation to the modes of practice identified in the five dimensions. Table 12.1 gives a list of theoretical advances necessary in relation to five cognitive needs in nursing practice in relation to the five dimensions of nursing practice in terms of the primary mode of practice for each dimension.

The modes of practice identified in the five dimensions are delineated out *analytically* as specific modes in this model, as these modes do not exist in practice as separate forms of actions but are integrated together to represent what nurses do in practice. However, it is necessary to use this analytical formulation as the basis for developing knowledge as the first approach because it is possible to raise epistemic questions more specifically to develop theories. As shown in this table, the five different cognitive needs point to different types of theories developed for these modes of practice. It is when we have a comprehensive set of knowledge regarding all five modes of practice in terms of all five types of cognitive needs that it is possible for nurses to design and act responsibly and be knowledge based in their practice.

The second approach is to examine the need for knowledge development to meet these five cognitive needs in relation to various phenomena in

**TABLE 12.2 Examples of Phenomena in the Practice Domain for Knowledge Development**

| ANALYTIC FOCUS | LEVEL OF CONCEPT DESCRIPTION | |
|---|---|---|
| | HOLISTIC (INCLUDES GENERAL NURSING TOOLS) | PARTICULARISTIC (INCLUDES GENERAL NURSING TOOLS) |
| **Holistic Focus** | Clinical competence<br>Clinical expertise<br>Clinical leadership<br>Innovation adoption<br>Knowing the patient<br>Knowledge utilization<br>Nursing process<br>Quality of practice<br>Specialization | |
| **Deliberation Focus** | Clinical decision making<br>Clinical reflection<br>Critical path development<br>Information processing<br>Nursing care planning<br>Program development | Clinical inferencing<br>Nursing diagnosis<br>Outcomes evaluation<br>Priority setting<br>Surveillance<br>Professional vigilance |
| **Enactment Focus** | Caring<br>Client advocacy<br>Consultation<br>Culture brokerage<br>Delegation<br>Empowerment<br>Ethical practice<br>Nursing aesthetics<br>Nurturing<br>Palliative care<br>Patient care management<br>Referral<br>Role modeling<br>Skillful comportment<br>Support<br>Transition care | Active listening<br>Anticipatory guidance<br>Client–nurse alliance<br>Client safety management<br>Comforting<br>Delegation<br>Environmental management<br>Nursing assessment<br>Nursing description<br>Nursing documentation<br>Nursing handover<br>Presence<br>Protection<br>Ritualization<br>Scaffolding<br>Security enhancement<br>Supportive counseling<br>Symptom management<br>Tailoring<br>Teaching<br>Technical competence |

Adapted from Kim (2010).

the practice domain. Table 12.2 gives a list of essential phenomena for which knowledge needs to be developed.

Knowledge development for each phenomenon has to be addressed to fulfill the five cognitive needs (see Figure 4.3 in Chapter 4). That is, knowledge development for phenomena in nursing practice has to be in the forms of generalized knowledge for the inferential cognitive needs, situated hermeneutic knowledge for the referential cognitive needs, critical hermeneutic knowledge for the transformative cognitive needs, ethical knowledge for the normative cognitive needs, and aesthetic knowledge for the desiderative cognitive needs. It means that there has to be these various types of knowledge developed for the phenomena in order to have a comprehensive base for nursing practice. For some of these phenomena, there is a rich base of knowledge developed already, especially in relation to the inferential and normative cognitive needs. However, there is a paucity of knowledge especially in relation to the referential, transformative, and aesthetic cognitive needs. In order for nursing practice to rely on knowledge comprehensively, it is necessary to develop knowledge in relation to all five cognitive needs.

## SUMMARY AND QUESTIONS FOR REFLECTION AND FURTHER DELIBERATION

A vision regarding nursing practice in the 21st century and beyond calls for a model of nursing practice that can be used to frame a movement toward a more "responsible" and increasingly effective, meaningful practice. With a proposed model of nursing practice, approaches to making nursing practice what it ought to be have been addressed in this book. We have been lacking a comprehensive model for nurses to both fashion and examine their practice, and the model proposed here is an attempt to show nurses what their practice is constituted of and how they may make their practice be "intentionally" good, effective, and meaningful to them as well as to clients and to the society. By systematically teasing out what goes into nursing practice from its foundations (i.e., the nursing frames, the knowledge, and the philosophies of practice) to the workings in practice (i.e., the dimensions of practice and the processes of practice), it has been shown that nursing has to be "designed" intentionally to produce "good" practice. There has been a great deal of discussion during the past three decades regarding how to conceptualize nursing practice from logicoscientific orientations to existential, phenomenological orientations. I do not believe that nursing practice can be described, explained, and proscribed from a one-dimensional perspective (i.e., either logicoscientific or as existential–phenomenological), as nursing practice integrates the "human practice" aspect, encompassing the existential, phenomenological, and interpretive meanings, and at the same time the "human service practice" aspect, encompassing the orientations in goal attainment, intentionality, and other-oriented responsibility. What it means is that nursing practice as human phenomena can be conceptualized and described as "living," "existing," and "experiencing" in a generic sense, but that this is not enough to understand and explain what "ought" to happen in nursing practice fully. As with all goal-directed systems, nursing practice as a goal-oriented system has to be guided by a framework that gives credence to actualizations that are framed, designed, and organized to accomplish its goals. The details offered in the preceding chapters provide guidelines for understanding, describing, and explaining what nursing practice "ought" to be from this perspective. The approach applied in this book is *analytical,* in that the levels, components, and details identified and discussed in the presentation of this model are analytically identified and discussed for a greater understanding of nursing practice. The details in the exposition are tentative, and require further investigations and discussions.

- Does the model of nursing practice provide analytically rich understanding about the essence and nature of nursing practice as presented in this book?
- Can the model of nursing practice be applied to evaluate qualitative differences in nursing practice?
- Can the model of nursing practice be applied as the frame to extract key questions for knowledge development to advance nursing practice?
- What are specific research questions associated with the epistemic questions presented in this chapter for advancing nursing practice?

# Bibliography

Abdellah, F. G., Beland, I. L., Martin, A., & Matheney, R. V. (1960). *Patient-centered approaches to nursing*. New York, NY: Macmillan.

Abel, E., & Nelson, M. (Eds.). (1990). *Circles of care: Work and identity in women's lives*. New York, NY: State University of New York Press.

Abma, T. A., & Broese, E. W. (2010). Patient participation as dialogue: Setting research agendas. *Health Expectations, 13*, 160–173.

Agency for Healthcare Research and Quality (AHRQ). (2005). *Systems to rate the strength of scientific evidence*. AHRQ Evidence Report #47. AHRQ Publication No. 02-E016. AHRQ; 2002. Retrieved from http://www.ahrq.gov/clinic/tp/strengthtp.htm

Agency for Healthcare Research and Quality (AHRQ). (2013). *2012 National Healthcare Quality Report*. AHRQ Publication No. 13-0002. Retrieved from www.ahrq.gov/research/findings/nhqrdr/index.html

Aguilar, J., & Buckareff, A. (Eds.). (2009). *Philosophy of action: 5 questions*. London, UK: Automatic Press/VIP.

Aiken, L. H., Clarke, S. P., Sloane, D. M., Lake, E. T., & Cheney, T. (2008). Effects of hospital care environment on patient mortality and nurse outcomes. *Journal of Nursing Administration, 38*, 223–229.

Aiken, L. H., Havens, D. S., & Sloane, D. M. (2000). The Magnet nursing service recognition program. *American Journal of Nursing, 100(3)*, 26–35.

Alexander, T. M. (1987). *John Dewey's theory of art, experience, and nature: The horizons of feeling*. Albany, NY: State University of New York Press.

Algase, D. L. (2008). Studying nursing practice. *Research and Theory for Nursing Practice: An International Journal, 22*, 3–4.

Allen, D. (2007). What do you do at work? Profession building and doing nursing. *International Nursing Review, 54*, 41–48.

Allen, D. E., Bockenhauer, B., Egan, C., & Kinnaird, L. S. (2006). Relating otucomes to excellent nursing practice. *Journal of Nursing Administration, 36*, 140–147.

Alligood, M. R. (2011). Theory-based practice in a major medical centre. *Journal of Nursing Management, 19*, 981–988.

Alt-White, A. C., Charns, M., & Strayer, R. (1983). Personal, organizational and managerial factors related to nurse-physician collaboration. *Nursing Administration Quarterly, 8*(1), 1–18.

American Association of Colleges of Nursing (AACN). (2006). *The essentials of doctoral education for advanced nursing practice.* Washington, DC: Author.

American Association of Colleges of Nursing (AACN). (2008). *The essentials of baccalaureate education for professional nursing practice.* Washington, DC: Author.

American Association of Colleges of Nursing (AACN). (2013). *Competencies and curriculum expectations for clinical nurse leader education and practice.* Washington, DC: Author.

American Nurses Association (ANA). (1980). *Nursing: A social policy statement.* Kansas City, MO: Author.

American Nurses Association (ANA). (1988). *Nursing practice in the 21st century.* Kansas City, MO: Author.

American Nurses Association (ANA). (2001). *Code of ethics for nurses with interpretive statements.* Kansas City, MO: Author.

American Nurses Association (ANA). (2003). *Nursing's social policy statement* (2nd ed.). Silver Spring, MD: NursesBooks.org.

American Nurses Association (ANA). (2008). *Professional role competence position statement.* Retrieved from http://nursingworld.org/MainMenuCategories/Healthcareand-Policy Issues/ANAPositionStatements/practice/PositionStatementProfessional-RoleCompetence.aspx

American Nurses Association (ANA). (2010a). *ANA's principles of nursing documentation: Guidance for registered nurses.* Silver Spring, MD: Author.

American Nurses Association (ANA). (2010b). *Nursing: Scope and standards of practice* (2nd ed.). Silver Spring, MD: Nursesbooks.org.

American Nurses Association (ANA). (2010c). *Nursing's social policy statement. The essence of the profession* (2010 edition). Silver Spring, MD: Nursesbooks.org

American Nurses Association (ANA). (2012a). *ANA's principles of delegation by registered nurses to unlicensed assistive personnel.* Silver Spring, MD: Nurses books.org

American Nurses Association (ANA). (2012b). Care coordination and registered nurses' essential role. Retrieved from http://nursingworld.org/MainMenuCategories/Policy-Advocacy/Positions-and-Resolutions/ANAPositionStatements/Position-Statements-Alphabetically/Care-Coordination-and-Registered-Nurses-Essential-Role.html

American Nurses Association (ANA). (2015). *Code of ethics for nurses with interpretive statements.* Silver Spring, MD: Nursesbooks.org.

American Nurses Credentialing Center (ANCC). (2008). *The Magnet model components and sources of evidence.* Silver Spring, MD: American Nurses Credentialing Center.

American Nurses Credentialing Center (ANCC). (2014). *Magnet recognition program model.* Retrieved http://www.nursecredentialing.org/Magnet/ProgramOverview/New-Magnet-Model

American Psychological Association. (2006). *APA task force on the assessment of competence in professional psychology: Final report.* Retrieved from http://www.apa.org/ed/resources/competency-revised.pdf

Ames, Van M. (1947). Expression and aesthetic expression. *Journal of Aesthetics and Art Criticism, 6* (2), 172–179.

Anderson, H. (2012). Collaborative practice: A way of being "with." *Psychotherapy and Politics International, 10*(2), 130–145.

Anderson, H., & Gehart, D. (Eds.). (2007). *Collaborative therapy: Relationships that make a difference.* New York, NY: Routledge.

Anderson, K. N. (Ed.). (1998). *Mosby's medical, nursing and allied health dictionary* (5th ed.). London, UK: Mosby.

Apel, K. O. (1980). *Towards a transformation of philosophy: The a priori of the communication community.* (G. Adey & D. Frisby, Trans.). London, UK: Routledge. (Original work published 1976.)

Archibald, M. M. (2012). The holism of aesthetic knowing in nursing. *Nursing Philosophy, 13,* 179–188.

Arendt, H. (1998). *The human condition* (2nd ed.). Chicago, IL: University of Chicago Press.

Argyris, C. (1980). *Inner contradictions of rigorous research.* San Diego, CA: Academic Press.

Argyris, C. (1993). *Knowledge for action.* San Francisco, CA: Jossey-Bass.

Argyris, C. (2002). Double-loop learning. Teaching and research. *Learning & Education, 1,* 206–219.

Argyris, C., Putnam, R., & Smith, D. M. (1985). *Action science: Concepts, methods, and skills for research and intervention.* San Francisco, CA: Jossey-Bass.

Argyris, C., & Schön, D. A. (1974). *Theory in practice.* San Francisco, CA: Jossey-Bass.

Argyris, C., & Schön, D. A. (1996). *Organizational learning II: Theory, method, and practice.* Reading, MA: Addision-Wesley.

Aristotle/Barnes, J. (1984). *The complete works of Aristotle: The revised Oxford translation* (J. Barnes, Trans.). Vol. 2. Princeton, NJ: Princeton University Press.

Aristotle/Butcher, S. H. (2011). *Poetics.* (S. H. Butcher, Trans.). Retrieved from http://classics.mit.edu//Aristotle/poetics.html

Aristotle/Ross, D. (1980). *The Nicomachean ethics* (D. Ross, Trans.). Oxford, UK: Oxford University Press.

Aristotle/Ross, W. D. (2011). *Metaphysics.* (W. D. Ross, Trans.). Retrieved from http://classics.mit.edu//Aristotle/metaphysics.html

Armstrong, A. E. (2006). Towards a strong virtue ethics for nursing practice. *Nursing Philosophy, 7,* 110–124.

Armstrong, K., Laschinger, H., & Wong, C. (2009). Workplace empowerment and Magnet hospital characteristics as predictors of patient safety climate. *Journal of Nursing Care Quality, 24,* 55–62.

Arries, E. (2006). Practice standards for quality clinical decision-making in nursing. *Curationis, 29,* 62–72.

Astedt-Kurki, P., & Haggman-Laitila, A. (1992). Good nursing practice as perceived by clients: A starting point for the development of professional nursing. *Journal of Advanced Nursing, 17,* 1195–1199.

Atkinson, P. (1995). *Medical talk and medical work. The liturgy of the clinic.* Thousand Oaks, CA: Sage Publications.

Audi, R. (1991). *Practical reasoning*. London, UK: Routledge.

Austgard, K. I. (2008). What characterises nursing care? A hermeneutical philosophical inquiry. *Scandinavian Journal of Caring Science, 22,* 314–319.

Austin, W. J. (2011). The incommensurability of nursing as a practice and the customer service model: An evolutionary threat to the discipline. *Nursing Philosophy, 12,* 158–166.

Baer, E. D., & Gordon, S. (1994). Money managers are unraveling the tapestry of nursing. *American Journal of Nursing, 94* (10), 38–40.

Baggs, J. G., & Schmitt, M. H. (1997). Nurses' and resident physicians' perceptions of the process of collaboration in an MICU. *Research in Nursing & Health, 20,* 71–80.

Bakken, S., Currie, L. M., Lee, N. J., Roberts, W. D., Collins, S. A., & Cimino, J. J. (2008). Integrating evidence into clinical information systems for nursing decision support. *International Journal of Medical Informatics, 77,* 413–120.

Bala, N., & Bromwich, R. J. (2002). Context and inclusivity in Canada's evolving definition of the family. *International Journal of Law, Policy and the Family, 16,* 145–180.

Baldwin, M. A. (2003). Patient advocacy: A concept analysis. *Nursing Standard, 17* (21), 33–39.

Banfield, B. E. (2011). Nursing agency: The link between practical nursing science and nursing practice. *Nursing Science Quarterly, 24,* 42–47.

Banfield, V., & Lackie, K. (2009). Performance-based competencies for culturally responsive interprofessional collaborative practice. *Journal of Interprofessional Care, 23,* 611–620.

Banning, M. (2008). A review of clinical decision making models and current research. *Journal of Clinical Nursing, 17,* 187–195.

Barrett, W. (1962). *Irrational man: A study in existential philosophy.* Garden City, NY: Doubleday.

Barsevick, A. M., & Johnson, J. E. (1990). Preference for information and involvement, information-seeking and emotional responses of women undergoing colposcopy. *Research in Nursing & Health, 13,* 1–7.

Batens, D. (1978). Rationality and ethical rationality. *Philosophica, 22,* 23–46.

Beauchamp, T. L. (2001). Internal and external standards for medical morality. *Journal of Medicine and Philosophy, 26,* 601–619.

Beauchamp, T. L., & Childress, J. F. (2012). *Principles of biomedical ethics* (7th ed.). New York, NY: Oxford University Press.

Beauvoir, S. (1989). *The second sex* (H. M. Parshley, Trans.). New York, NY: Vintage Books. (Original work published 1949.)

Beckwith, S., Dickinson, A., & Kendall, S. (2010). Exploring understanding of the term nursing assessment: A mixed method review of the literature. *Worldviews on Evidence-Based Nursing, 7,* 98–110.

Bedwell, W. L., Wildman, J. L., DiazGrandados, D., Salazer, M., Kramer, W. S., & Salas, E. (2012). Collaboration at work: An integrative multilevel conceptualization. *Human Resource Management Review, 22,* 128–145.

Bellack, J. P., & O'Neil, E. H. (2000). Recreating nursing practice for a new century. recommendations and implications of the Pew Health Professions Commission's final report. *Nursing & Health Care Perspectives, 21*, 14–21.

Benner, P. (1984). *From novice to expert: Excellence and power in clinical nursing practice.* Menlo Park, CA: Addison-Wesley.

Benner, P. (1991). The role of experience, narrative and community in skilled ethical comportment. *Advances in Nursing Science, 14*(2), 1–21.

Benner, P. (Ed.). (1994). *Interpretive phenomenology. Embodiment, caring, and ethics in health and illness*. Thousand Oaks, CA: Sage Publications.

Benner, P. (2000). The wisdom of caring practice. *Nursing Management, 6*, 32–37.

Benner, P. (2004). Designing formal classification systems to better articulate knowledge, skills, and meanings in nursing practice. *American Journal of Critical Care, 13*, 426–430.

Benner, P. (2009). *From novice to expert: Excellence and power in clinical nursing practice* (Commemorative edition). Englewood Cliffs, NJ: Prentice-Hall.

Benner, P., Hughes, R. G., & Sutphen, M. (2008). Clinical reasoning, decision making, and action: Thinking critically and clinically. In R. G. Hughes (Ed.), *Patient safety and quality: An evidence-based handbook for nurses* (Chapter 6). Rockville, MD: Agency for Healthcare Research and Quality, USDHHS. AHRQ Publication No. 08-0043.

Benner, P., Sutphen, M., Leonard-Kahn, V., & Day, L. (2008). Formation and everyday ethical comportment. *American Journal of Critical Care, 17*, 473–476.

Benner, P., Tanner, C. A., & Chesla, C. A. (2009). *Expertise in nursing practice: Caring, clinical judgment, and ethics* (2nd ed.). New York, NY: Springer Publishing.

Benner, P., & Wrubel, J. (1989). *The primacy of caring*. Menlo Park, CA: Addison-Wesley.

Benoist, J., & Cathebras, P. (1993). The body: From an immateriality to another. *Social Science and Medicine, 36*, 857–865.

Bent, K., Moscatel, S., Baize, T., & McCabe, J. (2007). Theory of human caring in 2050. *Nursing Science Quarterly, 20*, 331.

Berleant, A. (1991). *Art and engagement*. Philadelphia, PA: Temple University Press.

Bernstein, R. J. (1971). *Praxis and action: Contemporary philosophies of human activity*. Philadelphia, PA: University of Pennsylvania Press.

Bernstein, R. J. (1983). *Beyond objectivism and relativism: Science, hermeneutics, and praxis*. Philadelphia, PA: University of Pennsylvania Press.

Bhaskar, R. (1986). *Scientific realism and human emancipation*. London, UK: Verso.

Bhaskar, R. (1991). *Philosophy and the idea of freedom*. Oxford, UK: Blackwell.

Bishop, A. H., & Scudder, J. R., Jr. (Eds.). (1985). *Caring, curing, coping*. Tuscaloosa, AL: University of Alabama Press.

Bishop, A. H., & Scudder, J. R., Jr. (1990). *The practical, moral, and personal sense of nursing: A phenomenological philosophy of practice*. Albany, NY: State University of New York Press.

Bishop, A. H., & Scudder, J. R., Jr. (1999). A philosophical interpretation of nursing. *Scholarly Inquiry for Nursing Practice: An International Journal, 13*, 17–27.

Bishop, A. H., & Scudder, J. R., Jr. (2003). Gadow's contribution to our philosophical interpretation of nursing. *Nursing Philosophy, 4,* 104–110.

Björnsdöttir, K. (2001). Language, research and nursing practice. *Journal of Advanced Nursing, 33,* 159–166.

Björnsdöttir, K. (2013). Philosophy in the nurse's world: Politics of nursing practice II. *Nursing Philosophy, 14,* 238–239.

Blau, P. (1964). *Exchange and power in social life.* New York, NY: John Wiley and Sons, Inc.

Bleakley, A., & Bligh, J. (2009). Who can resist Foucault? *Journal of Medicine and Philosophy, 34,* 368–383.

Boh, W. F., Ren, Y., Kiesler, S., & Bussjaeger, R. (2007). Expertise and collaboration in the geographically dispersed organization. *Organization Science, 18,* 595–612.

Borrill, C., & West, M. (2002). *Team working and effectiveness in health care: Findings from the Healthcare Team Effectiveness Project.* Birmingham, UK: Aston Centre for Health Service Organisation Research.

Bourdieu, P. (1977). *Outline of a theory of practice.* Cambridge, UK: Cambridge University Press.

Bourdieu, P. (1990). *The logic of practice* (R. Nice, Trans.). Stanford, CA: Stanford University Press.

Bourdieu, P., & Wacquant, L. J. D. (1992). *An invitation to reflexive sociology.* Chicago, IL and London: University of Chicago Press.

Bowers, A. C., & Thompson, J. M. (1988). *Clinical manual of health assessment* (3rd ed.). St Louis, MO: Mosby.

Bradbury-Jones, C., & Sambrook, S. (2008). Power and empowerment in nursing: A fourth theoretical approach. *Journal of Advanced Nursing, 62,* 258–66.

Bradford, R. (1989). Obstacles to collaborative practice. *Nursing Management, 20*(4), 72I, 72L-72M, 72P.

Braveman, P., & Egerter, S. (2008). Overcoming obstacles to health. Princeton, NJ: Robert Wood Johnson Foundation. Retrieved from http://www.rwjf.org/content/dam/farm/reports/reports/2008/rwjf22441

Brilowski, G. A., & Wendler, M. C. (2005). An evolutionary concept analysis of caring. *Journal of Advanced Nursing, 50,* 641–650.

Bronstein, L. (2003). A model for interdisciplinary collaboration. *Social Work, 48,* 297–306.

Brown, P., Zavestoski, S., McCormick, S., Mayer, B., & Morello-Frosch, R. (2004). Embodied health movements: New approaches to social movements in health, *Sociology of Health & Illness, 26,* 50–80.

Brown, S. J. (1992). Tailoring nursing care to the individual client: Empirical challenge of a theoretical concept. *Research in Nursing & Health, 15,* 39–46.

Brown, S. J. (1994). Communicating strategies used by an expert nurse. *Clinical Nursing Research, 3,* 43–56.

Brown, S. J. (2013). *Evidence-based nursing: The research-practice connection* (3rd ed.). Burlington, MA: Jones & Bartlett Learning.

Bryant-Lukosius, D., Dicenso, A., Browne, G., & Pinelli, J. (2004). Advanced practice nursing roles: Development, implementation and evaluation. *Journal of Advanced Nursing, 48,* 519–529.

Bu, X., & Jezewski, A. (2007). Developing a mid-range theory of patient advocacy through concept analysis. *Journal of Advanced Nursing, 57,* 101–110.

Buber, M. (1970). *I and Thou* (W. Kaufmann, Trans.). New York, NY: Scribner. (Original work published 1923.)

Bulechek, G., Butcher, H., Dochterman, J., & Wagner, C. (Eds.). (2013). *Nursing interventions classification (NIC)* (6th ed.). St. Louis, MO: Elsevier.

Bury, M. (1982). Chronic illness as biographical disruption. *Sociology of Health and Illness,* 4(2), 167–182.

Buse, K., & Harmer, A. M. (2007). Seven habits of highly effective global public-private health partnerships: Practice and potential. *Social Science & Medicine, 64,* 259–271.

Butler, J. (1990). *Gender trouble: Feminism and the subversion of identity.* New York, NY: Routledge.

Cahill, J. (1996). Patient participation: A concept analysis. *Journal of Advanced Nursing, 24,* 561–571.

Calhoun, C., LiPuma, E., & Postone, M. (Eds.). (1993). *Bourdieu: Critical perspective.* Chicago, IL: The University of Chicago Press.

Campbell, J. D. (1997). Collaborative practice in the 1980s. In T. J. Sullivan (Ed.), *Collaboration: A health care imperative* (pp. 107–206). New York, NY: McGraw-Hill.

Canadian Interprofessional Health Collaborative. (2007). *Interprofessional Education & Core Competencies. Literature Review.* Vancouver: Author.

Carmel, S. (2013). The craft of intensive care medicine. *Sociology of Health & Illness, 35,* 731–745.

Carnevale, F. A. (2013). Charles Taylor, hermeneutics and social imaginaries: A framework for ethics research. *Nursing Philosophy, 14,* 86–95.

Carper, B. A. (1978). Fundamental patterns of knowing in nursing. *Advances in Nursing Science, 1*(1), 13–23.

Carr, D. (1986). *Time, narrative, and history.* Bloomington, IN: Indiana University Press.

Carr, W., & Kemmis, S. (1986). *Becoming critical: Education, knowledge and action research.* Basingstoke, UK: Falmer Press.

Cash, K. (1995). Benner and expertise in nursing: A critique. *International Journal of Nursing Studies, 32,* 527–534.

Cassirer, E. (1955). *The philosophy of symbolic forms. Volume 1: Language.* New Haven, CT: Yale University Press.

Cavanaugh, M. (1982). A modest proposal. *The Philosophy of the Social Sciences, 12,* 289–301.

Centre for the Advancement of Interprofessional Education (CAIPE). (2002). *Interprofessional education—A definition.* London: Author. Retrieved from: http://www.caipe.org.uk/about-us/defining-ipe

Centre for the Advancement of Interprofessional Education (CAIPE). (2002). *Interprofessional education—A definition.* London: Centre for the Advancement of Interprofessional Education. Retrieved from http://www.caipe.org.uk/about-us/defining-ipe

Chater, K. (1999). Risk and representation. Older people and noncompliance. *Nursing Inquiry, 6,* 132–138.

Cheung, R. B., Aiken, L. H., Clarke, S. P., & Sloane, D. M. (2008). Nursing care and patient outcomes: International evidence. *Enfermia Clinica,18*(1), 35–40.

Chinn, P. L. (2001). Toward a theory of nursing art. In N. Chaska (Ed.), *The nursing profession: Tomorrow and beyond* (pp. 287–298). Thousand Oaks, CA: Sage Publications.

Chinn, P. L. (2007). Challenge to action. In C. Roy & D. A. Jones (Eds.), *Nursing knowledge development and clinical practice* (pp. 93–101). New York, NY: Springer Publishing.

Chinn, P. L., & Kramer, M. K. (2007). *Integrated theory and knowledge development in nursing* (7th ed.). St. Louis, MO: Elsevier.

Christensen, M., & Hewitt-Taylor, J. (2006). From expert to tasks, expert nursing practice redefined? *Journal of Clinical Nursing, 15*, 1531–1539.

Clarke, A., Shim, J. K., Mamo, L., Fosket, J. R., & Fishman, J. (2003). Biomedicalization: Theorizing technoscientific transformation of health, illness, and U.S. biomedicine. *American Sociological Review, 68*, 161–194.

Clarke, H. F., & Mass, H. (1998). Comox Valley Nursing Centre: From collaboration to empowerment. *Public Health Nursing, 15*, 216–224.

Clarke, M. (1986). Action and reflection: Practice and theory in nursing. *Journal of Advanced Nursing, 11*, 3–11.

Clickner, D. A., & Shirey, M. R. (2013). Professional comportment: The missing element in nursing practice. *Nursing Forum, 48*, 106–113.

Clifton-Soderstrom, M. (2003). Levinas and the patient as other: The ethical foundation of medicine. *Journal of Medicine and Philosophy, 28*, 447–460.

Coffman, M. J. (2004). Cultural caring in nursing practice: A meta-synthesis of qualitative research. *Journal of Cultural Diversity, 11*, 100–109.

Collins, H. M. (1993). The structure of knowledge. *Social Research, 60*, 95–116.

Condon, E. H. (1992). Nursing and the caring metaphor: Gender and political influences on an ethics of care. *Nursing Outlook, 40*, 14–19.

Connor, M. J. (2004). Practical discourse in philosophy and nursing: An exploration of linkages and shifts in the evolution of praxis. *Nursing Philosophy, 5*, 54–66.

Conrick, M. (2005). The international classification for nursing practice: A tool to support nursing practice? *Collegian: Journal of the Royal College of Nursing, Australia, 12*, 9–13.

Cooper, D. (1999). *Existentialism*. Oxford, UK: Blackwell.

Coulter, A. (2002). After Bristol: Putting patients at the center. *Quality & Safety in Health Care, 11*, 186–188.

Council on Linkages Between Academia and Public Health Practice (COL). (2014). *Core competencies for public health professionals*. Washington, DC: Author. Retrieved from http://www.phf.org/resourcestools/Documents/Core_Competencies_for_Public_Health_Professionals_2014June.pdf

Cowan, D. T., Norman, I., & Coopamah, V. P. (2005). Competence in nursing practice: A controversial concept—A focused review of literature. *Nursing Education Today, 25*, 355–362.

Cowling, W. R. (2000). Healing as appreciating wholeness. *Advances in Nursing Science, 22*(3), 16–32.

Cowling, W. R., Chinn, P. L., & Hagedorn, S. (2000). A nursing manifesto: A call to conscience and action. Retrieved from http://www.nursemanifest.com/manifesto_num.htm

Cox, C. L. (1982). An interaction model of client health behavior: Theoretical prescription for nursing. *Advances in Nursing Science*, *5*(1), 41–56.

Craven, M. A., & Bland, R. (2006). Better practices in collaborative mental health care: An analysis of the evidence base. *Canadian Journal of Psychiatry*, *51* (Supplement 1), 1s–72s.

Crawford Shearer, N. B., & Reed, P. G. (2004). Empowerment: reformulation of a non-Rogerian concept. *Nursing Science Quarterly*, *17*, 253–259.

Croker, A., Trede, F., & Higgs, J. (2012). Collaboration: What is it like?—Phenomenological interpretation of the experience of collaborating within rehabilitation teams. *Journal of Interprofessional Care*, *26*, 13–20.

Cronenwett, L., Sherwood, G., Barnsteiner, J., Disch, J., Johnson, J., Mitchell, P., ... Warren, J. (2007). Quality and safety education for nurses. *Nursing Outlook*, *55*, 122–131.

Cronenwett, L., Sherwood, G., & Gelmon, S. B. (2009). Improving quality and safety education: The QSEN Learning Collaborative. *Nursing Outlook*, *57*, 304–312.

Cronenwett, L., Sherwood, G., Pohl, J., Barnsteiner, J., Moore, S., Sullivan, D. T., ... Warren, J. (2009). Quality and safety education for advanced nursing practice. *Nursing Outlook*, *57*, 338–348.

Crowell, S. (2001). *Husserl, Heidegger, and the space of meaning: Paths toward transcendental phenomenology*. Evanston, IL: Northwestern University Press.

Crowell, S. (2010). Existentialism. In E. N. Zalta (Ed.), *The Stanford encyclopedia of philosophy* (Winter 2010 Edition). Retrieved from http://plato.stanford.edu/archives/win2010/entries/existentialism

Crowley, A. A., & Sabatelli, R. M. (2008). Collaborative childcare health consultation: A conceptual model. *Journal for Specialists in Pediatric Nursing*, *13*, 74–88.

CURN project. (1983). *Using research to improve nursing practice: A guide*. New York, NY: Grune & Stratton.

Curtis, E., & Nicholl, H. (2004). Delegation: A key function to nursing. *Nursing Management*, *11*(4), 26.

Dale, A. E. (2005). Evidence-based practice; compatibility with nursing. *Nursing Standard (Royal College of Nursing)*, *19*, 48–53.

D'Amour, D., Ferrada-Videla, M., San Martin-Rodriguez, L., & Beaulieu, M. (2005). The conceptual basis for interprofessional collaboration: Core concepts and theoretical frameworks. *Journal of Interprofessional Care* (Supplement 1), 116–131.

D'Amour, D., & Oandasan, I. (2005). Interprofessionality as the field of interprofessional practice and interprofessional education: An emerging concept. *Journal of Interprofessional Care*, *19* (Supplement 1), 8–20.

Davidson, D. (1982). *Essays on actions and events*. Oxford, UK: Clarendon Press.

Davies, K., Gray, M., & Webb, S. A. (2014). Putting the parity into service-user participation: An integrated model of social justice. *International Journal of Social Welfare*, *23*, 119–124.

Department of Health. (1999). *Making a difference*. London, UK: Author.

de Stampa, M., Vedel, I., Bergman, H., Novella, J., Lechowski, L., Ankri, J., & Lapointe, L. (2012). Opening the black box of clinical collaboration in integrated care models for frail, elderly patients. *The Gerontologist, 53*, 313–325.

Dewey, J. (1957). *Human nature and conduct: An introduction to social psychology*. New York, NY: The Modern Library. (Originally published 1922.)

Dewey, J. (1987). Aesthetic experience. In J. A. Boydston & H. F. Simon (Eds.), *John Dewey: The later works, 1925–1953. Volume 10: 1934*. Carbondale, IL: Southern Illinois University Press. (Original work published 1934.)

Dhillon, J. K. (2009). The role of social capital in sustaining partnership. *British Educational Research Journal, 35*, 687–703.

Dias, P. (2011). Aesthetics and ethics in engineering: Insights from Polanyi. *Science and Engineering Ethics, 17*, 233–243.

Ditmyer, S., Coepsell, B., Branum, V., Davis, P., & Lush, M. T. (1998). Developing a nursing outcomes measurement tool. *Journal of Nursing Administration, 28*, 10–16.

Doane, G., Pauly, B., Brown, H., & McPherson, G. (2004). Exploring the heart of ethical nursing practice: Implications for ethics education. *Nursing Ethics: An International Journal for Health Care Professionals, 11*, 240–253.

Doane, G. A. (2002). Beyond behavioral skills to human-involved processes: Relational nursing practice and interpretive pedagogy. *Journal of Nursing Education, 41*, 400–404.

Doane, G. H., & Varcoe, C. (2008). Knowledge translation in everyday nursing: From evidence-based to inquiry-based practice. *Advances in Nursing Science, 31*, 283–295.

Dodd, M., Janson, S., Facione, N., Faucett, J., Froelicher, E., Humphreys, J., ... Taylor, D. (2001). Advancing the science of symptom management. *Journal of Advanced Nursing, 33*, 668–676.

Dombeck, M.-T. (2003). Work narratives: Gender and race on professional personhood. *Research in Nursing & Health, 26*, 351–365.

Donabedian, A. (1988). The quality of care. *Journal of the American Medical Association, 260*, 1743–1748.

Donagan, A. (1987). *Choice: The essential element in human action*. London, UK: Routledge & Keegan Paul.

Donaldson, S. K., & Crowley, D. M. (1978). The discipline of nursing. *Nursing Outlook, 26*, 113–120.

Donnelly, G. (2003). Clinical expertise in advanced practice nursing: A Canadian perspective. *Nursing Education Today, 23*, 168–173.

Doody, O. (2014). The role and development of consultancy in nursing practice. *British Journal of Nursing, 23*, 32–39.

Doucet, T. J., & Merlin, M. D. (2014). Conceptualizations of health in nursing practice. *Nursing Science Quarterly, 27*, 118–125.

Dow, A. Q., DiazGranados, D., Mazmanian, P. E, & Retchin, S. M. (2013). Applying organizational science to health care: A framework for collaborative practice. *Academic Medicine: Journal of the Association of American Medical Colleges, 88*, 952–957.

Downie, J., Orb, A., Wynaden, D., McGowan, S., Zeeman, Z., & Ogilvie, S. (2001). A practice-research model for collaborative partnership. *Collegian (Royal College of Nursing Australia), 8*(4), 27–32.

Dreyfus, H. (1979). *What computers can't do: The limits of artificial intelligence.* New York, NY: Harper Colophon.

Dreyfus, H. (1992). *What computers still can't do.* Cambridge, MA: MIT Press.

Dreyfus, H. L., & Dreyfus, S. E. (1986). *Mind over machine: The power of human intuition and expertise in the era of the computer.* New York, NY: Free Press.

Dreyfus, H., & Wrathall, M. A. (Eds.). (2008). *A companion to phenomenology and existentialism.* Hoboken, NJ: Wiley-Blackwell.

Dudley, S. K., & Carr, J. M. (2004). Vigilance: The experience of parents staying at the bedside of hospitalized children. *Journal of Pediatric Nursing, 19,* 267–275.

Duffy, J. R., & Hoskins, L. M. (2003). The Quality-Caring Model: Blending dual paradigms. *Advances in Nursing Science, 26,* 77–88.

Dunlop, M. J. (1994). Is a science of caring possible? In P. Benner (Ed.), *Interpretive phenomenology: Embodiment, caring, and ethics in health and illness* (pp. 27–42). Thousand Oaks, CA: Sage Publications.

Dunne, J. (1993). *Back to the rough ground: "Phronesis" and "techné" in modern philosophy and in Aristotle.* Notre Dame, IN: University of Notre Dame Press.

Dunne, J. (1999). Virtue, phronesis and learning. In D. Carr & J. Steutel (Eds.), *Virtue ethics and moral education* (pp. 49–63). London, UK: Routledge.

Dunne, J. (2003). Arguing for teaching as a practice: A reply to Alasdair MacIntyre. *Journal of Philosophy of Education, 37,* 353–369.

Eason, F. R. (2000). The four A's of delegation. *Advance for Nurses Carolina/Georgia,* 2(23), 11–13.

Edgar, A., & Pattison, S. (2011). Integrity and the moral complexity of professional practice. *Nursing Philosophy, 12,* 94–106.

Edwards, S. D. (1996). What are the limits to the obligations of the nurse? *Journal of Medical Ethics, 22,* 90–94.

Edwards, S. D. (1998). The art of nursing. *Nursing Ethics, 5,* 393–400.

Edwards, S. D. (2001). Benner and Wrubel on caring in nursing. *Journal of Advanced Nursing, 33,* 167–171.

Edwards, S. D. (2009). Three versions of an ethics of care. *Nursing Philosophy, 10,* 231–240.

Edwards, S. D. (2011). Is there a distinctive care ethics? *Nursing Ethics,18,* 184–191.

Ellefsen, B. (2004). Frames and perspectives in clinical nursing practice: A study of Norwegian nurses in acute care settings. *Research & Theory for Nursing Practice, 18,* 95–109.

Ellefsen, B., & Kim, H. S. (2004). Nurses' construction of clinical situations: A study conducted in an acute-care setting in Norway. *Canadian Journal of Nursing Research, 36,* 115–131.

Ellefsen, B., & Kim, H. S. (2005). Nurses' clinical engagement: A study from an acute-care setting in Norway. *Research and Theory for Nursing Practice: An International Journal, 19,* 297–313.

Ellefsen, B., Kim, H. S., & Han, K. J. (2007). Nursing gaze as framework for nursing practice: A study from acute-care settings in Korea, Norway and the USA. *Scandinavian Journal of Caring Science, 21,* 98–105.

Elstein, A. S., Shulman, L. S., & Sprafka, S. A. (1978). *Medical problem solving: An analysis of clinical reasoning.* Cambridge, MA: Harvard University Press.

Enburg, C. B. L., Klein, C., Abdur-Rahman, V. A., Spencer, T., & Boyer, S. (2009). The COPA model: A comprehensive framework designed to promote quality care and competence for patient safety. *Nursing Education Perspectives, 30,* 312–317.

Engebretson, J., & Littleton, L. Y. (2001). Cultural negotiation: A constructivist-based model for nursing practice. *Nursing Outlook, 49,* 223–230.

Epstein, R. M., & Hundert, E. M. (2002). Defining and assessing professional competence. *Journal of the American Medical Association, 287,* 226–235.

Eraut, M. (1994). *Developing professional knowledge and competence.* London, UK: Falmer Press.

Eriksson, K. (1987). *Vårdandets idé [The idea of caring].* Stockholm, Sweden: Almqvist & Wiksell.

Evans, J. A. (1994). The role of the nurse manager in creating an environment for collaborative practice. *Holistic Nursing Practice, 8*(3), 22–31.

Evans, R. J., & Donnelly, G. W. (2006). A model to describe the relationship between knowledge, skill, and judgment in nursing practice. *Nursing Forum, 41,* 150–157.

Fackenheim, E. (1961). *Metaphysics and historicity.* Milwaukee, WI: Marquette University Press.

Fagermoen, M. S. (1997). Professional identity: Values embedded in meaningful nursing practice. *Journal of Advanced Nursing, 25,* 434–441.

Fagermoen, M. S. (2006). Humanism in nursing theory: A focus on caring. In H. S. Kim & I. Kollak (Eds.), *Nursing theories: Conceptual and philosophical foundations* (pp. 157–183). New York, NY: Springer Publishing.

Fairhurst, K., & May, C. (2001). Knowing patients and knowledge about patients: Evidence of modes of reasoning in the consultation? *Family Practice, 18,* 501–505.

Fasnacht, P. H. (2003). Creativity: A refinement of the concept for nursing practice. *Journal of Advanced Nursing, 41,* 195–202.

Fealy, G. M. (1995). Professional caring: The moral dimension. *Journal of Advanced Nursing, 22,* 1135–1140.

Fealy, G. M. (1997). The theory-practice relationship in nursing: An exploration of contemporary discourse. *Journal of Advanced Nursing, 25,* 1061–1069.

Felder, A. J., & Robbins, B. D. (2011). A cultural-existential approach to therapy: Merleau-Ponty's phenomenology of embodiment and its implications for practice. *Theory & Psychology, 21,* 355–376.

Fell, J. (1979). *Heidegger and Sartre: An essay on being and place.* New York, NY: Columbia University Press.

Finfgeld-Connett, D. (2006). Meta-synthesis of presence in nursing. *Journal of Advanced Nursing, 55,* 708–714.

Finfgeld-Connett, D. (2008a). Concept synthesis of the art of nursing. *Journal of Advanced Nursing, 62,* 381–388.

Finfgeld-Connett, D. (2008b). Meta-synthesis of caring in nursing. *Journal of Clinical Nursing, 17*, 196–204.

Finfgeld-Connett, D. (2008c). Qualitative comparison and synthesis of nursing presence and caring. *International Journal of Nursing Terminologies and Classifications, 19*, 111–119.

Flaming, D. (2001). Using phronesis instead of "research based practice" as the guiding light for nursing practice. *Nursing Philosophy, 2*, 251–258.

Forchuk, C., Martin, M. L., Jensen, E., Ouseley, S., Sealy, P., Beal, G., ... Sharkey, S. (2013). Integrating an evidence-based intervention into clinical practice: "Transitional relationship model." *Journal of Psychiatric and Mental Health Nursing, 20*, 584–594.

Fordor, J. (1981). *Representations*. Cambridge, MA: Bradford Books/MIT Press.

Fordor, J. (2000). *The mind doesn't work that way*. Cambridge, MA: MIT Press.

Foster, M., & Tilse, C. (2003). Referral to rehabilitation following traumatic brain injury: A model for understanding inequities in access. *Social Science & Medicine, 56*, 2201–2210.

Foucault, M. (1973a). *The birth of the clinic* (A. M. Sheridan Smith, Trans.). London, UK: Tavistock Publications. (Originally published 1963.)

Foucault, M. (1973b). *The order of things* (A. M. Sheridan Smith, Trans.). New York, NY: Vintage. (Originally published 1966.)

Fowler, M. D. (Ed.). (2008). *Guide to the Code of Ethics for nurses: Interpretation and application*. Silver Spring, MD: Nursesbooks.org

Fraenkel, P. (2006). Engaging families as experts: Collaborative family program development. *Family Process, 45*, 237–257.

Frank, J. R. (Ed). (2005). *The CanMEDS 2005 physician competency framework. Better standards. Better physicians. Better care.* Ottawa: The Royal College of Physicians and Surgeons of Canada.

Freire, P. (1985). *The politics of education*. South Hadley, MA: Bergin & Garvey Publishers.

Freire, P. (1992). *Pedagogy of the oppressed* (M. B. Ramos, Trans.). New York, NY: Continuum. (Original work published 1970.)

Freire, P. (1998). *Pedagogy of freedom: Ethics, democracy, and civic courage*. Lanham, MD: Rowman & Littlefield.

Frenk, J., Chen, L., Bhutta, Z. A., Cohen, J., Crisp, N., Evans, T., ... Zurayk, H. (2010). Health professionals for a new century: Transforming education to strengthen health systems in an interdependent world. *Lancet, 376*, 1923–1958.

Fu, M. R., LeMone, P., & McDaniel, R. W. (2004). An integrated approach to an analysis of symptom management in patients with cancer. *Oncology Forum, 31*, 65–70.

Funk, L. M., Stajduhar, K. I., & Purkis, M. E. (2011). An exploration of empowerment discourse within home-care nurses' accounts of practice. *Nursing Inquiry, 18*, 66–76.

Gadamer, H. (1992). *On education, poetry, and history*. Albany, NY: State University of New York Press.

Gadotti, M. (2002). *General theme: The possible dream. Paulo Freire and the future of humanity*. Paper presented at the Third International Paulo Freire Forum, Los Angeles, September 18–21, 2002.

Gadow, S. (1980). Body and self: A dialectic. *Journal of Medicine and Philosophy, 5,* 172–185.

Gadow, S. (1990). *Existential advocacy: Philosophical foundations of nursing. NLN Publications* (20-2294) (pp. 41–51). New York, NY: National League for Nursing.

Gadow, S. (1994). Whose body? Whose story? The question about narrative in women's health care. *Soundings, 77,* 295–307.

Gadow, S. (1995a). Clinical epistemology: A dialectic of nursing assessment. *Canadian Journal of Nursing Research [Revue Canadienne De Recherche En Sciences Infirmieres], 27,* 25–34.

Gadow, S. (1995b). Narrative and exploration: Toward a poetics of knowledge in nursing. *Nursing Inquiry, 2,* 211–214.

Gadow, S. (1996). Ethical narratives in practice. *Nursing Science Quarterly, 9,* 8–9.

Gadow, S. (1999). Relational narrative: The postmodern turn in nursing ethics. *Scholarly Inquiry for Nursing Practice, 13,* 57–70.

Gadow, S. (2003). Restorative nursing: Toward a philosophy of postmodern punishment. *Nursing Philosophy, 4,* 161–167.

Gage, M. (1998). Ten steps to a patient-driven interdisciplinary care plan. *Aspen Advisory Nurse Executive, 13,* 6–8.

Gardner, D. B., & Cary, A. (1999). Collaboration, conflict, and power: Lessons for care managers. *Family & Community Health, 22*(3), 64–77.

Gardner, G., Chang, A., & Duffield, C. (2007). Making nursing work: Breaking through the role confusion of advanced practice nursing. *Journal of Advanced Nursing, 57,* 382–391.

Gardner, S. (1999). *Beyond collaboration to results: Hard choices in the future of services to children and families.* Phoenix, AZ: Arizona Prevention Resource Center, the Center for Collaboration for Children.

Gavin, J. N. (1997). Nursing ideology and the "generic carer." *Journal of Advanced Nursing, 26,* 692–697.

Gibson, C. H. (1991). A concept analysis of empowerment. *Journal of Advanced Nursing, 16,* 354–361.

Giddens, A. (1984). *The constitution of society: Outline of the theory of structuration.* Berkeley, CA: University of California Press.

Gilligan, C. (1982). *In a different voice.* Cambridge, MA: Harvard University Press.

Glen, S. (1998). The key to quality of nursing care: Towards a model of personal and professional development. *Nursing Ethics, 5,* 95–102.

Gobbi, M. (2005). Nursing practice as bricoleur activity: A concept explored. *Nursing Inquiry, 12,* 117–125.

Good, B. J. (1994). *Medicine, rationality, and experience: An anthropological perspective.* Cambridge, UK: Cambridge University Press.

Goodwin, D. (2010). Sensing the way: Embodied dimensions of diagnostic work. In M. Buscher, D. Goodwin, & J. Mesman (Eds.). *Ethnographies of diagnostic work: Dimensions of transformative practice* (pp. 73–94). Basingstoke, UK: Palgrave Macmillan.

Gordon, M. (2007). *Manual of nursing diagnosis* (11th ed.). Boston, MA: Jones & Bartlett.

Gordon, S. (1997). *Life support: Three nurses on the front lines.* Boston, MA: Little, Brown and Company.

Green, C. (2009). A comprehensive theory of the human person from philosophy and nursing. *Nursing Philosophy, 10,* 263–274.

Greiner, A. C., & Knebel, E. (Eds.). (2003). *Health professions education: A bridge to quality.* Washington, DC: Institute of Medicine, the National Academies Press.

Gustad, J. W. (1953). The definition of counseling. In R. F. Berdie (Ed.), *Roles and relationships in counseling* (pp. 3–39). Minneapolis, MN: University of Minnesota Press.

Habermas, J. (1984). *Theory of communicative action. Volume One: Reason and rationalization of society* (T. A. McCarthy, Trans.). Boston, MA: Beacon Press. (Original publication 1981.)

Habermas, J. (1986). *Knowledge and human interests.* Cambridge, UK: Polity.

Habermas, J. (1987). *Theory of communicative action. Volume Two: Liveworld and system: A critique of functionalist reason* (T. A. McCarthy, Trans.). Boston, MA: Beacon Press. (Original publication 1981.)

Habermas, J. (1988). *On the logic of the social science* (S. W. Nicholsen & J. A. Stark, Trans.). Cambridge, MA: The MIT Press.

Habermas, J. (1990). *Moral consciousness and communicative action* (C. Lenhardt & S. W. Nicholsen, Trans.). Cambridge, MA: MIT Press (Original work published 1983.)

Hadorn, D. C. (1997). Kinds of patients. *Journal of Medicine and Philosophy, 22,* 567–587.

Hage, A. M., & Lorensen, M. (2005). A philosophical analysis of the concept empowerment: The fundament of an education-programme to the frail elderly. *Nursing Philosophy: An International Journal for Healthcare Professionals, 6,* 235–246.

Haggerty, L. A., & Grace, P. (2008). Clinical wisdom: The essential foundation of "good" nursing care. *Journal of Professional Nursing, 24,* 235–240.

Hansson, S. O. (2007). Values in pure and applied science. *Foundations of Science, 12,* 257–268.

Hansten, R. I., & Jackson, M. (2009). *Clinical delegation skills: A handbook for professional practice* (4th ed.). Burlington, MA: Jones & Bartlett Learning.

Hardy, C., Phillips, N., & Lawrence, T. (2003). Resources, knowledge and influence: The organizational effects of interorganizational collaboration. *Journal of Management Studies, 40,* 321–347.

Hardy, S., Titchen, A., & Manley, K. (2007). Patient narratives in the investigation and development of nursing practice expertise: A potential for transformation. *Nursing Inquiry, 14,* 80–88.

Hardy, S., Titchen, A., Manley, K., & McCormack, B. (2006). Re-defining nursing expertise in the United Kingdom. *Nursing Science Quarterly, 19,* 260–264.

Harmer, B., & Henderson, V. (1955). *Textbook of the principles and practices of nursing.* New York, NY: Macmillan.

Harris, M. D. (1992). Outcomes of care from the professional's perspective. *Home Healthcare Nurse, 10*(6), 48–49.

Harris, V. (2008). Mediators or partners? Practitioner perspectives on partnership. *Development in Practice, 18,* 701–712.

Hart, G. (1990). Peer consultation and review. *Australian Journal of Advanced Nursing, 7*, 40–46.

Hartrick, D. G., Storch, J. L., & Pauly, B. (2009). Ethical nursing practice: Inquiry-in-action. *Nursing Inquiry, 16*, 232–240.

Harvey, T. S. (2008). Where there is no patient: An anthropological treatment of a biomedical category. *Culture, Medicine and Psychiatry, 32*, 577–606.

Hasseler, M. (2006). Evidence-based nursing for practice and science. In H. S. Kim & I. Kollak (Eds.), *Nursing theories: Conceptual and philosophical foundations* (2nd ed.) (pp. 215–235). New York, NY: Springer Publishing.

Havens, D. S., Wood, S. O., & Leeman, J. (2006). Improving nursing practice and patient care: Building capacity with appreciative inquiry. *The Journal of Nursing Administration, 36*, 463–470.

Health Canada. (2004). *Interprofessional education for collaborative patient-centred practice. Health Canada. Health human resources strategy—Interprofessional education*. Retrieved from http://www.hcsc. gc.ca/hcs-sss/hhr-rhs/strateg/interprof/accomp-9_e.html

Heidegger, M. (1962). *Being and time* (J. Macquarrie & E. Robinson, Trans.). New York, NY: Harper and Row. (Original work published 1927.)

Hellesø, R., Sorensen, L., & Lorensen, M. (2005). Nurses' information management across complex health care organizations. *International Journal of Medical Informatics, 74*, 960–972.

Henderson, A. (1994). Power and knowledge in nursing practice: The contribution of Foucault. *Journal of Advanced Nursing, 20*, 935–939.

Henderson, D., Sealover, P., Sharrer, V., Fusner, S., Fones, S., Sweet, S., & Blake, T. (2006). Nursing EDGE: Evaluating delegation guidelines in education. *International Journal of Nursing Education Scholarship, 3*, 1–10. doi: 10.2202/1548-923X.1197

Henderson, V. (1961). *Basic principles of nursing care*. London, UK: International Council of Nurses.

Henderson, V. (1966). *The nature of nursing: A definition and its implications for practice, research, and education*. New York, NY: Macmillan.

Henderson, V. A. (1991). *The nature of nursing: A definition and its implications for practice, research, and education: Reflections after 25 years*. NLN Publication No. 15-2346. New York, NY: National League for Nursing Press.

Henneman, E. A., Gawlinski, A., & Giuliano, K. K. (2012). Surveillance: A strategy for improving patient safety in acute and critical care units. *Critical Care Nurse, 32*, e9-e18. Retrieved from www.ccnonline.org

Henneman, E., Lee, J., & Cohen, J. (1995). Collaboration: A concept analysis. *Journal of Advanced Nursing, 21*, 103–109.

Herdman, T. H. (Ed.). (2009). *NANDA International nursing diagnoses: Definitions & classification, 2009–2011*. Oxford, UK: Wiley-Blackwell.

Hermansson, E., & Martensson, L. (2011). Empowerment in the midwifery context—A concept analysis. *Midwifery, 27*, 811–816.

Hess, J. D. (2003). Gadow's relational narrative: An elaboration. *Nursing Philosophy, 4*, 137–148.

Hewitt, A. (2005). *Social choreography: Ideology as performance in dance and everyday movement*. Durham, NC: Duke University Press.

Hinds, P. J., & Kiesler, S. (Eds.). (2002). *Distributed work*. Cambridge, MA: The MIT Press.

Holmes, C., & Warelow, P. (2000). Nursing as normative praxis. *Nursing Inquiry, 7*, 175–181.

Holmes, C. A. (1992). The drama of nursing. *Journal of Advanced Nursing, 17*, 941–950.

Holmes, D., & Gastaldo, D. (2004). Rhizomatic thought in nursing: An alternative path for the development of the discipline. *Nursing Philosophy, 5*, 258–267.

Holmstrom, I., & Larsson, J. (2005). A tension between genuine care and other duties: Swedish nursing students' views of their future work. *Nurse Education Today, 25*, 148–155.

Holmström, I., & Röing, M. (2010). The relation between patient-centeredness and patient empowerment: A discussion on concepts. *Patient Education and Counseling, 79*, 167–172.

Hornby, S., & Atkins, J. (2000). *Collaborative care: Interprofessional, interagency and interpersonal*. Oxford, UK: Blackwell Science Ltd.

Horst, S. (2011). The computational theory of mind. In E. N. Zalta (Ed.), *The Stanford encyclopedia of philosophy*. Retrieved from http://plato.stanford.edu/archives/spr2011/entries/computational-mind

Hughes, R. G. (Ed.). (2008). *Patient safety and quality: An evidence-based handbook for nurses*. Rockville, MD: Agency for Healthcare Research and Quality, USDHHS. AHRQ Publication No. 08-0043.

Hull, C. S., & O'Rourke, M. E. (2007). Oncology-critial care nursing collaboration: Recommendations for optimizing continuity of care of critically patients with cancer. *Clinical Journal of Oncology Nursing, 11*, 925–927.

Hunt, J. M. (1996). Barriers to research utilization. *Journal of Advanced Nursing, 23*, 423–425.

Hunter, B. (2005). Emotion work and boundary maintenance in hospital-based midwifery. *Midwifery, 21*, 253–266.

Hunter, D. (2007). Am I my brother's gatekeeper? Professional ethics and the prioritisation of healthcare. *Journal of Medical Ethics, 33*, 522–526.

Hussey, T. (2012). Just caring. *Nursing Philosophy, 13*, 6–14.

Hyde, A., Treacy, M., Scott, P. A., Butler, M., Drennan, J., Irving, K., … Hanrahan, M. (2005). Modes of rationality in nursing documentation: Biology, biography and the "voice of nursing." *Nursing Inquiry, 12*, 66–77.

Institute of Medicine (IOM). (2001b). *Envisioning the National Health Care Quality Report*. Washington, DC: The National Academies Press.

Institute of Medicine (IOM). (2003a). *Priority areas for national action: Transforming health care quality*. Washington, DC: The National Academies Press.

Institute of Medicine (IOM). (2003b). *Unequal treatment: Confronting racial and ethnic disparities in health care*. Washington, DC: The National Academies Press.

Institute of Medicine (IOM). (2003c). *The future of the public's health in the twenty-first century*. Washington, DC: The National Academies Press.

Institute of Medicine (IOM). (2004a). *Health literacy: A prescription to end confusion*. Washington, DC: The National Academies Press.

Institute of Medicine (IOM). (2004b). *Measuring what matters: Allocation, planning, and quality assessment for the Ryan White CARE Act*. Washington, DC: The National Academies Press.

Institute of Medicine (IOM). (2008). *Retooling for an aging America: Building the health care workforce*. Washington, DC: The National Academies Press.

Institute of Medicine (IOM). (2009). *The healthcare imperative: Lowering costs and improving outcomes: Brief summary of a workshop*. Washington, DC: The National Academies Press.

Institute of Medicine (IOM). (2010a). *The future of nursing. Focus on scope of practice*. Washington, DC: The National Academies Press.

Institute of Medicine (IOM). (2010b). *A summary of the December 2009 Forum on the Future of Nursing: Care in the community*. Washington, DC: The National Academies Press.

Institute of Medicine (IOM). (2012). *Best care at lower cost. The path to continuously learning health care in America*. Washington, DC: The National Academies Press.

Institute of Medicine (IOM). (2014). *Interprofessional education for collaboration: Learning how to improve health from interprofessional models across the continuum of education to practice*. Workshop summary of the Global Forum on Innovation in Health Professional Education. Board on Global Health, National Research Council of the National Academies. Washington, DC: The National Academies Press.

Institute of Medicine (IOM) Committee on the Robert Wood Johnson Foundation Initiative on the Future of Nursing. (2014). *The future of nursing: Leading change, advancing health*. Washington, DC: The National Academies Press.

Institute of Medicine (IOM) Roundtable on evidence-based medicine. (2008). *Learning healthcare system concepts, v. 2008*. Washington, DC: The National Academies Press.

International Council of Nurses (ICN). (2006). *The ICN code of ethics for nurses*. Geneva, Switzerland: Author.

International Council of Nurses (ICN). (2014). *Definition of nursing*. Retrieved from http://www.icn.ch/about-icn/icn-definition-of-nursing

Interprofessional Education Collaborative Expert Panel. (2011). *Core competencies for interprofessional collaborative practice: Report of an expert panel*. Washington, DC: Author.

Jackson, K. (2002). *Assessment made incredibly easy* (2nd ed.). Philadelphia, PA: Springhouse.

Jacobs, B. B. (2001). Respect for human dignity: A central phenomenon to philosophically unite nursing theory and practice through consilience of knowledge. *Advances in Nursing Science, 24*, 17–35.

Jacobs, B. B., Fontana, J. S., Kehoe, M. H., Matarese, C., & Chinn, P. L. (2005). An emancipatory study of contemporary nursing practice. *Nursing Outlook, 53*, 6–14.

James, I., Andershed, B., Gustavsson, B., & Ternestedt, B. (2010). Knowledge constructions in nursing practice: Understanding and integrating different forms of knowledge. *Qualitative Health Research, 20*, 1500–1518.

Jansen, Y. J. F. M., de Bont, A., Foets, M., Bruijnzeels, M., & Bal, R. (2007). Tailoring intervention procedures to routine primary health care practice: An ethnographic process evaluation. *BMC Health Services Research, 7*, 125–132. Retrieved from http://www.biomedcentral.com/1472-6963/7/125

Jasper, M. A. (1994). Expert: A discussion of the implications of the concept as used in nursing. *Journal of Advanced Nurisng, 20*, 769–776.

Jaspers, K. (1955). *Reason and existenz* (W. Earle, Trans.). New York, NY: Noonday Press. (Original work published 1935.)

Jefferies D., Johnson M., & Griffiths R. (2010). A meta-study of the essentials of quality nursing documentation. *International Journal of Nursing Practice, 16*, 112–124.

Jeffs, L., Sidani, S., Rose, D., Espin, S., Smith, O., Martin, K., ... Ferris, E. (2013). Using theory and evidence to drive measurement of patient, nurse and organizational outcomes of professional nursing practice. *International Journal of Nursing Practice, 19*, 141–148.

Jennings, B. M., & Staggers, N. (1998). The language of outcomes. *Advances in Nursing Science, 20*, 72–80.

Jenny, J., & Logan, J. (1992). Knowing the patient: One aspect of clinical knowledge. *Image: The Journal of Nursing Scholarship, 24*, 254–258.

Jezewski, M. A. (1990). Culture brokering in migrant farm worker health care. *Western Journal of Nursing Research, 12*, 497–513.

Jezewski, M. A., & Sotnik, P. (2001). *Culture brokering: Providing culturally competent rehabilitation services to foreign-born persons*. Buffalo, NY: Center for International Rehabilitation Research Information and Exchange. Retrieved from http://cirrie.buffalo.edu/monographs/cb.pdf

Johnson, L. J., Zorn D., Tam B. K. Y., LaMontagne M., & Johnson, S. A. (2003). Stakeholders' views of factors that impact successful interagency collaboration. *Exceptional Children. 69*, 195–209.

Joint Commission on Accreditation of Healthcare Organizations (JCAHO). (Ed.). (1997). *Nursing practice and outcome measurement*. Oakbrook Terrace, IL: Author.

Jonas, H. (1979). Toward a philosophy of technology. *Hastings Center Report, 9*, 34–43.

Jonsdottir, H., Litchfield, M., & Pharris, M. D. (2004). The relational core of nursing practice as partnership. *Journal of Advanced Nursing, 47*, 241–248.

Jormsri, P., Kunaviktikul, W., Ketefian, S., & Chaowalit, A. (2005). Moral competence in nursing practice. *Nursing Ethics, 12*, 582–594.

Kagan, P. N., Smith, M. C., Cowling, W. R., & Chinn, P. L. (2009). A nursing manifesto: An emancipatory call for knowledge development, conscience, and praxis. *Nursing Philosophy, 11*, 67–84.

Kahn, R. L., & Prager, D. J. (1994). Collaborations are a scientific and social imperative. *Scientist, 8*(14), 12.

Kahneman, D., Tversky, A., & Slovic, P. (Eds.). (1982). *Judgment under uncertainty: Heuristics & biases*. Cambridge, UK, Cambridge University Press.

Kelly, L., & Vincent, D. (2011). The dimensions of nursing surveillance: A concept analysis. *Journal of Advanced Nursing, 67*, 651–662.

Kelly-Heidenthal, P., & Marthaler, M. T. (2005). *Delegation of nursing care*. New York, NY: Thomson Delmar Learning.

Kendall, J. (1992). Fighting back: Promoting emancipatory nursing actions. *Advances in Nursing Science, 15*(2), 1–15.

Kendrick, K. D., & Robinson, S. (2002). "Tender loving care" as a relational ethic in nursing practice. *Nursing Ethics, 9*, 291–300.

Kennedy, H. (1999). *Linking midwifery practice to outcomes: A Delphi study*. PhD Dissertation. Kingston, RI: University of Rhode Island.

Khushf, G. (1999). The aesthetics of clinical judgment: Exploring the link between diagnostic elegance and effective resource utilization. *Medicine, Health Care, and Philosophy, 2*, 141–159.

Kiesler, S., & Cummings, J. N. (2002). What do we know about proximity and distance in work groups? A legacy of research. In P. Hinds & S. Kiesler (Eds.), *Distributed work* (pp. 57–80). Cambridge, MA: MIT Press, Cambridge.

Kim, H. S. (1983). Collaborative decision making in nursing practice: A theoretical framework. In P. Chinn (Ed.), *Advances in nursing theory development* (pp. 271–283). Washington, DC: Aspen Systems.

Kim, H. S. (1993). Putting theory into practice: Problems and prospects. *Journal of Advanced Nursing, 18*, 1632–1639.

Kim, H. S. (1994a). Action science as an approach to develop knowledge for nursing practice. *Nursing Science Quarterly, 7*, 134–138.

Kim, H. S. (1994b). Practice theories in nursing and a science of nursing practice. *Scholarly Inquiry for Nursing Practice: An International Journal, 8*, 123–137.

Kim, H. S. (1997). Terminology in structuring and developing nursing knowledge. In I. M. King & J. Fawcett (Eds.), *The langauge of nursing theory and metatheory* (pp. 27–36). Indianapolis, IN: Sigma Theta Tau International Center Nursing Press.

Kim, H. S. (1999). Critical reflective inquiry for knowledge development in nursing practice. *Journal of Advanced Nursing, 29*, 1205–1212.

Kim, H. S. (2000). An integrative framework for conceptualizing clients: A proposal for a nursing perspective in the new century. *Nursing Science Quarterly, 13*, 37–44.

Kim, H. S. (2006a). Knowledge synthesis and use in practice—debunking "evidence-based." *Klinisk sygepleje, 20*(Nr. 2), 24–34.

Kim, H. S. (2006b). The core of nursing profession. In U. Zeitler (Ed.), *Perspectives on nursing profession* (pp. 19–37). Aarhus, Denmark: The Centre for Innovation in Nursing Education.

Kim, H. S. (2006c). The concept of holism. In H. S. Kim & I. Kollak (Eds.), *Nursing theories: Conceptual and philosophical foundations* (pp. 89–108). New York, NY: Springer Publishing.

Kim, H. S. (2007a). Critical narrative epistemology. In C. Roy & D. A. Jones (Eds.), *Nursing knowledge development and clinical practice* (pp. 201–213). New York, NY: Springer Publishing.

Kim, H. S. (2007b). Toward an integrated epistemology for nursing. In C. Roy & D. A. Jones (Eds.), *Nursing knowledge development and clinical practice* (pp. 181–190). New York, NY: Springer Publishing.

Kim, H. S. (2010). *The nature of theoretical thinking in nursing* (3rd ed.). New York, NY: Springer Publishing.

Kim, H. S., & Kollak, I. (Eds.). (2006). *Nursing theories: Conceptual and philosophical foundations* (2nd ed.). New York, NY: Springer Publishing.

Kim, H. S., Ellefsen, B., Han, K. J., & Alves, S. L. (2008). Clinical constructions by nurses in Korea, Norway, and the United States. *Western Journal of Nursing Research, 30*, 54–72.

Kim, H. S., Holter, I. M., Lorensen, M., Inayoshi, M., Shimaguchi, S., Shimazaki-Ryder, R., ... Munkki-Utunen, M. (1993). Patient–nurse collaboration: A comparison of Patients' and nurses' attitudes in Finland, Japan, Norway, and the U.S.A. *International Journal of Nursing Studies, 30*, 387–401.

Kim, H. S., Lauzon Clabo, M. M., Burbank, P., Leveillee, M., & Martins, D. (2010). Application of critical reflective inquiry in nursing education. In N. Lyons (Ed.), *Handbook of reflection and reflective inquiry: Mapping a way of knowing for professional reflective inquiry* (pp. 159–172). New York, NY: Springer Publishing.

Kim, H. S., Sjöström, B., & Schwartz-Barcott, D. (2006). Pain assessment in the perspective of action science. *Research and Theory for Nursing Practice: An International Journal, 20*, 215–228.

Kinsella, E. A. (2009). Professional knowledge and the epistemology of reflective practice. *Nursing Philosophy, 11*, 3–14.

Kitson, A. (1986). Indicators of quality in nursing care—An alternative approach. *Journal of Advanced Nursing, 11*, 133–144.

Kitson, A. (1997). Johns Hopkins address: Does nursing have a future? *Image: The Journal of Nursing Scholarship, 29*, 111–115.

Kitson, A. (1998). Research utilization: Knowledge for practice. *Proceedings of the 9th Biennial Conference of the Workgroup of European Nurse Researchers* (pp. 52–64). Helsinki, Finland, July, 1998.

Kitson, A. (1999). The essence of nursing. *Nursing standard (Royal College of Nursing), 13*(23), 42–46.

Kitson, A., Ahmed, L. B., Harvey, G., Seers, K., & Thompson, D. R. (1996). From research to practice: One organizational model for promoting research-based practice. *Journal of Advanced Nursing, 23*, 430–440.

Kitwood, T. (1997). On being a person. In T. Kitwood (Ed.), *The person comes first* (pp. 7–19). Milton Keynes: Open University Press.

Kleinman, A. (1988). *The illness narratives: Suffering, healing, and the human condition.* New York, NY: Basic Books.

Kohn, L., Corrigan, J., & Donaldson, M. (Eds.). (2000). *To err is human: Building a safer health system.* Report of the Institute of Medicine, Committee on Quality of Health Care in America. Washington, DC: The National Academies Press.

Kooker, B. M., Shoultz, J., & Codier, E. E. (2007). Identifying emotional intelligence in professional nursing practice. *Journal of Professional Nursing: Official Journal of the American Association of Colleges of Nursing, 23*, 30–36.

Korsgaard, C. (1996). *The sources of normativity*. Cambridge UK: Cambridge University Press.

Kosnoski, J. (2005). Artful discussion. John Dewey's classroom as a model of deliberative association. *Political Theory, 33*, 654–677.

Kristjánsson, K. (2005). Smoothing it: Some Aristotelian misgivings about the phronesis-praxis perspective on education. *Educational Philosophy and Theory, 37*, 455–473.

Krouse, H. J., & Roberts, S. J. (1989). Nurse-patient interative styles, power, control, and satisfaction. *Western Journal of Nursing Research, 11*, 717–725.

Kubsch, S. M., Handerson, C., & Ghoorahoo, R. (2005). Content analysis of holistic ethics. *Complementary Therapies in Clinical Practice, 11*, 51–57.

Kuokkanen, L., & Leino-Kilpi, H. (2000). Power and empowerment in nursing: Three theoretical approaches. *Journal of Advanced Nursing, 31*, 235–241.

Lacey, S. R., Cox, K. S., Lorfing, K. C., Teasley, S. L., Carroll, C. A., & Sexton, K. (2007). Nursing support, workload, and intent to stay in Magnet, Magnet-aspiring, and non-Magnet hospitals. *Journal of Nursing Administration, 37*, 199–205.

Landzelius, K. (2006). Introduction: Patient organization movements and new metamorphoses in patienthood. *Social Science & Medicine, 62*, 529–537.

Lane, M. R. (2006). Arts in health care: A new paradigm for holistic nursing practice. *Journal of Holistic Nursing, 24*, 70–75.

Lang, N. M., & Marek, K. D. (1992). Outcomes that reflect clinical practice. In National Institutes of Health (Ed.), *Patient outcomes research: Examining the effectiveness of nursing practice* (pp. 27–38). NIH Publication No. 93-3411. Washington, DC: DHHS.

Lange, B. (2006). Mutual moral caring actions: A framework for community nursing practice. *Advances in Nursing Science, 29*, E45–55.

Lantz, G. (2000). Applied ethics: What kind of ethics and what kind of ethicist? *Journal of Applied Philosophy, 17*, 21–28.

Larrabee, M. J (Ed.). (1993). *An ethic of care: Feminist and interdisciplinary perspectives.* New York, NY: Routeledge.

Laschinger, H. K. S. (2008). Effect of empowerment on professional practice environments, work satisfaction, and patient care quality: Further testing the nursing work-life model. *Journal of Nursing Care Quality, 23*, 322–330.

Lauder, W. (1994). Beyond reflection: Practical wisdom and the practical syllogism. *Nursing Education Today, 14*, 91–98.

Lauzon Clabo, L. M. (2008). An ethnography of pain assessment and the role of social context on two postoperative units. *Journal of Advanced Nursing, 61*, 531–539.

Lawler, M. C. (2003). Gazing anew: The shift from a clinical gaze to an ethnographic lens. *American Journal of Occupational Therapy, 57*, 29–39.

Lee, I., Lee, E., Kim, H. S., Park, Y. S., Song, M., & Park, Y H. (2004). Concept development of family resilience: A study of Korean families with a chronically ill child. *Journal of Clinical Nursing, 13,* 636–645.

Lee, Y. S., Huang, Y. C., & Kao, Y. H. (2005). Physical activities and correlates of clinical nurses in Taipei municipal hospitals. *Journal of Nursing Research, 13,* 281–292.

Lees, G. D., Richman, J., Salauroo, M. A., & Warden, S. (1987). Quality assurance: Is it professional insurance? *Journal of Advanced Nursing, 12,* 719–727.

Légaré, F., Ratté, S., Stacey, D., Kryworuchko, J., Gravel, K., Graham, I. D., & Turcotte, S. (2010). Interventions for improving the adoption of shared decision making by healthcare professionals. *The Cochrane Collaboration.* doi: 10.1002/14651858.CD006732.pub2

Leino-Kilpi, H. (1991). Good nursing care: The relationship between client and nurse. *Hoitotiede, 3,* 200–207.

Lekka-Kowalik, A. (2010). Why science cannot be value-free. Understanding the rationality and responsibility of science. *Science and Engineering, Ethics, 16,* 33–41.

Lenz, E. R., Pugh, L. C., Milligan, R., Gift, A. G., & Suppe, F. (1997). The middle-range theory of unpleasant symptoms: An update. *Advances in Nursing Science, 19*(3), 14–27.

Lenz, E. R., Suppe, F., Gift, A. G., Pugh, L. C., & Milligan, R. (1995). Collaborative development of middle-range nursing theories: Toward a theory of unpleasant symptoms. *Advances in Nursing Science, 17*(3), 1–13.

Leplege, A., Gzil, F., Cammelli, M., Lefeve, C., Pachoud, B., & Ville, I. (2007). Person-centredness: Conceptual and historical perspectives. *Disability and Rehabilitation, 29,* 1555–1565.

Levin, M. E. (1966). Adaptation and assessment: A rationale for nursing intervention. *American Journal of Nursing, 66,* 2450–2454.

Levinas, E. (1998). *On thinking-of-the-other. Entre nous* (M. B. Smith & B. Harshav, Trans.). New York, NY: Columbia University Press. (Originally published in 1991.)

Lewis, T. E. (2008). Revolutionary leadership ↔ revolutionary pedagogy: Reevaluating the links and disjunctions between Lukacs and Freire. In B. S. Stengel (Ed.), *The philosophy of education 2007* (pp. 285–293 ). Urbana-Champaign, IL: University of Illinois at Urbana-Champaign.

Lewis, T. E. (2009). Education in the realm of the senses: Understanding Paulo Freire's aesthetic unconscious through Jacques Rancière. *Journal of Philosophy of Education, 43,* 285–299.

Liaschenko, J. (1994). The moral geography of home care. *Advances in Nursing Science, 17,* 16–26.

Liaschenko, J. (1995). Ethics in the work of acting for clients. *Advances in Nursing Science, 18,* 1–12.

Liaschenko, J. (1997). Knowing the patient? In S. E. Thorne & V. E. Hayes (Eds.), *Nursing praxis: Knowledge and action* (pp. 23–38). Thousand Oaks, CA: Sage Publications.

Liaschenko, J. (1998). The shift from the closed to the open body—Ramifications for nursing testimony. In S. D. Edwards (Ed.), *Philosophical issues in nursing* (pp. 11–30). London, UK: Macmillan Press.

Liedtka, J. M., & Whitten, E. (1998). Enhancing care delivery through cross-disciplinary collaboration: A case study. *Journal of Healthcare Management, 43*, 185–205.

Liimatainen, L., Poskiparta, M., Kahlia, P., & Sjögren, A. (2001). The development of reflective learning in the context of health counseling and health promotion during nurse education. *Journal of Advanced Nursing, 34*, 648–658.

Lindahl, B., & Sandman, P. O. (1998). The role of advocacy in critical care nursing: A caring response to another. *Intensive & Critical Care Nursing: The Official Journal of the British Association of Critical Care Nurses, 14*, 179–186.

Lipscomb, M. (2012). Social justice—special issue. *Nursing Philosophy, 13*, 1–5.

Lobkowicz, N. (1967). *Theory and practice: A history of a concept from Aristotle to Marx*. Notre Dame, IN: University of Notre Dame Press.

Louch, A. R. (1966). *Explanation and human action*. Berkeley, CA: University of California Press.

Luhmann, N. (2000). *Art as social system*. Standford, CA: Stanford University Press.

Luker, K. A., & Chalmers, K. I. (1989). The referral process in health visiting. *International Journal of Nursing Studies, 26*, 173–185.

Lundmark, V. A. (2008). Magnet environments for professional nursing practice. In R. G. Hughes (Ed.), *Patient safety and quality. An evidence-based handbook for nurses* (Chapter 46). Rockville, MD: U.S. Department of Health and Human Services. AHRQ Publication No. 08-0043.

Lunney, M. (2009). Assessment, clinical judgment, and nursing diagnoses: How to determine accurate diagnoses. In T. H. Herdman (Ed.), *NANDA International nursing diagnoses: Definitions & classification 2009-2011* (pp. 3–17). Chichester, UK: WIley-Blackwell.

Lutz, B. J., & Bowers, B. J. (2000). Patient-centered care: Understanding its interpretation and implementation in health care. *Scholarly Inquiry for Nursing Practice, 14*, 165–183.

Lyneham, J., Parkinson, C., & Denholm, C. (2009). Expert nursing practice: A mathematical explanation of Benner's 5th stage of practice development. *Journal of Advanced Nursing, 65*, 2477–2484.

MacDonald, J. A., Herbert, R., & Thibeault, C. (2006). Advanced practice nursing: Unification through a common identity. *Journal of Professional Nursing: Official Journal of the American Association of Colleges of Nursing, 22*, 172–179.

Mahler, H. I., & Kulik, J. A. (1990). Preferences for health care involvement, perceived control and surgical recovery: A prospective study. *Social Science & Medicine, 31*, 743–751.

Manley, K. Hills, V., & Marriot, S. (2011). Person-centred care: Principle of nursing practice D. *Nursing Standard (Royal College of Nursing), 25*(31), 35–37.

Manojlovich, M., & Laschinger, H. (2007). The nursing work-life model: Extending and refining a new theory. *Journal of Nursing Management, 15*, 256–263.

Manojlovich, M. (2005). Predictors of professional nursing practice behaviors in hospital settings. *Nursing Research, 54*, 41–47.

Manojlovich, M., & DeCicco, B. (2007). Healthy work environments, nurse-physician communication, and patients' outcomes. *American Journal of Critical Care, 16*, 536–543.

Mantzoukas, S., & Watkinson, S. (2007). Review of advanced nursing practice: The international literature and developing the generic features. *Journal of Clinical Nursing, 16*, 28–37.

Marcel, G. (1964). *Creative fidelity* (R. Rosthal, Trans.). New York, NY: Farrar, Strauss and Company.

Marcel, G. (1968). *The philosophy of existentialism*. New York, NY: Citadel Press.

March, B., Todd, P. M., & Gigerenzer, G. (2004). Cognitive heuristics: Reasoning the fast & frugal way. In J. P. Leighton & R. J. Stemberg (Eds.), *The nature of reasoning* (pp. 273–287). New York, NY: Cambridge University Press.

Mark, B. A., Slayer, J., & Wan, T. T. (2003). Professional nursing practice: Impact on organizational and patient outcomes. *Journal of Nursing Administration, 33*, 224–234.

Marsden, J., Farrell, M., Bradbury, C., Dale-Perera, A., Eastwood, B., Roxburgh, M., & Taylor, S. (2008). Development of the treatment outcomes profile. *Addiction, 103*, 1450–1460.

Martinsen, K. (2006). *Care and vulnerabilitty*. Oslo, Norway: Akribe.

Matthew-Maich, N., Ploeg, J., Dobbins, M., & Jack, S. (2013). Supporting the uptake of nursing guidelines: What you really need to know to move nursing guidelines into practice. *Worldviews on Evidence-Based Nursing/Sigma Theta Tau International, Honor Society of Nursing, 10*, 104–115.

Mattingly, C. (1994). The concept of therapeutic "emplotment." *Social Science & Medicine, 38*, 811–822.

May, C. (1990). Research on nurse-patient relationships: Problems of theory, problems of practice. *Journal of Advanced Nursing, 15*, 307–315.

May, C. (1992). Nursing work, nurses' knowledge, and the subjectification of the patient. *Sociology of Health & Illness, 14*, 472–487.

May, C. (1993). Subjectivity and culpability in the constitution of nurse-patient relationships. *International Journal of Nursing Studies, 30*, 181–192.

May, C. (1995a). Patient autonomy and the politics of professional relationships. *Journal of Advanced Nursing, 21*, 83–87.

May, C. (1995b). "To call it work somehow demeans it": The social construction of talk in the care of terminally ill patients. *Journal of Advanced Nursing, 22*, 556–561.

May, C., & Fleming, C. (1997). The professional imagination: Narrative and the symbolic boundaries between medicine and nursing. *Journal of Advanced Nursing, 25*, 1094–1100.

May, T., Craig, J. M., May, C., & Tomkowiak, J. (2005). Quality of life, justice, and the demands of hospital-based nursing. *Public Affairs Quarterly, 19*, 213–225.

McAllister, J. W. (2002). Recent work on aesthetics of science. *International Studies in the Philosophy of Science, 16*, 7–11.

McAllister, M. (2003). Doing practice differently: Solution-focused nursing. *Journal of Advanced Nursing, 41*, 528–535.

McCance, T. V. (2003). Caring in nursing practice: The development of a conceptual framework. *Research and Theory for Nursing Practice: An International Journal, 17*, 101–116.

McCance, T., McCormack, B., & Dewing, J. (2011). An exploration of person-centredness in practice. *OJIN: The Online Journal of Issues in Nursing, 16*(2). Manuscript 1. Retrieved from http://nursingworld.org/MainMenuCategories/ANAMarketplace/ANAPeriodicals/OJIN/TableofContents/Vol-16-2011/No2-May-2011/Person-Centredness-in-Practice.aspx

McCarthy, J. (2006). A pluralist view of nursing ethics. *Nursing Philosophy, 7*, 157–164.

McCloskey, D. J. (2008). Nurses' perceptions of research utilization in corporate healthcare system. *Journal of Nursing Scholarship, 40*, 39–45.

McClure, M. L., Poulin, M. A., Sovic, M. D., & Wandelt, M. (1983). *Magnet hospitals: Attraction and retention of professional nurses*. Washington, DC: American Nurses Association.

McClure, M. L. (2005). Magnet hospitals. Insights and issues. *Nursing Administration Quarterly, 29*, 198–201.

McCormack, B. (2003). Researching nursing practice: Does person-centredness matter? *Nursing Philosophy, 4*, 179–188.

McCormack, B. (2004). Person-centredness in gerontological nursing: An overview of the literature. *International Journal of Older People Nursing (in association with the Journal of Clinical Nursing), 13*(3A), 31–38.

McCormack, B., Karlsson, B., Dewing, J., & Lerdal, A. (2010). Exploring person-centredness: A qualitative metasynthesis of four studies. *Scandinavian Journal of Caring Science, 24*, 620–634.

McCormack, B., & McCance, T. V. (2006). Development of a framework for person-centred nursing. *Journal of Advanced Nursing, 56*, 472–479.

McCullough-Zander, K. (Ed.). (2000). *Caring across cultures: The provider's guide to cross-cultural health* (2nd ed.). Minneapolis, MN: The Center for Cross-Cultural Health.

McCurry, M. K., Revell, S. M., & Roy, S. C. (2010). Knowledge for the good of the individual and society: Linking philosophy, disciplinary goals, theory, and practice. *Nursing Philosophy, 11*, 42–52.

McGillis Hall, L., & Kiesners, D. (2005). A narrative approach to understanding the nursing work environment in Canada. *Social Science & Medicine, 61*, 2482–2491.

McHugh, M. D., Kelly, L. A., Smith, H. L., Wu, E. S., Vanak, J. M., & Aiken, L. H. (2013). Lower mortality in Magnet hospitals. *Medical Care, 51*, 382–388.

McIver, D., Lengnick-Hall, C. A., Lengnick-Hall, M. L., & Ramachandran, I. (2012). Integrating knowledge and knowing: A framework for understanding knowledge-in-practice. *Human Resource Management Review, 22*, 86–99.

McLeish, K. N., & Oxoby, R. J. (2011). Social interactions and the salience of social identity. *Journal of Economic Psychology, 32*, 172–178.

McMahon, R. (1998). Therapeutic nursing: Theory, issues, and practice. In R. McMahon & A. Pearson (Eds.), *Nursing as therapy* (2nd ed.) (pp. 1–20). London, UK: Stanley Thomas Publishers, Ltd.

McMahon, R., & Pearson, A. (Eds.). (1998). *Nursing as therapy* (2nd ed.). London, UK: Stanley Thomas Publishers, Ltd.

Mead, N., & Bower, P. (2000). Patient-centredness: A conceptual framework and review of the empirical literature. *Social Science & Medicine, 51*, 1087–1110.

Meehan, T. C. (2003). Careful nursing: A model for contemporary nursing practice. *Journal of Advanced Nursing, 44*, 99–107.

Meehan, T. C. (2012). The careful nursing philosophy and professional practice model. *Journal of Clinical Nursing, 21*, 2905–2916.

Mele, A., & Sverdlik, S. (1996). Intention, intentional action, and moral responsibility. *Philosophical Studies, 82*, 265–287.

Mele, A. (1997). *The philosophy of action*. Oxford, UK: Oxford University Press.

Meleis, A. I. (2011). *Theoretical nursing: Development and progress* (5th ed.). Philadelphia, PA: Lippincott Williams & Wilkins.

Melville-Smith, J., & Kendal, G. E. (2011). Importance of effective collaboration between health professionals for the facilitation of optimal community diabetes care. *Australian Journal of Primary Health, 17*, 150–155.

Meretoja, R., Isoaho, H., & Leino-Kilpi, H. (2004). Nurse Competence Scale: Development and psychometric testing. *Journal of Advanced Nursing, 47*, 124–133.

Merleau-Ponty, M. (1962). *Phenomenology of perception* (C. Smith, Trans.). New York, NY: Routledge and Kegan Paul. (Original work published 1945.)

Metzler, M. M., Higgins, D. L., Beeker, C. G., Freudenberg, N., Lantz, P. M., Sneturia, K. D., … Softley, D. (2003). Addressing urban health in Detroit, New York City, and Seattle through community-based participatory research partnerships. *American Journal of Public Health, 93*, 903–911.

Meyer, G., & Lavin, M. A. (2005). Vigilance: the essence of nursing. *Online Journal of Issues in Nursing, 10*(3), 38–51.

Mickan, S. M. (2005). Evaluating the effectiveness of health care teams. *Australian Health Review, 29*, 211–217.

Mickan, S., Hoffman, S. J., & Nasmith, L. (2010). Collaborative practice in a global health context: Common themes from developed and developing countries. *Journal of Interprofessional Care 24*, 492–502.

Millard, L., Hallett, C., & Luker, K. (2006). Nurse-patient interaction and decision-making in care: Patient involvement in community nursing. *Journal of Advanced Nursing, 55*, 142–150.

Miller, K. L., & Kontos, P. C. (2013). The intraprofessional and interprofessional relations of neurorehabilitation nurses: A negotiated order perspective. *Journal of Advanced Nursing, 69*, 1797–1807.

Miller, M., & Kearney, N. (2004). Guidelines for clinical practice: Development, dissemination and implementation. *International Journal of Nursing Studies, 41*, 813–821.

Miller, W. D., Pollack, C. E., & Williams, D. R. (2011). Healthy homes and communities: Putting the pieces together. *American Journal of Preventive Medicine, 40*(1S1), S48–S57.

Mitchell, G. J. (1995). Reflection: The key to breaking with tradition. *Nursing Science Quarterly, 8,* 57.

Mokros, H. B., Mullins, L. S., & Saracevic, T. (1995). Practice and personhood in professional interaction: Social identities and information needs. *Library & Information Science Research, 17,* 237–257.

Mol, A. (2002). *The body multiple: Ontology in medical practice.* Durham, NC: Duke University Press.

Moody, R. C., & Pesut, D. J. (2006). The motivation to care: Application and extension of motivation theory to professional nursing work. *Journal of Health Organization and Management, 20,* 15–48.

Moore, J., & Prentice, D. (2013). Collaboration among nurse practitioners and registered nurses in outpatient oncology settings in Canada. *Journal of Advanced Nursing, 69,* 1574–1583.

Moore, S. M., & Duffy, E. (2007). Maintaining vigilance to promote best outcomes for hospitalized elders. *Critical Care Nursing Clinics of North America, 19,* 313–319, vi–vii.

Moorhead, S., Johnson, M., & Maas, M. (2004). *Nursing outcomes classification (NOC)* (3rd ed.). St. Louis, MO: Mosby.

Moorhead, S., Johnson, M., Maas, M. L., & Swanson, E. C. (2013). *Nursing outcomes classification (NOC)* (5th ed.). St. Louis, MO: Mosby.

Moran, R. (2001). *Authority and estrangement: An essay on self knowledge.* Princeton, NJ: Princeton University Press.

Morgan, S., & Yoder, L. H. (2012). A concept analysis of person-centered care. *Journal of Holistic Nursing, 30,* 6–15.

Morkros, H. B., Mullins, L. S., & Saracevic, T. (1995). Practice and personhood in professional interaction: Social identities and information needs. *Library & Information Science Research, 17,* 237–257.

Morrison, S. M., & Symes, L. (2011). An integrative review of expert nursing practice. *Journal of Nursing Scholarship, 43,* 163–170.

Morse, J. M. (1992). Comfort: The refocusing of nursing care. *Clinical Nursing Research, 1,* 91–106.

Mort, M., & Smith, A. (2009). Beyond information: Intimate relations in sociotechnical practice. *Sociology, 43,* 215–231.

Moshman, D. (1995). The construction of moral rationality. *Human Development, 38,* 265–281.

Moules, N. J. (2002). Nursing on paper: Therapeutic letters in nursing practice. *Nursing Inquiry, 9,* 104–113.

Moya, C. J. (1990). *The philosophy of action: An introduction.* Oxford, UK: Polity Press.

Müller-Staub, M., Lavin, M. A., Needham, I., & Van Achterberg, T. (2006). Nursing diagnoses, interventions and outcomes—Application and impact on nursing practice: Systematic review. *Journal of Advanced Nursing, 56,* 514–531.

Murphy, M., Hinch, B., Llewellyn, J., Dillon, P. J., & Carlson, E. (2011). Promoting professional nursing practice: Linking a professional practice model to performance expectations. *The Nursing Clinics of North America, 46,* 67–79.

Myhrvold, T. (2006). The different other—towards an including ethics of care. *Nursing Philosophy, 7*, 125–136.

Myrick, F., Yonge, O., & Billay, D. (2010). Preceptorship and practical wisdom: A process of engaging in authentic nursing practice. *Nurse Education in Practice, 10*, 82–87.

Natanson, M. (1968). *Literature, philosophy, and the social sciences*. The Hague: Martinus Nijhoff.

National Center for Cultural Competence. (2004). *Bridging the cultural divide in health care settings: The essential role of cultural broker programs*. Washington, DC: The National Health Service Corps (NHSC), Bureau of Health Professions (BHPr), Health Resources and Services Administration (HRSA), U.S. Department of Health and Human Services (DHHS). Retrieved from http://www11.georgetown.edu/research/gucchd/nccc/documents/Cultural_Broker_Guide_English.pdf

National Committee for Quality Assurance (NCQA). (2014). *2013 Special needs structure & process measures*. Washington, DC: Author. Retrieved from https://www.ncqa.org/Portals/0/Programs/SNP/2013_S&P_Measures_Final_2.6.14.pdf

National Council of State Boards of Nursing (NCSBN). (1995). Delegation: Concepts and decision-making process. *National Council Position Paper*.

National Panel for Psychiatric Mental Health NP Competencies. (2003). *Psychiatric-mental health nurse practitioner competencies*. Washington, DC: National Organization of Nurse Practitioner Faculties.

National Quality Forum. (2004). *National voluntary consensus standard for nursing-sensitive care: An initial performance measure set*. Washington, DC: Author.

Nehamas, A. (1998). *The art of living: Socratic reflections from Plato to Foucault*. Berkeley, CA: University of California Press.

Nelson, S., & Purkis, M. E. (2004). Mandatory reflection: The Canadian reconstitution of the competent nurse. *Nursing Inquiry, 11*, 247–257.

Ness, O., Karlsson, B., Borg, M., Biong, S., Sundet, R., McCormack, B., & Kim, H. S. (2014). A model for collaborative practice in community mental health care. *Scandinavian Psychologist, 1*, e6. http://dx.doi.org/10.15714/scandpsychol.1.e6

Neuman, B. (1998). *The Neuman systems model* (4th ed.). Norwalk, CT: Appleton & Lange.

Newman, M. A. (1992). Prevailing paradigms in nursing. *Nursing Outlook, 40*, 10–13, 32.

Newman, M. A. (1994). *Health as expanding consciousness* (2nd ed.). New York, NY: National League for Nursing.

Newman, M. A. (2002). The pattern that connects. *Advances in Nursing Science, 24*, 1–7.

Nightingale, F. (1859/1946). *Notes on nursing*. Philadelphia, PA: J. B. Lippincott.

Noddings, N. (1984). *Caring: A feminine approach to ethics and morals*. Berkeley, CA: University of California Press.

Nordenstam, T. (1981). Intention in art. In K. S. Johannessen & T. Nordenstam (Eds.), *Wittgenstein—Aesthetics and transcendental philosophy (Wittgenstein—Asthetik und transzendeltale philosophie)* (pp. 127–135). Vienna, Austria: Hölder-Pichler-Temsky.

Norman, I. (2013). The nursing practice environment. *International Journal of Nursing Studies, 50*, 1577–1579.

Nortvedt, P. (1998). Sensitive judgment: An inquiry into the foundations of nursing ethics. *Nursing Ethics, 5*, 385–392.

Nortvedt, P. (2001a). Clinical sensitivity: The inseparability of ethical perceptiveness and clinical knowledge. *Scholarly Inquiry for Nursing Practice, 15*, 25–43.

Nortvedt, P. (2001b). Needs, closeness and responsibilities: An inquiry into some rival moral considerations in nursing care. *Nursing Philosophy, 2*, 112–121.

Nortvedt, P. (2003). Immersed subjectivity and engaged narratives: Clinical epistemology and normative intricacy. *Nursing Philosophy, 4*, 129–136.

Nortvedt, P. (2011). An ethics of care: Normative challenges. *Nursing Ethics, 18*, 147–148.

Nortvedt, P., Hem, M. H., & Skirbekk, H. (2011). The ethics of care: Role obligations and moderate partiality in health care. *Nursing Ethics, 18*, 192–200.

Nursing and Midwifery Council (formerly UKCC). (2002). *Scope of professional practice*. London, UK: Author.

O'Brien-Pallas, L., Meyer, R. M., Hayes, L. J., & Wang, S. (2011). The patient care delivery model—An open system framework: Conceptualisation, literature review and analytical strategy. *Journal of Clinical Nursing, 20*, 1640–1650.

Olson, D. H., & Gorall, D. M. (2003). Circumplex model of marital and family systems. In F. Walsh (Ed.), *Normal Family Processes* (3rd ed.) (pp. 514–547). New York, NY: Guilford Press.

Olson, T. C. (1993). Laying claim to caring: Nursing and the language of training, 1915-1937. *Nursing Outlook, 41*, 68–72.

Orem, D. E. (1995). *Nursing: Concepts of practice* (5th ed.). St Louis, MO: Mosby.

Orlando, I. (1961). *The dynamic nurse-patient relationship: Function, process, and principle*. New York, NY: G. Putnam's Sons.

Organisation for Economic Co-operation and Development (OECD). (2005). *The definition and selection of key competencies: Executive summary*. Retrieved from http://www.oecd.org/pisa/35070367.pdf

Osterman, P., & Schwartz-Barcott, D. (1996). Presence: Four ways of being there. *Nursing Forum, 31*(2), 23–30.

Owen, J., & Grealish, L. (2006). Clinical education delivery—A collaborative, shared governance model proves a framework for planning, implementation and evaluation. *Collegian, 13*, 15–21.

Paavilainen, E., & Åstedt-Kurki, P. (1997). The client-nurse relationship as experienced by public health nurses: Toward better collaboration. *Public Health Nursing, 14*, 137–142.

Paganini, M. C., & Yoshikawa Egry, E. (2011). The ethical component of professional competence in nursing: An analysis. *Nursing Ethics, 18*, 571–582.

Paley, J. (2004a). Clinical cognition and embodiment. *International Journal of Nursing Studies, 41*, 1–13.

Paley, J. (2004b). Gadow's romanticism: Science, poetry and embodiment in postmodern nursing. *NursingPhilosophy, 5*, 112–126.

Paquin, S. O. (2011). Social justice advocacy in nurisng: What is it? How do we get there? *Creative Nursing, 17*, 63–67.

Park, E., McDaniel, A., & Jung, M. (2009). Computerized tailoring of health information. *CIN: Computers, Informatics, Nursing, 27*, 34–43.

Parse, R. R. (1987). *Nursing science: Major paradigms, theories, and critiques*. Philadelphia, PA: W. B. Saunders.

Parse, R. R. (1997). The human becoming theory: The was, is, and will be. *Nursing Science Quarterly, 10*, 32–38.

Parse, R. R. (1998). *The human becoming school of thought: A perspective for nurses and other health professionals*. Thousand Oaks, CA: Sage.

Parsons, T. (1951). *The social system*. New York, NY: The Free Press.

Patel, H., Pettitt, M., & Wilson, J. R. (2012). Factors of collaborative working: A framework for a collaboration model. *Applied Ergonomics, 43*, 1–28.

Pembroke, N. (2006). Marcelian charm in nursing practice: The unity of agape and eros as the foundation of an ethic of care. *Nursing Philosophy, 7*, 266–274.

Peplau, H. E. (1952). *Interpersonal relations in nursing*. New York, NY: G. Putnam's Sons.

Perron, A., Fluet, C., & Holmes, D. (2005). Agents of care and agents of the state: Biopower and nursing practice. *Journal of Advanced Nursing, 50*, 536–544.

Petri, L. (2010). Concept analysis of interdisciplinary collaboration. *Nursing Forum, 45*, 73–82.

Phillips, J. (2005). Knowledge is power: Using nursing information management and leadership interventions to improve services to patients, clients and users. *Journal of Nursing Management, 13*, 524–536.

Philpin, S. (2006). "Handing over": Transmission of information between nurses in an intensive therapy unit. *Nursing in Critical Care, 11*, 86–93.

Pike, M. A. (2004). Aesthetic teaching. *Journal of Aesthetic Education, 38* (2), 20–37.

Pink, T. (2007). Normativity and reason. *Journal of Moral Philosphy, 4*, 406–431.

Pinker, S. (1997). *How the mind works*. New York, NY: W. W. Norton.

Piper, A. M. S. (2008a). *Rationality and the structure of the self. Volume I: The Humean conception*. Berlin, Germany: Adrian Piper Research Archive.

Piper, A. M. S. (2008b). *Rationality and the structure of the self. Volume II: The Kantian conception*. Berlin, Germany: Adrian Piper Research Archive.

Piper, S. (2010). Patient empowerment: Emancipatory or technological practice? *Patient Education and Counseling, 79*, 173–177.

Powers, P. (2003). Empowerment as treatment and the role of health professionals. *Advances in Nursing Science, 26*, 227–237

Pridham, K. F. (1993). Anticipatory guidance of parents of new infants: Potential contribution of the internal working model construct. *Image: The Journal of Nursing Scholarship, 25*, 49–56.

Probandari, A., Utarin, A., Lindholm, L., & Hurtig, A. (2011). Life of a partnership: The process of collaboration between the National Tuberculosis Program and the hospitals in Yogyakarta, Indonesia. *Social Science & Medicine, 73*, 1386–1394.

Pullon, S. (2008). Competence, respect and trust: Key features of successful interprofessional nurse-doctor relationships. *Journal of Interprofessional Care, 22*, 133–147.

Purkis, M. E., & Bjornsdottir, K. (2006). Intelligent nursing: Accounting for knowledge as action in practice. *Nursing Philosophy: An International Journal for Healthcare Professionals, 7*, 247–256.

Putnam, R. (1999). Transforming social practice: An action science perspective. *Management Learning, 30*, 177–187.

Quad Council of the Public Health Nursing Organizations. (2011). *Quad Council competencies for public health nurses*. Retrieved from http://www.resourcenter.net/images/ACHNE/Files/QuadCouncilCompetenciesForPublicHealthNurses_Summer2011.pdf

Radwin, L. (2000). Oncology patients' perceptions of quality of nursing care. *Research in Nursing & Health, 23*, 179–190.

Radwin, L. E. (1996). "Knowing the patient": A review of research on an emerging concept. *Journal of Advanced Nursing, 23*, 1142–1146.

Rafferty, A. M., Allcock, N., & Lathlean, J. (1996). The theory/practice "gap": Taking issue with the issue. *Journal of Advanced Nursing, 23*, 685–691.

Raines, D. A. (2010). Nursing practice competency of accelerated Bachelor of Science in nursing program students. *Journal of Professional Nursing, 26*, 162–167.

Ranciére, J. (2006). *The politics of aesthetics* (G. Rockhill, Trans.). London, UK: Continuum.

Rashotte, J. (2005). Dwelling with stories that haunt us: Building a meaningful nursing practice. *Nursing Inquiry, 12*, 34–42.

Reckwitz, A. (2002). Toward a theory of social justice: A development in culturalist theorizing. *European Journal of Social Theory, 5*, 243–263.

Redman, R. W., & Lynn, M. R. (2005). Assessment of patient expectations for care. *Research and Theory for Nursing Practice: An International Journal, 19*, 275–285.

Reed, L., Blegen, M. A., & Goode, C. S. (1998). Adverse patient occurrences as a measure of nursing care quality. *Journal of Nursing Administration, 28*(5), 62–69.

Reed, P. G. (2011). The spiral path of nursing knowledge. In P. G. Reed & N. B. Crawford Shearer (Eds.), *Nursing knowledge and theory innovation: Advancing the science of practice* (pp. 1–35). New York, NY: Springer Publishing.

Reed, P. G., & Crawford Shearer, N. B. (Eds.). (2011). *Nursing knowledge and theory innovation: Advancing the science of practice*. New York, NY: Springer Publishing.

Reese, D., & Sontag, M. (2001). Successful interprofessional collaboration on the hospice team. *Health and Social Work, 26*(3), 167–175.

Reeves, J., Lloyd-Williams, M., Payne, S., & Dowrick, C. (2010). Revisiting biographical disruption: Exploring individual embodied illness experience in people with terminal cancer. *Health, 14*, 178–195.

Reilly, T. (2008). Collaboration in action. *Administration in social work, 25*(1), 53–74.

Ren, Y., Kiesler, S., & Fussell, S. (2008). Multiple group coordination in complex and dynamic task environments: Interruptions, coping mechanisms, and technology recommendations. *Journal of Management Information Systems, 25*, 107–133.

Rescher, N. (1987). Rationality and moral obligation. *Synthese, 72*, 29–43.

Richards, D. A. J. (1987). Moral rationality. *Synthese, 72*, 91–101.

Ricoeur, P. (1992). *Oneself as another* (K. Blamey, Trans.). Chicago, IL: University of Chicago Press.

Ring, N., Malcolm, C., Coull, A., Murphy-Black, T., & Watterson, A. (2005). Nursing best practice statements: An exploration of their implementation in clinical practice. *Journal of Clinical Nursing, 14*, 1048–1058.

Rischel, V., Larsen, K., & Jackson, K. (2008). Embodied dispositions or experience? Identifying new patterns of professional competence. *Journal of Advanced Nursing, 61*, 512–521.

Robert Wood Johnson Foundation Commission to Build a Healthier America. (2008). *Overcoming obstacles to health.* Princeton, NJ: The Robert Wood Johnson Foundation.

Robert Wood Johnson Foundation Commission to Build a Healthier America. (2009). *Beyond health care: New directions to a healthier America; recommendations.* Princeton, NJ: Author. Retrieved from http://www.rwjf.org/content/dam/farm/reports/reports/2009/rwjf40483

Roberts, D. (2013). The clinical viva: An assessment of clinical thinking. *Nurse Education Today, 33*, 402–406.

Rodney, P., Varcoe, C., Storch, J. L., McPherson, G., Mahoney, K., Brown, H., ... Starzomski, R. (2009). Navigating toward a moral horizon: A multisite qualitative study of ethical practice in nursing. *Canadian Journal of Nursing Research, 41*, 292–319.

Rogers, E. M. (1983). *Diffusion of innovations.* New York, NY: Free Press.

Rogers, M. E. (1970). An introduction to the theoretical basis of nursing. Philadelphia, PA: F.A. Davis.

Rogers, M. E. (1989). Nursing: A science of unitary human beings. In J. Riehl-Sisca (Ed.), *Conceptual models for nursing practice* (3rd ed.) (pp. 181–188). Norwalk, CT: Appleton & Lange.

Rogers, M. E. (1990). Nursing: Science of unitary, irreducible, human beings: Update 1990. In E. A. M. Barrett (Ed.), *Visions of Rogers' science-based nursing* (pp. 5–11). New York, NY: National League for Nursing.

Rogers, M. E. (1992). Nursing science and the space age. *Nursing Science Quarterly, 5*, 27–34.

Rogers, M. E. (1994). The science of unitary human beings. *Nursing Science Quarterly, 7*, 33–35.

Rolfe, G. (1996). Going extreme: Action research, grounded practice and theory-practice gap in nursing. *Journal of Advanced Nursing, 24*, 1315–1320.

Rolfe, G. (1997a). Nursing praxis: A zealot responds. *Journal of Advanced Nursing, 25*, 426–427.

Rolfe, G. (1997b). Science, abduction and the fuzzy nurse: An exploration of expertise. *Journal of Advanced Nursing, 25*, 1070–1075.

Rolfe, G. (1998). The theory-practice gap in nursing: From research-based practice to practitioner-based research. *Journal of Advanced Nursing, 28*, 672–679.

Rolfe, G. (2005). The deconstructing angel: Nursing, reflection and evidence-based practice. *Nursing Inquiry, 12*, 78–86.

Rolfe, G. (2006). Nursing praxis and the science of the critique. *Nursing Science Quarterly, 19*, 39–43.

Rolfe, G. (2011). Practitioner-centered research: Nursing praxis and the science of the unique. In P. M. Reed & N. B. Crawford Shearer (Eds.), *Nursing knowledge and theory innovation: Advancing the science of practice* (pp. 59–74). New York, NY: Springer Publishing.

Rolfe, G., & Freshwater, D. (2005). "To save the honour of thinking": A slightly petulant response to Griffiths. *International Journal of Nursing Studies, 42*, 363–369.

Rotegaard, A. K., Moore, S. M., Fagermoen, M. S., & Ruland, C. M. (2010). Health assets: A concept analysis. *International Journal of Nursing Studies, 47*, 513–525.

Rotegaard, A,. K., & Ruland, C. M. (2010). Patient centeredness in terminologies: Coverage of health assets concepts in the International Classification of Nursing Practice. *Journal of Biomedical Informatics, 43*, 805–811.

Rothenberg, D. (1993). *Hand's end: Technology and the limits of nature*. Berkeley, CA: University of California Press.

Roy, C., & Andrews, H. A. (1991). *The Roy adaptation model: A definitive statement*. Norwalk, CT: Appleton & Lange.

Roy, C. (2007). Advances in nursing knowledge and the challenge for transforming practice. In C. Roy & D. A. Jones (Eds.), *Nursing knowledge development and clinical practice* (pp. 3–37). New York, NY: Springer Publishing.

Roy, C., & Jones, D. A. (Eds.). (2007). *Nursing knowledge development and clinical practice*. New York, NY: Springer Publishing.

Royal College of Nursing (RCN). (2004). *Nursing assessment and older people. A Royal College of Nursing toolkit*. London, UK: Author.

Rudolph, J. W., Taylor, S. S., & Foldy, E. G. (2001). Collaborative off-line reflection: A way to develop skill in action science and action inquiry. In P. Reason & H. Bradbury (Eds.), *Handbook of action research: Participative inquiry and practice* (pp. 405–412). London, UK: Sage Publications.

Ruesch, C., Mossakowski, J., Forrest, J., Hayes, M., Jahrsdoerfer, M., Comeau, E., Singleton, M. (2012). Using nursing expertise and telemedicine to increase nursing collaboration and improve patient outcomes. *Telemedicine journal and e-health: The official journal of the American Telemedicine Association, 18*(8), 591–595.

Ryan, A. E. (1997). A fresh perspective. *Nursing, 27*(4), 77.

Ryan, S. N., & Lauver, D. R. (2002). The efficacy of tailored interventions. *Journal of Nursing Scholarship, 34*, 331–337.

Rychen, D. S., & Salganik, L. H. (Eds.). (2003). *Key competencies for a successful life and a well-functioning society*. New York, NY: Hogrefe & Huber Publications.

Rycroft-Malone, J., Seers, K., Titchen, A., Harvey, G., Ktson, A., & McCormack, B. (2004). What counts as evidence in evidence-based practice? *Journal of Advanced Nursing, 47*, 81–90.

Sackett, D. L., Straus, S. E., & Richardson, W. S. (2000). *Evidence-based medicine: How to practice and teach EBM* (2nd ed.). Edinburgh, Scotland: Churchill Livingstone.

Saettler, P. (1990). *The evolution of American educational technology*. Englewood, CO: Libraries Unlimited, Inc.

Salvage, J., & Smith, R. (2000). Doctors and nurses: Doing it differently. *British Medical Journal, 320,* 1019–1020.

San Martin-Rodriguez, L., Beaulieu, M., D'Amour, D., & Ferrada-Videla, M. (2005). The determinants of successful collaboration: A review of theoretical and empirical studies. *Journal of Interprofessional Care, Supplement 1,* 132–147.

Sartre, J. P. (1958). *Being and nothingness: An essay on phenomenological ontology* (H. Barnes, Trans.). London, UK: Methuen. (Original work published 1943.)

Sartre, J. P. (1962). *Being and time* (J. Macquarrie & E. Robinson, Trans.). Oxford, UK: Basil Blackwell. (Original work published 1927.)

Sasso, L., Stievano, A., Jurado, M. G., & Rocco, G. (2008). Code of ethics and conduct for European nursing. *Nursing Ethics, 15,* 821–836.

Schatzki, T. R. (1996). *Social practices: A Wittgensteinian approach to human activity and the social.* New York, NY: Cambridge University Press.

Scheffer, B., & Rubenfeld, M. G. (2000). A consensus statement on critical thinking in nursing. *Journal of Nursing Education, 39,* 352–359.

Schmidt, H. G., Norman, G. R., & Boshuizen, H. P. A. (1990). A cognitive perspective on medical expertise: Theory and implications. *Journal of the Association of American Medical Colleges, 65,* 611–621.

Schön, D. A. (1983). *Reflective practitioner: How professionals think in action.* New York, NY: Basic Books.

Schroeter, K. (2009). *Competence literature review.* Competency & Credentialing Institute. Retrieved from http://www.cc-institute.org/docs/default-document-library/2011/10/19/competence_lit_review.pdf

Schultz, D. S., & Flasher, L. V. (2011). Charles Taylor, phronesis, and medicine: Ethics and interpretation in illness narrative. *Journal of Medicine and Philosophy, 36,* 394–409.

Schwartz, D. G. (2007). Integrating knowledge transfer and computer-mediated communication: Categorizing barriers and possible responses. *Knowledge Management Research & Practice, 5,* 249–259.

Scott, S., Profetto-McGrath, J., Estabrooks, C. A., Winter, C., Wallin, L., & Lavis, J. N. (2010). Mapping the knowledge utilization field in nursing from 1945 to 2004: A bibliometric analysis. *Worldviews on Evidence-Based Nursing, 7,* 226–237.

Scruton, R. (2011). A bit of help from Wittgenstein. *British Journal of Aesthetics, 51,* 309–319.

Searle, J. (1992). *The rediscovery of mind.* Cambridge, MA: MIT Press.

Seidman, J. (2008). Caring and the boundary-driven structure of practical deliberation. *Journal of Ethics & Social Philosophy, 3,* 1–36.

Seidman, J. (2010). Caring and incapacity. *Philosophical Studies, 147,* 301–322.

Seikkula, J., Aaltonen, J., Alakare, B., Haarankangas, K., Keränen, J., & Lethinen, K. (2006). Five-year experience of first episode nonaffective psychosis in open dialogue approach: Treatment principles, follow-up outcomes and two case studies. *Psychotherapy Research, 16*(2), 214–228.

Seikkula, J., Aaltonen, J., Rasinkangas, A., Alakare, B., Holma, J., & Lethinen, V. (2003). Open dialogue approach: Treatment principles and preliminary results of a two-year follow-up on first episode schizophrenia. *Ethical and Human Sciences and Services*, *5*(3), 163–182.

Shapiro, J. (2002). (Re)examining the clinical gaze through the prism of literature. *Family System Health*, *20*, 161–70.

Shaw, H. K., & Degazon, C. (2008). Integrating the core professional values of nursing: A profession, not just a career. *Journal of Cultural Diversity*, *15*(1), 44–50.

Shealy, N. (1985). Restoring health. *Basal Facts*, *7*, 31–44.

Shor, I., & Freire, P. (1987). *A pedagogy for liberation: Dialogues on transforming education*. South Hadley, MA: Bergin & Garvey.

Shortell, S. M., Zukoski, A. P., Alexander, J. A., Bazzoli, G. J., Conrad, D. A., Hasnain-Wynia, R., ... Margolin, F. S. (2002). Evaluating partnerships for community health improvement: Tracking the footprints. *Journal of Health Politics, Policy and Law*, *27*, 49–91.

Shusterman, R. (2010). Dewey's art as experience. *Journal of Aesthetic Education*, *44*, 26–43.

Sicotte, C., D'Amour, D., & Moreault, M. (2002). Interdisciplinary collaboration within Quebec community health care centers. *Social Science & Medicine*, *55*, 991–1003.

Sidani, S. (2008). Effects of patient-centered care on patient outcomes: An evaluation. *Research and Theory for Nursing Practice: An International Journal*, *22*, 24–37

Simmons, B. (2010). Clinical reasoning: Concept analysis. *Journal of Advanced Nursing*, *66*, 1151–1158.

Simon, H. (1979). *Models of thoughts*. New Haven, CT: Yale University Press.

Skott, C. (2001). Caring narratives and the strategy of presence: Narrative communication in nursing practice and research. *Nursing Science Quarterly*, *14*, 249–254.

Smith, A. (1998). Learning about reflection. *Journal of Advanced Nursing*, *28*, 891–898.

Speed, S., & Luker, K. A. (2004). Changes in patterns of knowing the patient: The case of British district nurses. *International Journal of Nursing Studies*, *41*, 921–931.

Spiegelberg, H. (1984). *The phenomenological movement* (3rd ed.). The Hague: Martinus Nijhoff.

Spielman, A. I., Fulmer, T., Eisenber, E. S., & Alfano, M. C. (2005). Dentistry, nursing, and medicine: A comparison of core competencies. *Journal of Dental Education*, *69*, 1257–1271.

Squires, A. (2004). A dimensional analysis of role enactment of acute care nurses. *Journal of Nursing Scholarship: An Official Publication of Sigma Theta Tau*, *36*, 272–278.

Stanley, D., & Joseph, H. (2003). How a pyramid helps to unravel the stages of nursing assessment. *Professional Nurse*, *18*, 596–597.

Sterling, W. C. (2003). *Satisficing games and decision making: With applications for engineering and computer science*. Cambridge, UK: Cambridge University Press.

Stetler, C. B. (1994). Refinement of the Stetler/Marram model for application of research findings to practice. *Nursing Outlook*, *42*, 15–25.

Stetler, C. B. (2003). Role of organization in translating research into evidence-based practice. *Outcomes Management*, *7*, 97–129.

Stevenson, J. S., & Woods, N. F. (1986). Nursing science and contemporary science: Emerging paradigms. In American Academy of Nursing (Ed.), *Setting agenda for the year 2000: Knowledge development in nursing* (pp. 6–20). Kansas City, MO: American Academy of Nursing.

Stewart, M., Brown, J. B., Weston, W. W., McWhinney, I. R., McWilliam, C. L., & Freeman, T. R. (1995). *Patient-centred medicine transforming the clinical method*. Thousand Oaks, CA: Sage Publications.

Stichler, J. F. (1995). Professional interdependence: The art of collaboration. *Advanced Practice Nursing Quarterly, 1*(1), 53–61.

Stimpfel, A. W., Rosen, J. E., & McHugh, M. D. (2014). Understanding the role of the professional practice environment on quality of care in Magnet and non-Magnet hospitals. *Journal of Nursing Administration, 44*, 10–16.

Stone, P. W., Harrison, M. I., Feldman, P., Linzer, P., Peng, T., Roblin D., ... Williams, E. S. (2005). *Organizational climate of staff working conditions and safety—an integrative model*. Rockville, MD: Agency for Healthcare Research and Quality. AHRQ Publication No. 05-0021-2.

Stone, P. W., Hughes, R., & Dailey, M. (2008). Creating a safe and high-quality health care environment. In R. G. Hughes (Ed.), *Patient safety and quality: An evidence-based handbook for nurses* (Chapter 21). Rockville, MD: Agency for Healthcare Research and Quality (US). Retrieved from http://www.ncbi.nlm.nih.gov/books/NBK2634

Strati, A. (2003). Knowing in practice: Aesthetic understanding and tacit knowledge. In D. Nicoline, S. Giherardi, & D. Yanow (Eds.), *Knowing in organizations: A practice-based approach* (pp. 53–73). Aronk, NY: M. E. Sharpe, Inc.

Strickland, O. L. (1997). Challenges in measuring patient outcomes. *Nursing Clinics of North America, 32*, 495–512.

Stroud, S. R. (2011). John Dewey and the question of artful criticism. *Philosophy and Rhetoric, 44*, 27–51.

Sullivan, D. T., Hirst, D., & Cronenwett, L. (2009). Assessing quality and safety competencies of graduating prelicensure nursing students. *Nursing Outlook, 57*, 323–331.

Summers, J. A., Poston, D. J, Turnbull, A. P., Marquis, J., Hoffman, L., Mannan, H., & Wang, M. (2005). Conceptualizing and measuring family quality of life. *Journal of Intellectual Disability Research, 49*, 777–783.

Svenaeus, F. (2003). Hermeneutics of medicine in the wake of Gadamer: The issue of phronesis. *Theoretical Medicine and Bioethics, 24*, 407–431.

Sverdlik, S. (1986). Hume's key and aesthetic rationality. *Journal of Aesthetics and Art Criticism, 45*, 69–76.

Swanson, K. M. (1991). Empirical development of a middle range theory of caring. *Nursing Research, 40*, 161–166.

Takase, M., Kershaw, E., & Burt, L. (2001). Nurse-environment misfit and nursing practice. *Journal of Advanced Nursing, 35*, 819–826.

Takase, M., Maude, P., & Manias, E. (2005). Explaining nurses' work behaviour from their perception of the environment and work values. *International Journal of Nursing Studies, 42*, 889–898.

Tanner, C. A. (2006). Thinking like a nurse: A research-based model of clinical judgment in nursing. *Journal of Nursing Education, 45*, 204–211.

Tanner, C. A., Benner, P., Chesla, C., & Gordon, D. R. (1993). The phenomenology of knowing the patient. *Image: The Journal of Nursing Scholarship, 25*, 273–280.

Taylor, C. (1985a). *Human agency and language. Philosophical papers 1*. Cambridge, UK: Cambridge University Press.

Taylor, C. (1985b). *Human agency and the human sciences. Philosophical papers 2*. Cambridge, UK: Cambridge University Press.

Taylor, C. (1987). Interpretation and the sciences of man. In P. Rabinow & W. M. Sullivan (Eds.), *Interpretive social science: A second look* (pp. 33–81). Berkeley, CA: University of California Press.

Taylor, C. (1989). *Sources of the self: The making of the modern identity*. Cambridge MA: Harvard University Press.

Taylor, J. S. (1997). Nursing ideology: Identification and legitimation. *Journal of Advanced Nursing, 25*, 442–446.

Taylor, J., & Wros, P. (2007). Concept mapping: A nursing model for care planning. *Journal of Nursing Education, 46*, 211–216.

The Joint Commission. (2015). The National Patient Safety goals for 2015 [PowerPoint slides]. Retrieved from http://www.jointcommission.org/npsg-presentations

Thompson, C., & Dowding, D. (2001a). *Clinical decision-making and judgement in nursing*. London, UK: Churchill Livingstone.

Thompson, C., & Dowding, D. (2001b). Responding to uncertainty in nursing practice. *International Journal of Nursing Studies, 38*, 609–615.

Thompson, D., Socolar, R., Brown, L., & Haggerty J. (2002). Interagency collaboration in seven North Carolina counties. *Journal of Public Health Management and Practice, 8*(5), 55–64.

Thompson, J., Allen, D. G., & Rodrigues-Fisher, L. (Eds.). (1992). *Critique, resistance, and action: Working papers in the politics of nursing*. New York, NY: National League for Nursing. NLN Pub. No. 14-2504.

Thorne, S. E., & Hayes, V. E. (Eds.). (1997). *Nursing praxis: Knowledge and action*. Thousand Oaks, CA: Sage Publications.

Thoroddsen, A. (2005). Applicability of the nursing interventions classification to describe nursing. *Scandinavian Journal of Caring Sciences, 19*, 128–139.

Tianji, J. (1985). Scientific rationalty, formal or informal? *The British Journal for the Philosophy of Science, 36*, 409–423.

Tierney, A. J. (2001). Shaping nursing practice. The United Kngdom perspective. *Nursing Leadership Forum, 5*, 96–99.

Timm, S. E. (2003). Effectively delegating nursing activities in home care. *Home Healthcare Nurse, 21*, 260–265.

Timmins, F. (2006). Critical practice in nursing care: Analysis, action and reflexivity. *Nursing Standard (Royal College of Nursing Great Britain), 20*(39), 49–54.

Torbert, W. R. (1991). *The power of balance: Transforming self, society, and scientific inquiry*. Newbury Park, CA: Sage Publications.

Travelbee, J. (1964). *Interpersonal aspects of nursing*. Philadelphia, PA: F. A. Davis.

Tronto, J. C. (1994). *Moral boundaries: A political argument for an ethics of care*. New York, NY: Routledge.

Trost, J. (1990). Do we mean the same by the concept of family? *Communication Research, 17*, 431–443.

Twigg, J., Wolkowitz, C., Cohen, R. L., & Nettleton, S. (2011). Conceptualizing body work in health and social care. *Sociology of Health & Illness, 33*, 171–188.

Ulrich, W. (2007). Philosophy for professionals: Toward critical pragmatism. *Journal of the Operational Research Society, 58*, 1109–1113.

Vaartio, H., & Leino-Kilpi, H. (2005). Nursing advocacy—A review of the empirical research 1990-2003. *International Journal of Nursing Studies, 42*, 705–714.

Vaartio, H., Leino-Kilpi, H., Salantera, S., & Suominen, T. (2006). Nursing advocacy: How is it defined by patients and nurses, what does it involve and how is it experienced? *Scandinavian Journal of Caring Science, 20*, 282–292.

Van Bogaert, P., Kowalski, C., Weeks, S. M., Van Heusden, D., & Clarke, S. P. (2013). The relationship between nurse practice environment, nurse work characteristics, burnout and job outcome and quality of nursing care: A cross-sectional survey. *International Journal of Nursing Studies, 50*, 1667–1677.

Van der Zalm, J. E., & Bergum, V. (2000). Hermeneutic-phenomenology: Providing living knowledge for nursing practice. *Journal of Advanced Nursing, 31*, 211–218.

van Hooft, S. (2011). Caring, objectivity and justice: An integrative view. *Nursing Ethics, 18*, 149–160.

Varcoe, C., Doane, E. G., Pauly, B., Rodney, P., Storch, J. L., Mahoney, K., ... Starzomski, R. (2004). Ethical practice in nursing: Working the in-betweens. *Journal of Advanced Nursing, 45*, 316-325.

Verma, S., Broers, T., Paterson, M., Schroder, C., Medves, J. M., & Morrison, C. (2009). Core competencies: The next generation. Comparison of a common framework for multiple professions. *Journal of Allied Health, 38*, 47–53.

Verma, S., & Paterson, M. (2006). Core competencies for health care professionals: What medicine, nursing, occupational therapy, and physiotherapy share. *Journal of Allied Health, 35*, 109–115.

Vogel, A., Ransom, P., Wai, S., & Luisi, D. (2007). Integrating health and social services for older adults: a case study of interagency collaboration. *Journal of Health and Human Services Administration, 30*, 199–228.

Volker, D. L. (2003). Is there a unique nursing ethic? *Nursing Science Quarterly, 16*, 207–211.

von Neumann, J., & Morgenstern, O. (1953). *Theory of games and economic behavior*. Princeton, NJ: Princeton University Press.

Wallace, D. (1996). Experiential learning and critical thinking in nursing. *Nursing Standards (Royal College of Nursing), 10*(31), 43–47.

Walsh, K., Kitson, A., Cross, W., Thoms, D., Thornton, A., Moss, C., ... Graham, I. (2012). A conversation about practice development and knowledge translation as mechanisms to align the academic and clinical contexts for the advancement of nursing practice. *Collegian, 19*, 67–75.

Warburton, J., Everingham, J., Cuthill, M., Bartlett, H., & Underwood, M. (2011). More than just a talkfest: The process of developing collaborations in ageing across two different community types. *Urban Policy and Research, 19*, 183–200.

Warelow, P. J. (1996). Is caring the ethical ideal? *Journal of Advanced Nursing, 24*, 655–661.

Warren, M. L., Houston, S., & Luquire, R. (1998). Collaborative practice teams: From multidisciplinary to interdisciplinary. *Outcomes Management for Nursing Practice, 2*(3), 95–98.

Watson, F., & Rebair, A. (2014). The art of noticing: Essential to nursing practice. *British Journal of Nursing, 23*, 514–517.

Watson, J. (1996). Watson's theory of transpersonal caring. In P. H. Walker & B. Neuman (Eds.), *Blueprint for use of nursing models: Education, research, practice, & administration* (pp. 141–184). New York, NY: National League for Nursing Press.

Watson, J. (2012). *Nursing. Human caring science* (2nd ed.). Boston, MA: Jones & Bartlett.

Way, D. O., & Jones, L. M. (1994). The family physician-nurse practitioner dyad: Indications and guidelines. *Canadian Medical Association Journal [journal de l'Association medicale canadienne], 151*(1), 28–34.

Way, D. O., Jones, L., & Baskerville, N. B. (2001). *Improving the effectiveness of primary health care through nurse/family physician structured collaborative practice.* Ottawa, Canada: University of Ottawa.

Weisman, C. (1992). Nursing practice models: Research on patient outcomes. In National Institutes of Health (Ed.), *Patient outcomes research: Examining the effectiveness of nursing practice* (pp. 112–120). Proceedings of the State of the Science Conference sponsored by the National Center for Nursing Research. Bethesda, MD: DHHS, NIH Publication No. 93-3411.

Welch, J. R. (1994). Science and ethics: Toward a theory of ethical value. *Journal for General Philosophy of Science/Zeitschrift für allgemeineWissenschaftstheorie, 25*, 279–292.

Welsch, W. (1998). Rationality and reason today. In D. R. Gordon & J. Nitznik (Eds.), *Criticism and defense of rationality in contemporary philosophy* (pp. 17–31). Amsterdam: Rodopi.

Wenger, A. F. (1995). Cultural context, health and health care decision making. *Journal of Transcultural Nursing, 7*, 3–14.

Whittemore, R. (2000). Consequence of not "knowing the patient." *Clinical Nurse Specialist CNS, 14*, 75–81.

Wilkinson, J. E., Rycroft-Malone, J., Davies, T. O., & McCormack, B. (2012). A creative approach to the development of an agenda for knowledge utilization: Outputs from the 11th International Knowledge Utilization Colloquium (KU11). *Worldviews on Evidence-Based Nursing, 9*, 195–199.

Williams, A. M. (1998). The delivery of quality nursing care: A grounded theory study of the nurse's perspective. *Journal of Advanced Nursing, 27*, 808–816.

Wills, E. M. (1996). Nurse-client alliance: A pattern of home health caring. *Home Healthcare Nurse, 14*, 455–459.

Wolf, Z. R. (1986). *Nurses' work: The sacred and the profane.* Philadelphia, PA: University of Pennsylvania Press.

World Health Organization (WHO). (2010). *Framework for action on interprofessional education & collaborative practice.* Geneva, Switzerland: Author. Retrieved from http://www.who.int/hrh/resources/framework_action/en

World Health Organization (WHO) Expert Committee on Nursing Practice. (1996). *Nursing practice: Report of a WHO Expert Committee.* Geneva, Switzerland: World Health Organization.

Wozniak, R. H. (1995). *Mind and body: Rene Déscartes to William James.* Retrieved from http://serendip.brynmawr.edu/Mind/; Bryn Mawr College, Serendip. Originally published in 1992 at Bethesda, MD and Washington, DC by the National Library of Medicine and the American Psychological Association.

Wu, Y., Larrabee, J. H., & Putnam, H. P. (2006). Caring behavior inventory: A reduction of the 42-item instrument. *Nursing Research, 55,* 18–25.

Xyrichis, A., & Ream, E. (2008). Teamwork: A concept analysis. *Journal of Advanced Nursing, 61,* 232–241.

Yan, J., Gilbert, J. H. V., & Hoffman, S. J. (2007). World Health Organization Study Group on interprofessional education and collaborative practice. *Journal of Interprofessional Care, 21,* 587–589.

Yura, H., & Walsh, M. B. (1978). *The nursing process: Assessing, planning, implementing, evaluating.* New York, NY: Appleton-Century-Crofts.

Zaibert, L. (2006). The fitting, the deserving, and the beautiful. *Journal of Moral Philosophy, 3,* 331–350.

Zetzel, E. R. (2004). Current concepts of transference. In A. H. Esman (Ed.), *Essential papers on transference* (pp. 136–149). New York, NY: New York University Press.

Zwarenstein, M., Goldman, J., & Reeves, S. (2009). Interprofessional collaboration: Effects of practice-based interventions on professional practice and healthcare outcomes. *Cochrane Database of Systematic Reviews,* Issue 3. Art. No.: CD000072. doi: 10.1002/14651858.CD000072.pub2

# Index

Printed in the United States
By Bookmasters